Philadelphia London Toronto Mexico City Rio de Janeiro Sydney Tokyo
1983 W.B. Saunders Company

susan irving, r.n., m.s.
FORMERLY PSYCHIATRIC NURSING DIRECTOR
EASTERN STATE HOSPITAL
MEDICAL LAKE, WASHINGTON

THIRD EDITION

basic psychiatric nursing

W. B. Saunders Company: West Washington Square
Philadelphia, PA 19105

1 St. Anne's Road
Eastbourne, East Sussex BN21 3UN, England

1 Goldthorne Avenue
Toronto, Ontario M8Z 5T9, Canada

Apartado 26370—Cedro 512
Mexico 4, D.F., Mexico

Rua Coronel Cabrita, 8
Sao Cristovao Caixa Postal 21176
Rio de Janeiro, Brazil

9 Waltham Street
Artarmon, N.S.W. 2064, Australia

Ichibancho, Central Bldg., 22-1 Ichibancho
Chiyoda-Ku, Tokyo 102, Japan

Library of Congress Cataloging in Publication Data

Irving, Susan.

Basic psychiatric nursing.

Includes bibliographical references and index.
1. Psychiatric nursing. I. Title. [DNLM: 1. Psychiatric nursing.
WY 160 I72b]
RC440.I78 1983 610.73'68 82-40309
ISBN 0-7216-5049-X AACR2

Listed here is the latest translated edition of this book together with the language of the translation and the publisher.

Spanish (1st Edition)—Nueva Editorial Interamericana S.A.
Mexico D.F. Mexico

Portuguese (2nd Edition)—Editora Interamericana Ltda.
Rio de Janeiro, Brazil

Basic Psychiatric Nursing ISBN 0-7216-5049-x

Last digit is the print number: 9 8 7 6 5 4 3 2 1

This book is dedicated
To N.G.
and
All of My Students

Preface to the Third Edition

I hope the effort to make this third edition more helpful will be successful. I have tried to incorporate a number of suggestions from people who use this book, so that it may more nearly meet their needs. To this end, I have added a new chapter, Chapter 9, "Treatment and Care Planning," which includes information more specifically related to the nursing process and nursing care planning. All of the chapter references, case histories, and drug tables as well as the Glossary have been updated. Major sections of the following chapters have been revised to reflect current diagnosis and practice: Chapter 11, "Schizophrenic Reactions to Stress"; Chapter 12, "Manic-Depressive Reactions to Stress"; Chapter 14, "Sociopathic Reactions to Stress"; Chapter 15, "Neurotic Reactions to Stress"; and Chapter 16, "Psychosomatic Reactions to Stress."

I have most often referred to the patient as "he" and the nurse as "she," knowing full well that not all patients are male nor all nurses female. The terms refer to groups of people composed of both men and women and are used to make reading easier and meaning clearer. These terms are not meant in any way to be sexist, and I hope they will not be interpreted as such.

I am indebted as usual to a number of people for their help and support in preparing this third edition. I would like to name a few of them: Joanne Griffith, R.N., and Phyllis Cornwall, R.N., for supplying invaluable clinical data, critical advice, and essential support; Betty Adams, R.N., and Douglas Adams, M.D., for their sustaining support and encouragement; and Ilona Johnson, secretary, for typing and proofreading parts of the manuscript.

SUSAN IRVING

Preface to the First Edition

Because of the many changes in attitudes and approaches to mental health and illness in recent years, psychiatric nursing is in a period of transition. It is no longer acceptable for the nurse to give merely custodial care to the hospitalized patient. Nursing care is expected to be therapeutic, personalized, comprehensive, preventive, and rehabilitative. Such care requires increased knowledge and understanding of human behavior, and greater ability and skill in human relations on the part of all nurses.

This book is written in an effort to help the nurse learn ways of relating to all people effectively enough to relieve suffering, increase security, and promote health in her care of patients. Although the focus of the book is primarily upon psychiatric nursing and the care of hospitalized patients, the same principles apply in any field of human endeavor, and in all relationships between people. The material in the book is aimed toward acquainting the nurse with the dimensions of health and illness, the corresponding dimensions of care and treatment, and her place on the treatment team.

I do not mean to be presumptuous in offering answers to all kinds of nursing problems, but I do believe that effective patient care is based upon a successful relationship between the patient and some helping person. That helping person may or may not be the nurse. If it is to be the nurse, she must prepare herself for the task of helping others by increasing her knowledge, understanding, and skill in human relations. We all need to work toward closing the gap between our great scientific progress and the lack of personal involvement among people. Then, and only then, will our work, our lives, our world be made more safe and secure. In his prayer of thanksgiving for the safe return of the astronauts from the first moon landing, the chaplain of the recovery ship said it this way: "May we be inspired to move toward new horizons in the spirit of brotherhood, human concern, and mutual respect for all mankind."

Although I assume the responsibility for what is written here, the material does not belong only to me. Some of the thoughts and words are those of other people, but they have become so much a part of me and my teaching that I am no longer able to identify their origins. This book is a result of many rewarding personal interactions, both successful and unsuccessful, and the culmination of a life's ambition to be of service to other people. It is not possible for me to thank each person from whom I have gained something that has become a part of this book. However, I would like to thank certain individuals who have had a specific and identifiable part in its creation: Richard Fredericks, M.D.; Raymond L. Leidig, M.D.; Joy R. Joffe, M.D.; Mr. Robert Greene, Pharmacist; Mrs. Lois Brevik, Librarian; and secretaries Mrs. Lynn Starkovich and Mrs. Barbara Vincent.

I would like to express my special thanks to my friends and colleagues, Mrs. Phyllis Cornwall, R.N., and Mrs. Joanne Griffith, R.N., upon whom I relied for assistance and suggestions. Finally, I would like to give most of the credit for this book to the patients, instructors, and students with whom I have worked during the past twenty-five years, because without them it would never have been possible.

This book, like any other, will be only as good as it is useful to those who read it. So to those people who do read it let me quote a passage from Kahlil Gibran's *The Prophet*, which says much better than I can what is in my heart and mind:

> Then said a teacher, Speak to us of Teaching.
> And he said:
>
> No man can reveal to you aught but that which already lies half asleep in the dreaming of your knowledge.
>
> The teacher who walks in the shadow of the temple, among his followers, gives not of his wisdom but rather of his faith and his lovingness.
>
> If he is indeed wise he does not bid you enter the house of his wisdom, but rather leads you to the threshold of your own mind.
>
> The astronomer may speak to you of his understanding of space, but he cannot give you his understanding.
>
> The musician may sing to you of the rhythm which is in all space but he cannot give you the ear which arrests the rhythm nor the voice that echoes it.
>
> And he who is versed in the science of numbers can tell of the regions of weight and measure, but he cannot conduct you thither.

For the vision of one man lends not its wings to another man.

And even as each one of you stands alone in God's knowledge, so must each one of you be alone in his knowledge of God and in his understanding of the earth.

SUSAN IRVING

Contents

Chapter 1

Psychiatric Nursing

Patients are people in trouble, usually serious trouble when they come under the care of the nurse. They have often lost the ability to care for themselves, to meet their own needs, to live their own lives. They generally must depend upon somebody else for their very survival, for their most intimate personal needs, for their existence as individuals. The nurse may become that "somebody else" upon whom they depend for help. It is up to her, then, to provide a certain kind of relationship and a certain kind of environment that allows the patient to move in the direction of health.

Patients are looking essentially for two things when they come to the nurse for help: someone who really cares about them and someone who will be honest with them. This is particularly true of psychiatric patients, but it is true of other patients as well. Patients in an intensive care unit, who had come to one hospital with life-threatening illnesses, were asked what aspects of their treatment had made the biggest impression upon them. Do you know what the majority of them answered? Not the life-saving measures, not the efficiency of the staff, not the latest scientific breakthroughs, but the fact that the nursing staff *really cared about them.* When we are in trouble, that's what we look for—a person who really cares. Before you can put your trust in someone else, you have to feel the other person genuinely cares about you and will be honest with you. That is essential in establishing a trust relationship—the basis for successful nursing care.

Two major responsibilities of the nursing staff are the establishment of a therapeutic relationship with the individual patient and the establishment of a therapeutic environment for all patients. That means that everything we do as nurses must reflect two basic attitudes—caring and honesty. The routine ward schedule, the arrangement of the furniture, and the serving of meals must reflect these attitudes. How we care for patients—what we say and how we say it, what we do and how we do it—tells the patient whether or not we care about him and determines whether or not our nursing care is therapeutic, effective, and helpful.

In caring for patients, the nurse goes through the steps of the nursing process: assessment, planning, implementation, and evaluation. In other words, she applies the problem-solving technique to her nursing care. In assessment, she identifies and assigns priorities to the patient's needs, taking into consideration his condition, his circumstances, and his ability to meet his own needs. Then, with the patient, she designs a nursing care plan, which outlines long and short range goals for the patient and the nursing actions or interventions that are needed to help the patient reach those goals. She puts that plan into effect by using her own healthy personality in a therapeutic manner to help the patient move in the direction of health. She documents the patient's response to her care and modifies her nursing actions according to the results of that evaluation. Thus, each patient's care is individualized and directed toward the resolution of his particular problems.

Psychiatric nursing is different from, yet similar to, all other kinds of nursing. Some people think of psychiatric nursing as being the basis, the heart, the core, the very art of nursing itself. Others think of psychiatric nursing as being strictly limited to the care of patients diagnosed as mentally ill. Psychiatric nursing is definitely not a neat set of procedures or rituals that ends with a cure. It is rather an arduous, personal, human struggle toward health.

It can be generally agreed that psychiatric nursing is a process of human communication which involves two people, one a nurse and the other a patient, and their relationship, the sum of their interactions with one another. The primary purpose of their relationship is to help the patient find greater satisfaction of his basic needs and more effective ways of behaving in order to obtain that satisfaction—in other words, to help the patient find greater success in living. Furthermore, it is the responsibility of the nurse to establish, maintain, and terminate such a relationship. Whether or not that relationship is therapeutic, helpful, or even healthy can be measured very simply by the sense of well-being that the patient experiences as a result of it.

Often the nurse who is beginning her study or practice of psychiatric nursing is influenced by commonly held misconceptions regarding mentally ill patients, their treatment, and the nurse's contribution to their care. As a result, she may look at and approach the care of psychiatric patients with attitudes, feelings, and actions that are harmful rather than helpful. It is essential for the nurse to recognize, understand, and correct her approach if she is to deal therapeutically with the patient—all patients—and I believe all people. With this in mind, let us discuss some basic facts regarding the patient, the nurse, and their relationship, as well as mental illness and psychiatric treatment.

THE PATIENT

First of all, the patient is a person, a unique human being different from all others. He is not a category of illness, a kind of condition, or a set of symptoms. He is a person, an individual who is sick, in trouble, alone and afraid. He often becomes an alien, an outcast, a burden, a stranger in his own world, and may be met with fear, anger, suspicion, hostility, contempt, disgust, despair, or ridicule from those closest to him as well as those who don't even know him. When he can no longer tolerate the fear and loneliness, he turns to strangers for the love and acceptance he needs and he becomes a patient.

He is sick with a strange and frightening illness over which he has little or no control. He often knows inside himself that he shouldn't think and feel such things, let alone say or do them, but he can't seem to stop. He sees people look at him with fear or distrust, guilt or anger, disgust or embarrassment. He finds that things are getting worse for him instead of better, and he begins to experience an ever-increasing succession of failures and rejection. When he can no longer meet his own needs or direct his behavior appropriately, he seeks, by becoming a patient, to obtain comfort and relief from those who are prepared to help him.

THE NURSE

The nurse, too, is a person, a unique human being, different from all others. She is not a particular kind of personality, or set of attributes, or accumulation of special qualities. She is an individual, a product of her own life experiences, who has acquired specific knowledge and skills in caring for others. She has decided that her life's work will be spent in the service of others and she becomes a nurse.

She is a healthy adult, emotionally mature enough to be able to postpone the satisfaction of her own needs and allow the patient's needs to take precedence. She is able to tolerate frustration and stress effectively enough to handle her resulting feelings in constructive ways. She has sufficient self-awareness to appreciate the impact she has upon others, and she assumes responsibility for her behavior. She is flexible enough to be able to change and receptive enough to learn new ways of perceiving and responding to life. She is concerned about the welfare of others and does something about it by becoming a nurse.

THEIR RELATIONSHIP

The therapeutic relationship assumes that one person (the patient) is in need of and asking for help, and the other person (the nurse) is able and willing to give him that help. It consists of a series of interactions between these two people, nurse and patient, that leads them both in the direction of greater health and happiness. It is of necessity a human, individual, and very personal experience. I am convinced that one person cannot help another unless he cares enough about him to risk personal involvement and commitment, and unless he himself has had the experience of being helped in some way.

Too frequently we hear the nurse's comment, "I wish I had enough time to relate (or socialize or visit) with the patient." It may have something to do with the short length of time the nurse and patient are in direct contact. In these days of advanced medical science and technology, the time the patient is in the care of the nurse has been considerably shortened. Also, the nurse has many patients to care for, not just one, and treatment facilities are notoriously overcrowded.

But how long does it take to relate to another person? Sometimes a single look or touch initiates a deep and lasting relationship. At the same time, one can spend a lifetime with another person and never relate in more than the most superficial way. Many people who have shared a single crisis situation in life, such as occurs in war time, have established meaningful relationships that last a lifetime. Such a relationship is special, an event that is not based upon duration of contact, numbers of people, scientific principles, or even logic. It is based instead upon the underlying feelings of compassion, desire, need, and love for another human being. Certainly illness is a time of crisis for the patient, and the necessary interaction of the nurse with the patient puts the nurse in an ideal spot for developing a supportive relationship.

The nurse relates with the patient in a single exchange or a series of interactions or in prolonged contact, but the relationship almost always involves something of a highly personal, critical, and important nature. In any single interaction the nurse either meets the patient's needs and adds to his feelings of comfort, security, and well-being or she does not. The way in which she relates with the patient, then, is either helpful or harmful and it becomes the basis of her effectiveness as a nurse. A helpful relationship between nurse and patient can be characterized by its acceptance, honesty, understanding, and faith.

Acceptance. First of all, the relationship between nurse and patient must be an accepting one. That means that the nurse must be able to accept the patient, no matter what he says or does or where he comes from, not just because he is a patient, but because he is a person of essential worth and dignity, deserving of her love and respect. It does not mean that she must or should or even could approve of everything he does. She may have feelings of disapproval, dislike, even disgust for certain of his actions. It is necessary, however, that she be able to control and express her feelings in a constructive way, so as not to reject, punish, or ignore the patient. At the same time he needs to know what is expected, appropriate, acceptable behavior on his part, and he needs help in learning how to behave in such a fashion.

For example, if a patient repeatedly spits in the drinking fountain, it may be up to the nurse to let him know that this is not acceptable behavior, why it is not, and what he can do to correct it. It is not necessary to bawl him out, or send him to his room, or make fun of him in front of other patients. It may be that he cannot find the bathroom in order to spit in the toilet, or he thinks the fountain contains evil spirits that can only be kept in control if he spits on them.

Honesty. The relationship between nurse and patient must be an honest one. That means that the nurse must be genuinely concerned about the welfare of the patient and willing to help him do something about it. It means further that she must be certain that what she says and does in interaction with him agrees with and expresses that kind of human concern. There is no room for phoniness.

For example, a patient may continue to tease a nurse about her private life until she becomes angry. It is important to her relationship with the patient that she not deny that anger, but that she express it in such a way that she helps him understand how his behavior affects her and perhaps others and how he might change it. If she says in an angry voice, "I'm not angry," she has told the patient two things—not only that she is indeed angry but that she is also dishonest, which lessens her effectiveness in relating with the patient. How can he be expected to put his faith and trust in someone who cannot even admit that she is human enough to become angry?

On the other hand, it is important that the nurse not attach her feelings of frustration about other situations to her relationship with the patient. If she is angry with the doctor, or her husband, or the afternoon shift, it should not be the patient who takes the brunt of it. It is, therefore, necessary for the nurse to understand her own motives, be able to face up to them, and direct them toward a constructive resolution. For example, if she has had a trying morning with a group of visitors, she should not be short or ill-tempered with the patient who asks for assistance from her; or if she is, she should apologize to him and explain the reasons for her inappropriate behavior.

Understanding. The relationship between nurse and patient must be one of understanding. That means that the nurse must know the individual patient well enough to be able to understand how *he* feels in the situation that he is in, not how *she* might feel, or how others have felt in similar situations. That is the difference between empathy on the one hand, and sympathy on the other. Empathy in psychiatric terms is one of the nonverbal ways the nurse uses to communicate her care and concern for the patient. She must do more than make assumptions about how he feels—she needs to check with him to be sure that is how he really feels.

For example, a patient may be scheduled to have visitors but they do not show up, and later the nurse finds him crying in his room. She might assume he is sad and lonely, and feels deserted by his family. However, if she were to check with him, she might find out that he is relieved that they did not come because he did not know how to explain to his little girl that he would not be home for her birthday.

Faith. The relationship between nurse and patient must be one of mutual faith. That means that the nurse must have faith in her ability to help the patient and his ability to respond to her. It means also that the patient must have sufficient faith in the nurse's competence that he can put himself in her care. It means further that these two people, nurse and patient, must have sufficient faith in one another to sustain them in times of difficulty. No human relationship exists without strife or strain, and that includes the therapeutic relationship. Both people must be able to rise above human frailty and to forgive and forget one another's shortcomings, not hold each other forever accountable for human error. It was Pope who said, "To err is human, to forgive, divine," but I like to think of both erring and forgiving as human characteristics, which are necessary for successful relationships.

For example, a patient may be making great strides toward recovery and then unaccountably begin to slip back into his illness. The nurse, in her disappointment, may reprimand him or avoid contact with him. In so doing, she has violated the essential element of faith in her relationship with the patient, and sold them both short. This may make it difficult for the patient to turn to her when he most needs help.

MENTAL ILLNESS AND PSYCHIATRIC TREATMENT

Mental illness is different from all other kinds of illness. In the first place, it is neither mental nor illness in the usual sense. It is not a disease of the brain or intellect, although it affects both. It is not a disease of the body with physical symptoms, although it may include these. It is not a disease of the culture or society in which it occurs, although it may reflect both. In an attempt to lessen the strangeness of mental illness and promote greater acceptance and understanding of it, we have bent over backwards, perhaps too far, in insisting that it is like any other illness, "like breaking a leg," for instance. But it isn't a disease like any other.

It is instead a disease of adjustment, a faulty way of living, and its symptoms are expressed in the way one behaves. It is an inability or failure on the part of an individual to behave in accord with the expectations of his society. Mental illness affects the whole person, and all of his functions. He does not think, feel, act as he should, that is, in accord with reality. There may be disruptions in the physical, emotional, or social aspects of his being. The paradoxical, inappropriate, unacceptable, unrealistic ways in which he behaves are the symptoms of his illness.

The nurse, then, is faced with dealing therapeutically with behavioral rather than physical symptoms of illness, and this calls for much more knowledge, understanding, and skill on her part. For example, it is much easier to relieve the symptoms of fever or pain than it is to relieve the symptoms of hallucinations and delusions. The patient behaves as he does because of his illness —that very behavior is the expression of his illness. If he could behave differently, he would—indeed if he could be well he would not be sick.

First of all, the nurse must learn to accept the patient's behavior as a symptom or expression of his illness. Second, she must learn how to help him find more effective ways of behaving. Third, she must learn to handle her own feelings of anxiety, fear, despair, disgust, anger, disappointment, guilt in ways that promote her relationship with the patient rather than interfere with it. The nurse cannot control or change her behavior until she is able to recognize underlying feelings in reaction to the patient's behavior. To deny her feelings may be sufficiently unhealthy to cause deterrents to her effective interaction with the patient. She cannot change what she cannot accept as a part of herself. She cannot accept others unless she can accept herself. She cannot know or understand others unless she knows and understands herself. She cannot help others change their behavior unless she is able to change her own.

Contrary to what many of us have learned, it is not wrong or bad to experience feelings of anger, hatred, disgust, despair. The wrong comes about in the way we handle such feelings and act toward one another, particularly in relation to those who depend upon us for their very survival, like patients. If we as nurses take out our feelings of hostility on patients we are apt to add to their discomfort, anxiety, and illness. If, on the other hand, we as nurses can recognize our own angry feelings, try to understand why we feel as we do, and resolve such feelings in constructive ways, then we are not so apt to harm patients or each other. At the same time, we demonstrate to the patient how it can be done, and serve as a "treatment model" for him.

Patients' behavior and symptoms are not funny or sad, good or bad. It is important that the nurse not ridicule the patient for his strange behavior, or make value or moral judgments about the symptoms of his illness. To do so implies that the patient could be symptom-free (or well) merely if he wanted to be, and thus denies his illness and the legitimacy of his behavior. Anyone who has ever had insomnia knows that the more he tries to make himself go to sleep, the more wide awake he becomes. No matter how logical, appropriate, good, or even necessary it is that he get some sleep, telling himself or his wife so does not help him sleep. Anyone who has ever had a drinking problem knows that all the logic and good intentions in the world are not sufficient to keep him from drinking. Someone has said, "The road to hell is paved with good intentions." The alcoholic needs someone to help him withstand the torments of temptation, and this is the basis for the organization and success of Alcoholics Anonymous.

Very often the patient behaves in ways that are similar to, or reminiscent of, childhood patterns. Sometimes the nurse expects more of him than he is able to accomplish, and this can only make matters worse for him instead of better. Repeated failure, disapproval, rejection, or ridicule can only cause him increased discomfort, anxiety, and illness. To simply try to correct the patient's behavior (his symptoms) without remedying the underlying conditions or helping the sick person overcome his illness may be the emergency treatment of choice and it may provide temporary respite from the illness. Obviously, however, the best approach in the long run is to help the patient into a position whereby he himself can make whatever corrections are necessary, and that takes time and skill on the part of people with whom he interacts.

Despite the fact that mental illness affects the person, not his parts, patients have areas of healthy as well as sick functioning. Some patients function very well except for specific kinds of distortions in their thinking. For example, a patient may carry out the functions of motherhood perfectly well in her own home, but become highly excited and emotionally disturbed outside of her home. An elderly patient may get along fairly well when he is around familiar people and objects, but become noisy, agitated, disoriented when he is in strange surroundings.

It is often necessary for the nurse to confront the patient with his behavior and the effect that he has on others in an attempt to help him see the necessity for change. This can be done, however, without stripping the patient of his defenses, so that he stands naked and shivering in front of God and everybody in the world. A person can withstand almost any kind of suffering if he is fortunate enough to have someone who truly cares for him. Confrontation, correction, and reenforcement therapy work most effectively for the patient when the nurse has a compassionate, sustaining, therapeutic relationship with him.

Someone has described such a relationship in these words: "Oh, the comfort, the inexpressible comfort of feeling safe with a person, having neither to weigh thoughts nor measure words, but pouring them all right out, just as they are, chaff and grain together; certain that a faithful hand will take and sift them, keep what is worth keeping, and then with the breath of kindness blow the rest away."

If the nurse is to be helpful or therapeutic in her interactions with the patient she needs helpful and therapeutic relationships with her co-workers. She needs the opportunity to express and share her feelings, thoughts, and reactions with other nurses, physicians, and supervisors. This kind of accepting, sharing, democratic environment must be planned and fostered, as well as spontaneous and informal. It must permeate the entire atmosphere of the treatment facility.

Psychiatric treatment centers are noted for their frequent group and individual conferences. Planned meetings are held regularly for patients and staff. Such conferences may be focused upon problems in group living, ward government, nursing care, psychiatric treatment, plans for disposition and followup care. To be helpful, such conferences should encourage the participants to express themselves freely. However, they must be assured that if they expose themselves through free expression, they will be accepted, respected, and protected by the other members of the group. If people are going to be honest with one another, they need assistance in expressing themselves, listening to others, and identifying and resolving whatever problems exist. A physician, psychiatrist, or nursing supervisor often functions as the group leader for such a conference.

It is important to remember that if you encourage another person to be honest with you, you must be prepared to be honest with him in return, accept whatever feelings he expresses, and respect his right to feel as he does. Only then can you move on by helping him find ways of expressing his feelings more constructively, and even sometimes resolving the problems which inevitably surround such feelings.

A mentally ill patient is similar to, yet different from, every other person. The degree of his health or illness depends upon how well his interactions with people around him satisfy his basic human needs. The form his illness takes is related to the kind of person he is, the way he has learned to behave, and the amount of success he has had in his experiences with others. The success of his treatment is determined largely by how capably the people who care for him ascertain his needs, assess his ability to meet them, and supply whatever help is required in order for his needs to be met.

Effective psychiatric nursing requires that the nurse gain the knowledge, understanding, and skill necessary to be able to observe, analyze, and respond therapeutically to the patient's needs. She must expend continued effort to improve her self-awareness, perceptions of the world around her, and sensitive relationships with others. It is not something that comes to her naturally or automatically or magically. It requires hard work, practice, ongoing evaluation, and continued learning. It requires courage and humility and strength to tolerate the inevitable failure and frustration that accompanies service to other people. It requires sufficient sources of satisfaction to maintain her state of health and sense of security. But the knowledge that she has helped to make one person's life more tolerable, or comfortable, or successful makes all the effort worthwhile.

REFERENCES

Benton, Denise W.: "You want to be a what?" *Nursing Outlook*, 79 (June, 1979) pp. 388–393.

Blaney, Doris: "An opinion on the scope of nursing,' *American Journal of Nursing*, 79 (November, 1979) pp. 2000–2001.

Cannon, Maureen: "To Sharon, with love," *American Journal of Nursing*, 79 (April, 1979) pp. 642–643.

Garant, Carol: "Stalls in the therapeutic process," *American Journal of Nursing*, 80 (December, 1980) pp. 2166–2169.

Kauffman, Mary: "One way to teach students empathy," *American Journal of Nursing*, 78 (May, 1978) pp. 860–862.

Kohnke, Mary F.: "The nurse as advocate," *American Journal of Nursing, 80* (November, 1980) pp. 2038–2040.
McGoran, Saralee: "Teaching students self-awareness," *American Journal of Nursing, 78* (May, 1978) pp. 859–861.
Pilette, Patricia Chehy: "Caution: objectivity and specialization may be hazardous to your humanity," *American Journal of Nursing, 80* (September, 1980) pp. 1588–1590.
Robinson, Lisa: *Psychiatric Nursing As A Human Experience*, 2nd Edition, W. B. Saunders, Philadelphia, 1977.
Rogers, Carl: *On Becoming a Person*, Houghton-Mifflin, Boston, 1970.
Stacklum, Margaret M.: "New student in psychiatry," *American Journal of Nursing, 81* (April, 1981) p. 762.
Storlie, Frances J.: "Henry," *American Journal of Nursing, 78* (December, 1978) pp. 2071–2072.
Thompson, John D.: "The passionate humanist: from Nightingale to the new nurse," *Nursing Outlook, 80* (May, 1980) pp. 290–295.
Ziemer, Mary M.: "Sounding board: just what is simple nursing?" *Nursing Outlook, 79* (May, 1979) pp. 344–345.

Chapter 2

Basic Human Needs

To know how to help people who are sick, either physically or emotionally, nurses need to understand behavior—the patients' as well as their own. Nurses need to know why people behave as they do, and what they can do to help people behave more successfully.

There are many explanations as to why man behaves as he does, what underlies or motivates or guides his behavior. It is generally agreed, however, that all behavior is aimed towards the satisfaction of basic needs. When a person behaves in ways which generally achieve satisfaction for him, we say he is mentally healthy. However, when he behaves in ways which consistently fail to bring him satisfaction, and his behavior falls into certain patterns, we say he is mentally ill, or we call his behavior pathological, sick, maladjusted, or disturbed.

PHYSICAL NEEDS

Basic human needs fall into three categories—physical, emotional, and social. Physical needs are closely related to body function and are sometimes described as primary or physiological drives—such as the sex drive or the hunger drive. They are usually thought to be innate, needs with which we are born. The common physical needs are the person's need for *food* or sustenance, including water, oxygen, and elimination; *clothing* and *shelter* for body warmth and protection; and *activity*, or sensory and motor stimulation, including sexual pleasure, physical exercise, and rest.

Certain physical or body needs are directly felt. When our bodies need food or water, we feel hungry or thirsty. Some physical needs are felt only under certain conditions, such as interference of some kind. We gasp for air when our oxygen supply is reduced or cut off. Other physical needs are known to exist, but physical longing or desire or awareness does not accompany them. We know we need vitamins but we are only aware of the after-effects when we don't get them. We experience fatigue or night blindness as a result of the lack of vitamins A or B.

As with all needs, physical needs are satisfied in interaction with significant other people. In the infant, all physical needs may be satisfied during the feeding period. The food sustains him, the way he is held warms and protects him, cuddling or fondling satisfies his infant sexual drive. He exercises his legs and arms and body muscles, cries out in delight, has a bowel movement, and falls asleep. How his physical needs are met has a very powerful influence on the kind of adult he becomes. If, as an infant, his needs are met consistently and with respect, he will develop a sense of trust in himself and others and the world he lives in. He will feel that he is a person of some worth and importance. If, as an infant, his physical needs are not met or are not met properly, serious damage to his physical and mental health may result. He may develop vitamin deficiencies that cause physical disease, such as rickets. He may develop habits or ways of behaving that prevent successful interaction with others and may eventually lead to mental illness. For example, if his mother gets very angry with him when he cries to be fed, she conveys this to him in the way she picks him up, holds him, and talks to him. The infant may react to this by crying all the more, by becoming disinterested in eating altogether, or by regurgitating his food.

At each stage of development a person is expected to learn new ways of behaving, new ways of satisfying his needs. For example, infants satisfy their need for food by sucking and biting, adults by biting and chewing. As the child begins to get teeth, he finds his behavior is no longer acceptable to his mother. He must learn to bite and chew and swallow differently. He must learn to take food from a spoon and milk from a glass.

Also, as a person grows up he learns to expect certain actions from others in response to how he behaves. He learns that if he behaves in certain ways, the result will be pleasant, whereas if he behaves in other ways, the result will be unpleasant. Thus, guided by the responses of people around him, particularly his mother, he tends to develop patterns of behavior which result in pleasant feelings within him. A person's food and eating habits develop as a result of the interactions he has with significant other people, immediately before, during, and after the feeding period. If mealtime is repeatedly a hectic, unpleasant experience for a youngster, he may develop the habit of bolting his food so as to end the unhappy experience as rapidly as possible.

As an infant, his needs to be warm and protected are satisfied when his mother holds him, covers him, or changes him. Soon he discovers that he is expected to take care of himself. He is expected to control his sphincters and deposit his body wastes in a special container. He learns to cover himself, dress himself, protect himself from the cold and other hazards in the environment. How he does it depends upon what he learns from his experiences as he grows up.

As an infant, his sexual drive is diffuse, ill-defined. He gains satisfaction through physical exercise and sensory contact with his mother. Denied physical activity and sensory experiences as a child, he may have difficulty fulfilling his heterosexual role as an adult, a role which requires physical closeness, contact, and pleasure. Overstimulation as a child may make it difficult for him to find sufficient sexual satisfaction as an adult.

EMOTIONAL NEEDS

Emotional needs, like physical needs, play a part in motivating behavior, and frustration of them results in serious disturbances in behavior. It is difficult to identify separately emotional needs and their satisfaction because they are so closely interwoven with physical needs. For the infant, the focus of the mother-child relationship characteristically is the meeting of his physical needs. His emotional needs are either satisfied or frustrated by the way in which his mother cares for him physically.

The common emotional needs are a person's need for *love*—to be loved and then to love others—including approval and esteem; the need for *importance*, which includes recognition and respect; the need for *adequacy,* which includes self-sufficiency, and the need to be needed and wanted; the need for *productivity,* which includes work and creative pursuits.

Emotional needs, like physical needs, are met in interaction with significant other people. Mother is the first such person the infant learns to interact with, and the ways in which she interacts with him either satisfy his emotional needs or they do not. It is in this primary relationship between mother and infant that the stage is set for the development of the individual's patterns for satisfying his needs or interacting with others.

If the child is loved freely and openly by his parents, he develops a feeling of essential worth and dignity and reaches out to love others. If he is treated like the important person he is, he develops a feeling of self-respect and respect for the rights of others. If he is helped to deal adequately with problems in his environment, he develops a feeling of strength and security. If his ability to produce is recognized and encouraged, he develops a feeling of wholeness and integrity.

Emotional growth and development can only take place in an atmosphere of love and acceptance and exchange. From being loved, an individual develops a sense of trust in himself and others that is basic to successful relationships with others. When he is loved, he is more capable of surmounting the struggles and disappointments life is bound to hold for him. He must receive before he has anything to give, so he learns to love others as he himself is loved.

If the child does not grow up in a climate of adequate warmth and love, it may be difficult for him as an adult to achieve the intimate relations of marriage and family. He may suffer from feelings of isolation and loneliness. He may become cold, detached, aloof. In any case, the result will be difficulty in giving, receiving, and sharing love with another human being. Many people think that deprivation in this area is the basis for most of man's maladjusted or sick behavior.

Everyone needs to feel that he has acquired at least some of the traits that society regards as valuable so that he measures up to the fellow next to him. If he does not feel this way about himself, he may experience feelings of worthlessness, guilt, or shame. He may severely criticize others in a vain attempt to elevate his own standing. He may be overcome by defeat and discouragement and develop an attitude of apathy or indifference. Any serious undermining of his self-respect will be reflected in his lack of respect for others.

The child must learn how to cope successfully with the problems of his environment. He must be able to master the tasks he is expected to perform. He must feel capable of facing change and the uncertainty of the future. If he does not learn these things about himself and his environment, he will be unable to develop effective behavior patterns. He may become confused or disorganized when faced with threatening situations. He may develop overwhelming feelings of apprehension, panic, helplessness. At any rate, his lack of confidence in himself will seriously interfere with his effectiveness.

The need for productive or creative expression is present in each person and in all people. Sometimes it is covered by discouragement, disuse, or doubt, but it sets the stage for entrance into the work-a-day world of adult life. It starts at home as the child begins to lose interest in activities that are involved only with playthings. He wants to use real tools and make real things. It begins to grow and develop when he learns to compete, produce, and achieve in his schoolwork. It really blossoms with his first job for pay. Throughout childhood and adolescence he is preparing for his role in life as a worker, contributor, provider.

If he does not have an opportunity to learn how to gain pleasure from producing, he may be in for serious trouble within himself and with his environment. He may experience feelings of inferiority and give up in despair. He may never have an example of satisfying productivity, and so lack interest and investment in work. He may retreat from the painful experience of repeated failure by exhibiting a general lack of ambition, sometimes mistakenly called "laziness" or "shiftlessness." All of these conditions result in serious deviations from the expected independent, cooperative, goal-directed behavior of the healthy adult.

SOCIAL NEEDS

Social needs and ways of satisfying them grow out of the culture or society of which one is a member. They are also closely intertwined with physical and emotional needs, and often cannot really be separated from them. Mother is the first teacher of social customs, but the child learns as well from father, family, peers, and other members of his social group. The common social needs are a person's need for *identification* or belonging, *education* or learning, *religion* or worship, and *recreation* or play. Social needs, also, are met in interaction with significant other people, who include members of the community and social groups as well as the family. In a democratic country, the satisfaction of social needs is often partially guaranteed by social legislation, such as that enacted in our own country to protect civil rights regardless of race, the right to work, freedom of religion, aid to education, and recreational areas such as national parks.

The infant gets satisfaction of his need to belong from the way in which his physical and emotional needs are met in interaction with his mother. As a person grows up, other people become increasingly significant in the satisfaction of this need. Father and other family members provide the models for identification. Members of the peer group are especially influential during adolescence and young adulthood. As an adult, he joins organizations and belongs to various groups in his community. He adopts certain values, ways of wearing his clothes and hair, certain ways of building his house and regulating his life.

If a person is denied satisfaction of his need to identify with others, his social behavior may be seriously disturbed. He may be distant and aloof in his relationships. He may have grave difficulty carrying out his role as a contributing member of society. He may be so isolated from others that he is cast as a social misfit. He may have problems in assuming the masculine (or feminine) role which is expected of him as an adult.

The need for learning or education starts at birth and is closely related to a person's survival and security. Unless the need to learn is encouraged and gratified, an infant may not survive, let alone feel secure. He has myriad tasks to master in order to develop into a healthy adult. He must be provided with the opportunity to learn and be supported in his efforts when he fails. A person's attitude towards learning is set early in his life. If he is constantly discouraged, scolded, or ridiculed in his attempts to learn, he may develop disturbances in his behavior. He may find it difficult or even impossible to achieve the requirements in formal education. He may be unable to realize his own potential and thus not attain self-realization. He may develop misconceptions about knowledge, education, and learning that lead him to fear, disdain, or envy others more successful than he.

Everyone has religious or spiritual needs, but since people satisfy these needs in so many different ways it is difficult to find a common denominator. However, it is generally characteristic of human beings to believe in a force or forces outside themselves. It may be a divine power, such as God, Buddha, or Allah, worshipped in organized religion. It may be some natural phenomenon, such as fire or water, in primitive cultures. It may be mystical, existential, or materialistic in nature, depending upon the individual and the society from which he comes.

Whatever religious needs a person has, they are related to the cultural influences upon his life. As an infant, he soon learns that there are forces, powers, controls outside himself, usually stronger than he. He may grow up in a family where there are very strict religious beliefs and practices, or where there are apparently no outside controls, or where there is a more liberal form of worship. He may react to harsh restrictions with resentment and rebellion. He may lack understanding and compassion for others. He may be immoral or amoral in his social conduct.

The need for recreation is associated with relaxation, fun, enjoyment, and is an essential aspect of every person's life. An infant's need for recreation is satisfied by playing with his mother, himself, or his toys. As a person grows up, he learns how to play with others, how to enjoy himself in socially acceptable ways, how to attain pleasure. Adults in our culture spend a great deal of time, effort, and money in recreational pursuits such as big league baseball.

If he is not allowed to play, a person may become so serious that other people avoid his company because he is no fun. If he is allowed to play too much, he may not become serious enough to be a successful businessman, husband, or father. If he is punished for playing, or taught that it is sinful, he may feel guilty or anxious when he tries to enjoy recreation.

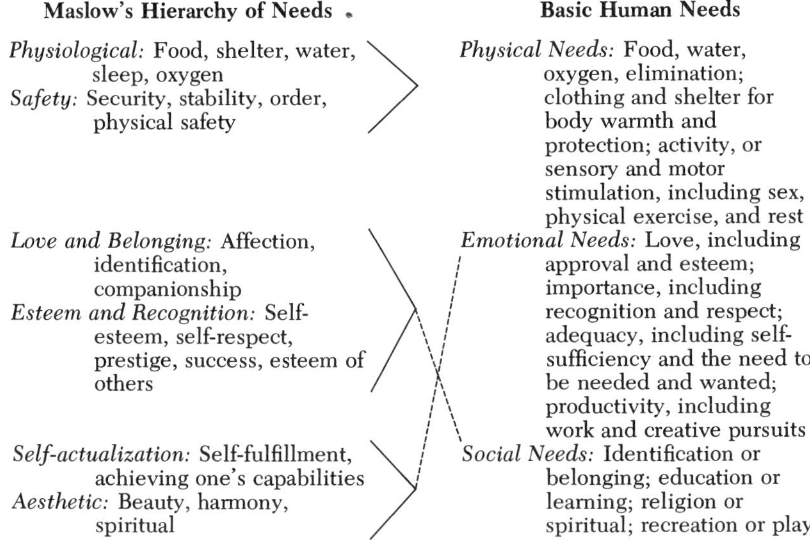

Figure 1. Comparison of Maslow's Hierarchy of Needs and Basic Human Needs.

Maslow describes needs in a slightly different way in comparison with the preceding description (Fig. 1). Further discussion of Maslow's hierarchy of needs may be found in his book *Motivation and Personality* and in *The Psychology of Human Behavior* by R. A. Kalish.

INTERRELATIONSHIP OF NEEDS

Needs are interwoven, interdependent, interrelated to such an extent that they cannot really be separated. They are fluid and changing—first one, then another, then a whole group taking priority. What may start out as a basic physical need for food takes on social and personal significance. In fact, so many basic needs may be satisfied by partaking of food that it has become a symbolic ritual of love and identification, strongly influenced by the family, church, and society of which one is a member. For example, the offering of refreshments becomes an expression of Southern hospitality. The consumption and enjoyment of whatever one is served becomes an expression of Oriental respect. Hamburgers and french fries are identified as the food of teenagers. Fried chicken and apple pie are considered typically American. Thus, certain foods, certain ways of preparing or serving food, certain table manners or eating habits are identified with the cultures from which they originate. Such habits or ways of behaving tend to persist since they gain for the individual the group approval which he seeks.

Thus, as a person grows up and learns to satisfy his needs in certain ways, and as these ways persist, they become incorporated into his personality. For example, if a child grows up in a home where mealtimes are a pleasant, satisfying experience, he tends to enjoy eating as an adult. If a child grows up in a home where mealtimes are surrounded by bickering and unpleasantness, he may find it difficult as an adult to enjoy food, even though the circumstances have changed for him. As long as such habits or ways of behaving result in satisfaction, security, and comfort for the person, any attempt to change them may be met with resistance because it is threatening to him.

Under stress, an individual may substitute the satisfaction of one need for the satisfaction of another. If he does not receive sufficient satisfaction in one area, he may try to make up for it in another. For example, a person who is unsuccessful in gaining the love he needs from other people may overeat in his attempt to find comfort and security. Unfortunately, such substitution often does not work, and instead of feeling better as a result of his action, he feels worse.

The frustration of one need may seriously interfere with the satisfaction of another. Various studies have been done regarding the effects of the lack of maternal love upon children, and all these demonstrate the powerful influence of this lack upon physical appearance and body functioning. Films of abandoned infants who were victims of the London blitz during World War II serve as classical examples. Despite the fact that the physical needs of the infants for food, clothing, shelter, and activity were met, many were malnourished, lethargic, and unresponsive. Most people have experienced the effect which frustration can have upon the appetite and the utilization of food.

Frustration

The satisfaction of basic needs results in a person's survival, security, and sense of well-being. Unmet needs produce physical tension and discomfort within an individual which must be relieved, so that the individual is propelled toward the goal of satisfaction. This internal condition is sometimes called motivation or drive, with the outward results hopefully being goal-directed behavior. When needs are not met, this tension results in a state of unbalance or disequilibrium within the person as well as between him and his environment. Balance, or homeostasis, must be restored in order for the person to feel safe, secure, and comfortable again, so he is forced to do something to resolve the situation.

Any interruption of a person's drive for satisfaction or interference with the satisfaction of one's basic needs results in frustration. If a person faces a threat to his survival and security he reacts accordingly. What he does depends upon how he has learned to behave in times of crisis or stress. The reaction to the experience of frustration has been generally characterized as fight or flight. Sometimes, however, the reaction may be paradoxical and not clearly defined. A person may become increasingly aggressive in his behavior in an attempt to gain satisfaction (fight). He may withdraw from the entire encounter, trying to pretend that it does not really matter anyway (flight). He may develop severe cramps in his digestive tract (paradoxical).

Consider the young bird who is pushed out of the nest by his mother and expected to change his source of satisfaction from mother and nest to the world around him. He is supposed to give up his successful way of living (dependent) for a new way that he has yet to master (independent). His survival and security are threatened. How does he react if someone approaches him? He may peck at his enemy—that's fight. He may try to get away—that's flight. He may open his mouth to be fed—and that's paradoxical.

Inside, a person may experience feelings of anger, despair, fear, guilt, or anxiety in reaction to a frustrating situation. To achieve successful adjustment, or mental health, an individual has to learn how to handle these feelings appropriately. If he turns these feelings inward upon himself, and feels guilty, we call that *introjection*. If he turns them outward upon the environment, and attributes them to others, we call that *projection*. If he recognizes the feeling and tries to find some productive way of expressing it, we call that *substitution* or *sublimation*, or working it through.

For example, an employee's supervisor may reprimand him in front of his co-workers for not doing his job properly. The action threatens his survival and security, and he feels angry. He may turn that anger inward upon himself, and experience feelings of shame or guilt or hurt (introjection). He may turn his anger outward and blame his co-workers for the job not being done properly (projection). He may go home and fight with his wife (substitution) or clean the garage (sublimation).

Deprivation

If the interference with a person's satisfaction is severe enough—that is, sufficiently prolonged, intense, and widespread—he will experience *deprivation*. Deprivation represents a serious threat to the survival and security of the individual and may result in serious disturbances in his behavior. The person's reaction varies in accordance with the severity of the deprivation, the ability of the person to successfully handle stress, and the circumstances in which he finds himself at the time.

One of the most serious kinds of deprivation is the loss of maternal love. Such deprivation can occur as a result of physical separation of mother and child, or can occur in situations where the relationship between mother and child is somehow deficient. The deficiency may occur when the child is not regarded as a person in his own right, and the mother interacts with him as an extension of herself, as in overprotectiveness. The deficiency may occur when the parent is so concerned with her own needs that she cannot supply the necessary satisfaction for the child, as in rejection.

No matter what the cause of the deprivation—physical separation or unsatisfactory mother-child relationship—the result may be disturbances in the person's behavior. As a child, he may exhibit learning difficulties, physical symptoms, compulsive eating, antisocial behavior, or withdrawn behavior. He may seemingly adjust in childhood, but disturbances in his behavior or adjustment may occur when he is faced with a severe threat in adult life. Or he may suffer no observable damage.

Conflict

Each person is engaged in a continual struggle to satisfy his needs, and this results in a psychological state which is called *conflict.* Conflict may result from internal or external forces. *Internal conflict* is a struggle within the individual between what he wants or needs, and what he believes to be right or possible. *External conflict* is a struggle between what an individual wants or needs, and what the physical environment and the people in it are willing and able to give him. Most conflict is a combination of internal and external forces at odds with one another.

Common causes of conflict are *ambivalence, trauma,* and *stress. Ambivalence* is the existence within the person of opposing emotions, impulses, or desires. For example, one may experience feelings of hate toward a person whom he loves, especially when there is a point of difference between them. *Trauma* is any experience that inflicts serious damage, physical or psychological, upon the person. Such injury or damage often results in maladjusted behavior. For example, a child who is repeatedly punished unfairly may develop such strong feelings of resentment towards authority that he begins to steal or set fires. *Stress* is any physical or psychological force that, when applied to a system, is sufficient to cause strain or distortion in the system, or when very great, to alter the system. For example, an athlete who runs the mile reacts physiologically to the demand made upon his circulatory system by compensatory enlargement of his heart. Similarly, persistent and prolonged psychological stress demands that the person change in some way in order to adjust. For example, if an individual holds a job which requires continual tact and diplomacy, he may have to repeatedly swallow his angry or aggressive feelings. Such a life situation may result in the formation of a peptic ulcer.

MEETING PATIENTS' NEEDS

Any treatment program or individual patient care plan is aimed toward the satisfaction of needs, and its effectiveness can be measured in terms of how well it meets the needs of those for whom it is intended. A lot has been said about the necessity for total patient care, meeting the patient's needs, treating the patient as an individual, and giving personalized care. Yet sometimes these phrases are used as if they were incantations, as if saying the words magically results in the realization of the task. The accomplishment of modern health care, particularly psychiatric treatment, takes more than magic words—it demands a special kind of comprehensive care aimed towards the satisfaction of the physical, emotional, and social needs of the person who is sick.

A patient has common human needs because he is a person, individual needs because he is unique, and special needs because he is sick. Illness poses a serious threat to his survival and security. It may also deprive him of his ability to care for himself by interfering with his functioning. It may remove him from his customary sources of satisfaction, such as home, job, and family, by requiring hospitalization. It may demand major changes in his life style by expecting him to be dependent rather than independent.

It is a nursing responsibility to supply the help that is required in order to meet a patient's needs. The nurse must determine a patient's needs, his ability to meet them by himself, and what must be supplied in the way of help from her. The nurse carries out this responsibility to the patient through her relationship with him.

Love is an essential part of helping others and the heart of any helping relationship. Erich Fromm, in *The Art of Loving*, describes that fundamental kind of love which underlies all others—the wish to further another human being's life—as brotherly love. He assigns four major qualities to that kind of love: care or concern for one's fellow man, respect for him as an individual, knowledge of him and his needs, and a sense of responsibility in helping him meet those needs. He says that like any art, love must be practiced, and this requires of the practitioner discipline, concentration, patience, and a supreme concern with the mastery of the art.

This kind of feeling for others, for one's fellow man, for one's patients, does not come automatically to the nurse. It requires hard work and conscious effort to establish and maintain a helping relationship. It isn't enough for the nurse to be a kind or tender or loving person (although that surely helps). She must know as well what is required of her, what is the most appropriate action for her to take, and what is the most skillful way for her to accomplish it. Any single interaction may satisfy a patient's basic needs and add to his comfort, security, and sense of well-being, or it may interfere with his satisfaction and result in discomfort, insecurity, and anxiety. Either result affects the individual's emotions, physiology, and behavior, and it has a direct effect upon the state of his health.

Most nurses at some time or other serve food to patients. How they serve the food can satisfy a patient's needs for food, love, and identification, or seriously interfere with the satisfaction of one or all three of these needs. If the food is arranged and served in an attractive manner, if the nurse is pleasant and friendly, if the group of patients eating together are congenial, then all three needs of the patient may be met. However, if the patient has arthritis and cannot use his hands, the nurse's action, to be effective, must change. The food may be arranged and served attractively, the nurse may be pleasant and friendly, and the group of patients may be congenial, but none of the three needs will be met if the nurse puts the tray down and walks out without cutting the meat, or opening the milk, or giving the patient whatever other assistance is required.

The patient's clothing should be warm and comfortable enough, as well as attractive and appropriate to the occasion. Letting a patient choose what he will wear may satisfy his need for importance. Showing him how to fasten his clothing himself, if he has lost the ability to do so, may satisfy his need for learning how to care for himself. Considering a patient's individual tastes in clothing will satisfy other emotional needs as well.

It is important for a blind patient or stroke victim to learn how to dress himself. Otherwise he is helplessly dependent upon others, his needs are not met, and he may feel himself a burden. The result may be that he functions below his capacity, is handicapped for the rest of his life, and remains less than healthy. It is often easier, or at least faster, to do for a patient, but if the nurse really cares about him, she will help him learn how to care for himself. Even though it hurts to use his arthritic fingers, even though it is painful to walk following a broken hip or abdominal surgery, it is necessary for a patient's sense of well-being to do as much for himself as he is able.

The patient's need for shelter, creativity, and religion can often be met by the nurse's careful attention to the immediate environment. So often an individual patient's needs and abilities are not taken into consideration. For some, a rosary, candles, and the Bible may be an essential part of life from which they derive great satisfaction. In some psychiatric hospitals, ward cleaning is scheduled for a particular day, such as Saturday or Sunday, and all patients are expected to take part. Working on the Sabbath may be contrary to the religious beliefs of a particular patient. As a result, the patient may find himself in conflict, and the nurse has thus contributed to his discomfort rather than helping him. Letting patients have a voice in the arrangement of the environment and allowing for individual differences will help to satisfy an individual patient's needs.

In socializing with patients, the nurse may satisfy or frustrate basic needs of the patients for activity, adequacy, and recreation. If the game or activity suggested is below the physical, emotional, or social level of a patient, he may feel insulted. If he is required to go to the movies every Wednesday night, he may no longer enjoy it. Activities imposed upon patients lose their benefit as sources of enjoyment.

For example, elderly patients with cardiac or circulatory difficulties may need to have restricted physical activity. Many elderly patients are not used to playing games and do not find them enjoyable. They may not be familiar with how the game is played so they feel inadequate or stupid. Sometimes nurses mistakenly think they will make the patient "feel good" by letting him win the game. However, an interaction of this sort may actually interfere with a patient's need to feel adequate. Most people do not find it fun to win when the other fellow throws the game, especially if they find they have been fooled into thinking they won legitimately.

People interact with others in an attempt to satisfy their basic needs. If a person's relationships are successful or healthy, his needs are satisfied, and he feels safe and secure. If his relationships fail, his needs are frustrated, and he experiences stress. He may react to stress with fight, flight, or paradoxical behavior.

It is up to the nurse to supply the help that is required in order for the patient's needs to be met. She carries out this responsibility through her relationship with the patient. A helping relationship must be based upon that fundamental love which underlies all others—the wish to further another human being's life.

REFERENCES

Barnes, Mary: *Two Accounts of a Journey Through Madness,* Harcourt Brace Jovanovich, New York, 1972.

Besch, Linda Briggs: "Informed consent: a patient's right," *Nursing Outlook, 79* (January, 1979) pp. 32–35.

Chamberlin, Adaline B.: "Shoes," *American Journal of Nursing, 80* (June, 1980) p. 1162.

Curtin, Leah L.: "Is there a right to health care?" *American Journal of Nursing, 80* (March, 1980) pp. 462–465.

D'Addio, Dina: "Reach out and touch," *American Journal of Nursing, 79* (June, 1979) p. 1081.

Francis, Gloria: "The therapeutic use of pets," *Nursing Outlook, 81* (June, 1981) pp. 369–370.

Fromm, Erich: *The Art of Loving,* Harper & Row, New York, 1974.

Hayter, Jean: "The rhythm of sleep," *American Journal of Nursing, 80* (March, 1980) pp. 457–461.

Kalish, Richard A.: *The Psychology of Human Behavior,* Wadsworth Publishing Co., Belmont, California, 1966.

Macrae, Janet: "Therapeutic touch in practice," *American Journal of Nursing, 79* (April, 1979) pp. 664-665.

Maslow, Abraham H.: *Motivation and Personality.* 2nd Edition, Harper & Row, New York, 1970.

Piche, Judith Coffman: "Tell me a story," *American Journal of Nursing, 78* (July, 1978) pp. 1188–1193.

Stillman, Margot J.: "Territoriality and personal space," *American Journal of Nursing, 78* (October, 1978) pp. 1670–1673.

Stoll, Ruth I.: "Guidelines for spiritual assessment," *American Journal of Nursing, 79* (September, 1979) pp. 1574–1577.

Tobiason, Sarah Jane Bradford: "Touching is for everyone," *American Journal of Nursing, 81* (April, 1981) pp. 728–730.

Towle, Charlotte: *Common Human Needs,* National Association of Social Workers, New York, 1965.

Chapter 3

Communication and Human Relations

There are many ways of explaining human interactions or human relations. One way is to look at them as a huge communication system. Part of the difficulty in making such an attempt is that the process of human communication is so complex that we do not even have adequate words to describe it. Nevertheless, to carry out our major responsibility to a patient in seeing that his needs are met, it is essential for nurses to have some understanding of how, what, and why people communicate with one another. Let us look at human interactions, then, particularly the nurse-patient relationship, as a complex communication system, realizing at the same time that the real process is by no means so simple.

Definition

Communication may be broadly defined as all the steps involved in a two-way relationship between the person and his environment. Human communication specifically involves the transmission of a message that touches off a response. We call it a process because it is a series of steps which are dynamic, fluid, continuous, and changing. It is like throwing a stone into a pool, so that the resulting circles go out farther and farther and become larger and larger.

Purpose

The major purpose of human communication is to satisfy basic needs. The effectiveness of a person's communication system can be measured by how well his needs and the needs of others with whom he is involved are satisfied. Communication also serves the purpose of correcting the information that a person has about himself and others, thereby helping to guide his behavior. For most people, there is the additional satisfaction or pleasure of expressing one's self.

Intrapersonal Process

Like systems used for transmitting messages by TV, radio, or telegraph, the human communication system is comprised of two essential components or parts—the sender and the receiver. The sender goes through a series of steps inside himself—*the intrapersonal process*—based upon his needs and his experience in life. First, he perceives himself and his environment—he gets a picture of what his needs are and what his situation in life is at the moment. Second, he evaluates these—he compares his internal strivings and external circumstances with his experiences in the past. Third, he decides to act accordingly—he decides upon a course of action he hopes will satisfy his needs. Fourth, he signals the receiver—a significant person from whom he hopes to obtain his satisfaction.

A person does not deliberately or consciously think out each step he takes in the communication process. A great deal of what happens to him and within him occurs outside his awareness. For example, a person feels hungry and asks for food or goes to the kitchen to get it, whichever has proved successful in the past. He feels uncomfortable and wants a glass of milk. He doesn't stop to figure out why, or perhaps he couldn't do so even if he tried. He does know that a glass of milk has made him feel better in similar circumstances in the past, so he tries to relieve his present discomfort in the same way.

Interpersonal Process

The sender transmits a message which sets into motion *the interpersonal process*. The message is divided into two layers—the outer layer is called the content, and the inner layer is called the intent. The outer layer, *the content,* is the covering on the message and may be compared to the husk on grain, the shell on a nut, or the peel on an apple. One can tell something about the inside layer, generally, from the look or feel or smell of the outside. For example, if a person drives past a field of grain, he may be able to recognize it as oats, timothy, barley, or wheat just from the size, shape, and color of the husk. One can tell an English walnut from a black walnut by looking at the shell, or a red delicious apple from a yellow transparent by looking at the peel.

The inside layer, *the intent,* is the meat or heart of the message. If the two layers are consistent, the message is more easily received and more readily understood. If the two are contradictory or unfamiliar or foreign, more strain is put upon the receiver to decode the message. For example, a common communication between friends is the greeting, "How are you?" The words on the outside, the *content,* do not accurately reflect the inside, the *intent.* The person transmitting the message does not usually want to know the state of the other person's health. Instead, he wants recognition from his friend, the satisfaction of his own needs. The closer the agreement between content and intent, the more straightforward the message, the easier it is for the receiver to understand and respond and the better are the chances for the sender's needs to be satisfied. In other words, the healthier the sender's intrapersonal process (perception, evaluation, decision, and signal), the more likely he is to communicate clearly, relate successfully, and satisfy his needs acceptably.

The message strikes the receiver with a force, called *impact.* It makes a connection which alerts the receiver that a message is coming in, and he should get ready to receive it. In accordance with his needs and experiences in life, the receiver in turn goes through the same series of steps as the sender—the intrapersonal process. He perceives himself in relation to his environment, evaluates both the internal and external circumstances in light of previous experiences, decides upon the best course of action, and signals the other person, the sender, from whom he hopes to obtain satisfaction. His signal is called *the response,* and it has the same two layers as the sender's message—content and intent. The response strikes the sender with a force called *feedback.* The response either results in satisfaction or frustration of the sender's needs, makes a correction or alteration in the sender's communication system, or asks for clarification or elaboration of the sender's message.

In successful communication, the receiver must correctly read the intent of the message as well as the content. For example, a person familiar with the intent of the greeting "How are you?" might very well respond, "I'm fine, how are you?" And again, he may not be fine nor is he inquiring about the state of the other person's health. It is instead a response to the first person's request for recognition, as well as a way of satisfying his own need for recognition.

The closer the agreement between content and intent and the more straightforward the response, the easier it is for the sender to understand, and the better the chances are that both sender and receiver will satisfy their needs in interaction with one another.

The receiver has great significance in any communication system, and no less so in human relations. Satisfaction of the sender's needs depends not only upon the sender's ability to communicate effectively, but also upon the receiver's ability to correctly observe, analyze, and respond to the sender's message. If the sender does not get the response he requires from a particular receiver, he may do a number of different things. He may alter his message and try again to communicate successfully, especially if the receiver is sufficiently significant to him as a major source of satisfaction. He may try to get what he needs from another receiver, especially if another is nearby. He may give up for the time being and postpone his satisfaction. Eventually, however, it is essential to the life, security, and health of the sender to get sufficient satisfaction of his basic needs. Any severe disturbance in his ability to communicate successfully may result in serious disturbances in his behavior.

Transactional Analysis

In the 1950s Eric Berne established a branch of social psychiatry called *transactional analysis*. TA, as it is called, has become increasingly popular, resulting in two bestsellers, *Games People Play* and *I'm OK–You're OK* (see References at end of chapter). The concepts of TA can be used in describing communication and human relations, growth and development, and reactions to stress and psychiatric treatment. Because it is another way of looking at communication, we will describe it briefly here.

In TA, the *stroke* is identified as the fundamental unit of social action, the basis for all human interaction. The stroke starts out as a physical necessity for survival. Without physical stimulation in the form of cuddling, patting, and stroking, the infant will not survive. In fact, Rene Spitz has reported on the death of infants who were adequately fed, but were not loved or stroked by those who cared for them. The stroke starts, then, as a physical necessity, but it is gradually replaced by more symbolic and socially acceptable approval or recognition. Nevertheless, the stroke continues throughout life to satisfy physical, emotional, and social needs of the individual. The stroke may be as frequent as the nightly applause for the performer or as rare as the honorary award for the scientist. It may be as remote as a military salute or as intimate as a kiss. An exchange of strokes between two people constitutes a *transaction*.

Every individual is made up of three different personalities; three different sets of ways of thinking, feeling, and doing; three different *ego states*, as they are described in TA. These are designated as the *Parent*, the *Adult*, and the *Child* in each of us. These are not roles that people play, but are existing realities within the individual. They are the result of his experiences and interactions with his environment and the significant people in it. You will see that there is a similarity between the Parent, Adult, and Child, and the three parts of the personality as we have described them in Chapter 5—the Conscience, Self, and Needs. Likewise, there is a similarity to the aspects of the personality as described by Sigmund Freud; that is, the superego, ego, and id.

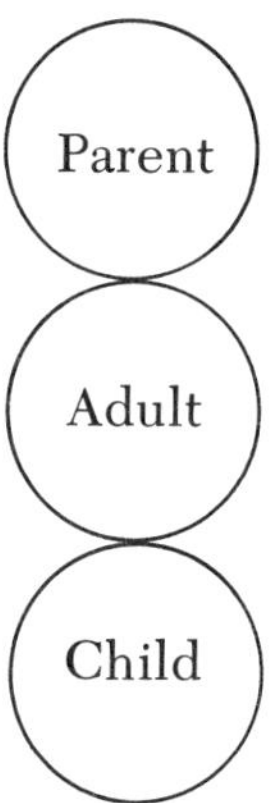

Parent. The Parent in each of us is a recording of what we see our own parents say and do. It is not necessarily an accurate recording—it is simply how we as children perceive our parents to be from the very earliest age on. Because an individual's experience begins before he understands words or before he understands why a parent does something, he simply incorporates into his Parent what he believes his parents think and feel and do. There are two distinct sets of attitudes that are generally part of the Parent in each of us. One is moralistic, critical, and forbidding; the other is nurturing, caring, and consoling. The one says "No, no, no. That's bad. Be a good boy." The other says, "You look tired. Let me rub your back." However, if a person has not experienced either of these kinds of parents, then his Parent will be different still.

Children have a Parent in them, just as they have an Adult and a Child in them. If you have ever watched children at play, you've seen the admonishing finger and the "No, no, no, no, no!"

Adult. The Adult is that part of us that looks at the facts and makes an appraisal. It is the practical, realistic, problem-solving part of the person. Its function is based upon the present, the here and now, and not upon the past. It is the mediator between the Child and the Parent, the compromiser. It is the computer, the data processing machine in us, that gathers the information from inside of the person and outside in the world in which he lives, in order to make a decision or a prediction or simply to store the information away for future use. The Adult part of us asks questions like "Why, What, How, When?" It says things like "Let's examine this further" or "I'm not quite sure we have all the facts" or "Maybe we don't quite understand" or "Let's give him the benefit of the doubt."

Child. The Child in us is a recording of our feeling reaction to what we saw and heard as we grew up, particularly from parents. It contains our creativity and spontaneity and pleasurable feelings, as well as our fears and anger and rebellion. Like the Parent, there are two sets of attitudes in the Child that result in very different kinds of behavior. The *adapted* Child modifies his behavior in response to the Parent by complying or withdrawing, in accord with what the Parent expects. The *natural* child is free and spontaneous, either in rebellion or joy, and expresses things in terms of his feelings or needs. The Child says things like "Wow" or "Yuk" or "I'm hungry" or "Let's have fun."

Each of the three—Parent, Adult, Child—is a legitimate, real, and respected part of the person. Each has its function and purpose. Each has a contribution to make toward the whole person and his self-realization. Each has its own part in creating a full, productive life for the individual. Only when there is a disturbance in the balance between them or a conflict in the way in which the person interacts with others is there a need for change and a transactional analysis.

Transactions. When two people meet they generally interact with one another. This can be a very simple stimulus and response (S-R) situation, or a very complex process of communication. The simplest kind of transaction is Adult to Adult, such as "Hi, how are you?" and "I'm fine, how are you?" As long as the transaction is complementary or parallel, the communication is successful: Adult to Adult, Child to Child, Parent to Parent; or Child to Parent and Parent to Child, Adult to Child and Child to Adult, Parent to Adult and Adult to Parent. (See Figure 2.)

When crossed transactions occur, then communication breaks down. The most common kind of crossed transaction, which also causes the most trouble, is if the stimulus is Adult to Adult and the response is Child to Parent. For example, if the husband comes home from work and asks his wife, "Is dinner ready?" that is an Adult to Adult stimulus, asking for information. If the wife interprets that as unjustified criticism, however, she may respond with hurt and anger: "Is that all you ever think about—eating? Don't you ever

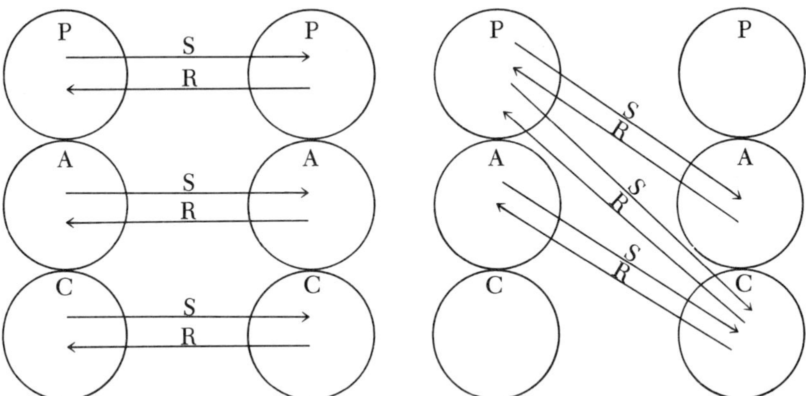

Figure 2. Complementary and parallel transactions.

think about me?" That is a Child to Parent response. (See Figure 3.) To resolve that situation, someone has to give. Either the husband has to switch to the consoling Parent, saying something like "There, there, honey, of course I care about you," or the wife has to switch to the cooperative Adult, saying "I'm sorry, I guess I'm just tired. Yes, dinner is almost ready." Otherwise, the communication ends and we have two adults glaring angrily and silently at one another. (See Figure 4.)

In summary, transactional analysis is another way of looking at behavior, communication, and human relations. The more aware a person becomes of how and why he is interacting with others, the

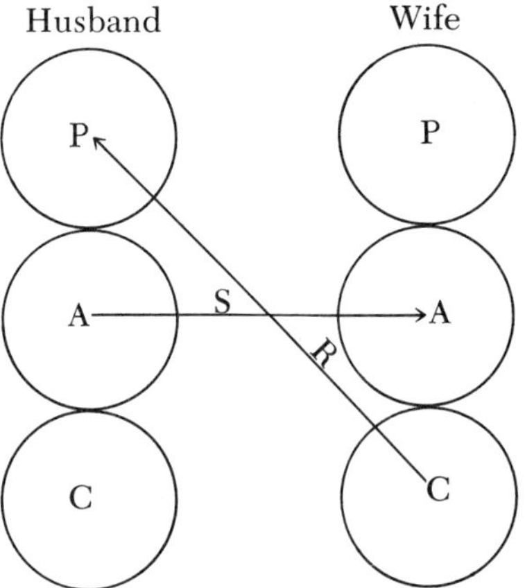

Figure 3. Crossed transaction.

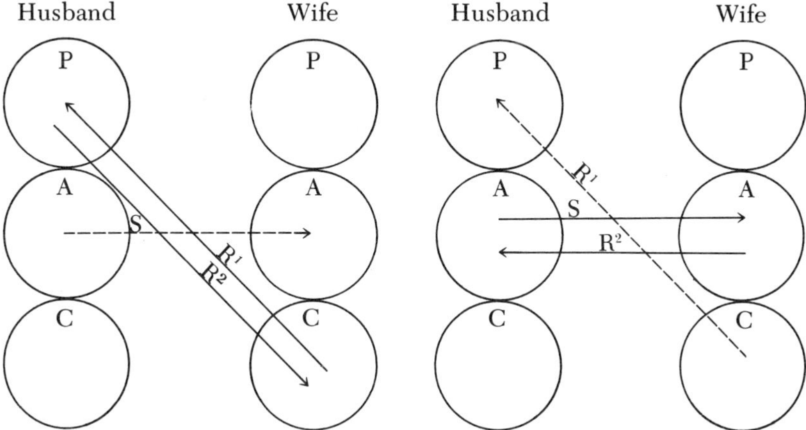

Figure 4. Corrected transactions.

more possible it is for him to control and correct his behavior and improve his effectiveness in his relationships. As Harris says in *I'm OK–You're OK*, we may not be able to erase what is recorded within each of us, but we can choose to turn it off.

METHODS OF COMMUNICATION

People involved in any interaction generally use both verbal and nonverbal methods of communication. The nonverbal methods which we will discuss first are extremely important in all communication but particularly so in the nurse-patient relationship.

Rapport. Rapport, a French word, is the harmonious feeling experienced by two people who hold one another in mutual respect, acceptance, and understanding. Popular expressions describe the experience as "being on the same wave length," "in tune with each other," "in touch," "I read you," or "I dig you." Sometimes one hears the statement about a nurse, "She has good rapport with her patients." However, there is no such thing as good or bad rapport. One either has rapport with someone or he does not.

Empathy. Empathy is that degree of understanding which allows one person to experience how another feels in a particular situation. Empathy is neither sympathy nor compassion, yet it combines a little of both. Sympathy usually implies feeling sorry for the other person, as in, "I'd feel bad if I were in his shoes." Compassion usually implies that quality of love or tenderness that causes one person to suffer along with another. Empathy implies knowledge and understanding of the other person's feelings, the situation he is in, and a positive feeling toward him. It is based upon the concept of brotherly love—concern for one's fellow man, respect for him as an individual, knowledge of him and his needs, and a sense of responsibility in helping him satisfy his needs. It is developed by learning how to read the nonverbal signs in another's behavior, and the intent of the message in the communication process.

Body Language. By means of body language we express ourselves physically by tone of voice, facial expression, gestures, touch or physical contact, posture, stance, walk, and so on. A person may express love and understanding by the way in which he looks at another person. A nurse may express her anxiety or irritation by the way she walks into a patient's room. A supervisor or physician may express disapproval by a frown or gesture. A patient can often tell whether the people caring for him respect him or not by the way in which they carry out physical tasks.

A patient often pays more attention to what is done than to what is said. He listens to the nurse's approaching footsteps, looks to see what her facial expression is, feels her touch as she turns him in bed—and in this way learns whether or not she really cares for him.

Silence. Through silence a person may express different feelings with varying degrees of helpfulness. It can range from an expression of love, respect, and empathy to destructive, hostile, anxiety-provoking communication. It may be a cold, rejecting, punishing kind of silence which greets a person when he is late getting home from work, or when he has forgotten an important anniversary. It may be the opposite kind of silence used to communicate the deepest love and respect—when words are often unnecessary.

Listening. In psychiatric nursing, you may hear the expression "listening with the third ear," which is taken from Theodor Reik's book of the same name. It is listening with an additional dimension of perception. It is "reading between the lines." It is picking up the underlying meaning of the message (intent), and not relying entirely upon the obvious or superficial meaning (content). There are many ways to measure one's ability to listen, and it is always amazing to discover how much or how little one person hears of what another person says. The parlor game of "gossip" really demonstrates the point. One person starts the game by whispering something to the person next to him, who in turn passes it on, until the last person to get the message announces aloud what he has heard. By the time the message has gone through less than half a dozen distortions, it is often no longer recognizable.

Spoken Word. The sixth way of communicating is verbal, that is, by the spoken word—a way which serves to acknowledge, amplify, confirm, contrast, or contradict other verbal and nonverbal messages. Verbal communication is always accompanied by nonverbal expression. In human relations, particularly successful relationships, people learn to rely upon more than the words themselves. It isn't just what is said, but how it is said—the speaker's tone of voice, facial expression, and gestures—which convey much of the meaning to the person listening. Patients are often less sophisticated and more like children so that they are more sensitive and particularly tuned to nonverbal communication.

In our society, however, verbal communication is extremely important to all people, sick or well. It is through verbal communication that a person attempts to share something of himself with a great many other people. It is the highest form of communication, as demonstrated in the complex process of learning, developing, and refining human speech.

THERAPEUTIC COMMUNICATION

The nurse's role is primarily composed of satisfying a patient's basic needs through her successful communication, relationship, or interaction with him. How effectively the nurse functions as the receiver in the nurse-patient communication system is a measure of her therapeutic ability.

In order to care effectively for a patient, the nurse must be able to correctly observe, evaluate, and respond to his communication. Such a role requires knowledge, understanding, and skill in human relations. First of all, to respond to a patient's communication in a therapeutic or helpful way, she must be able to decipher his message. She must know the particular patient well enough to discover the underlying meaning of his communication, the intent. He may ask for a drink of water or a bedpan when what he really wants is the comfort of the nurse's presence for a few minutes or the reassurance that someone cares about him. She must care enough about him to try to understand what he wants and needs. She must be able to express herself in such a way that his needs are met.

Second, if the nurse is to interpret correctly the incoming communication, her own receiving set must be in good working order. She must be sufficiently alert and perceptive to pick up the message. She must be realistic enough in her relationships with people to be able to avoid making assumptions or judgments about the patient's behavior.

Third, in order to meet the needs of the patient, the nurse must be emotionally mature enough to postpone the satisfaction of her own needs in preference to the patient's. It is essential that the nurse not meet her needs at the expense of the patient. That means that she must have other sources of satisfaction in addition to her relationships with patients so that she can tolerate the inevitable frustrations which occur in any relationship. She must allow a patient his own identity while she meets his dependent needs, and then release him for growth toward independence. A patient is dependent upon the nurse for love and care. If the nurse can meet his needs, the patient will reach out spontaneously to master his circumstances, since he is assured that he will be sustained during the failures and hurts which learning inevitably brings.

Psychiatric illness, or any illness for that matter, represents a disruption in a patient's ability to relate successfully with others. It is a primary nursing goal to help the psychiatric patient, not only to satisfy his basic needs, but to find more successful ways of doing so. The nurse, then, often becomes the model for a patient in psychiatric treatment, particularly in the hospital setting. In the position of receiver, she uses herself (her own healthy personality) to provide a continuous, corrective, nonevaluative feedback to the patient in the nurse-patient relationship. In this way she helps the patient correct his distortions and the faulty conclusions he has drawn about himself and others. She helps him improve the intra- as well as the interpersonal process in his communication with others. In so doing, she helps him relate more successfully, obtain greater satisfaction, and move in the direction of healthier behavior.

The most difficult part of the nurse's role in therapeutic communication is the necessity of looking at her own motivations, emotions, methods, and impact on others. Someone has said, "To gain in knowledge of self, one must have the courage to seek it, and the humility to accept what one may find."

The six methods of communication may be used as therapeutic tools by the nurse in her relationships with patients, since they are an essential part of any helping relationship. Marion Kalkman (*New Dimensions in Mental Health—Psychiatric Nursing, 1974*) lists similar methods as ways through which the nurse may alleviate a patient's anxiety—presence, touch, listening, and talking. The way in which a nurse uses the methods of communication—rapport, empathy, body language, silence, listening, and the spoken word—may either help a patient satisfy his needs and add to his sense of security, comfort, and well-being, or frustrate his needs and add to his state of anxiety, discomfort, and ill health.

The nurse establishes rapport with a patient when she respects him as an individual and accepts his right to be exactly as he is. Empathy stems from a feeling of compassion and concern for a patient, and is developed by the nurse in her effort to understand how he feels in his situation, not how she might feel.

Through her body language, the nurse conveys to a patient whether or not she really cares about him. The nurse must know when to be silent, and in her silence she communicates the love and acceptance a patient so greatly needs. By listening to a patient, the nurse increases her knowledge of him and his condition and at the same time communicates to him that she thinks what he has to say is important. Through the spoken words of explanation, direction, encouragement, the nurse makes it possible for a patient to master the strange and frightening world of illness. Thus, as the nurse meets a patient's physical needs through her nursing actions, she meets his emotional and social needs through her communication or relationship with him.

Frequently the importance and value of verbal communication is overemphasized while nonverbal expression is minimized. Often in nursing when we do not get the kind of verbal response or exchange we expect from patients, we feel uneasy or inadequate. In an effort to relieve our own anxiety, we turn the experience around, and mistakenly say, think, act as if the patient were out of contact. The patient may know what is going on around him, and at the same time be unable to communicate this to others. For example, a patient who has had a stroke may not be able to respond verbally, and yet he may be acutely aware of what others are saying to or about him. Patients who are not entirely conscious, for instance, before or after surgery or following a head injury, or who have a high fever or are under great stress, may be completely aware of others and what is going on around them without being able to communicate their awareness either verbally or nonverbally.

Patients who are unconscious or semi-conscious may experience sensations and respond to the way they are lifted, turned, or moved. For example, they may physically resist if they are frightened, angry, or hurt by the nurse's action. Patients and their conditions are sometimes discussed within earshot as if they did not exist as human beings but only as disease conditions. That kind of experience can be extremely traumatic to the patient, his family, and even innocent bystanders.

A patient suffering from mental illness may not be able to respond because his own world has temporarily replaced the real one, but he still knows what is said and how it is said, and he may respond nonverbally. Patients can often recount at length what has been said, how they have been treated, and the impact it had upon them, following their recovery from medical, surgical, or psychiatric illness. The patient's ability to realize what is going on around him should never be underestimated or discounted. Although he may not be able to respond or interact in the customary ways, chances are he has some awareness of what is happening to him and how people feel about him.

To a patient in a hospital, or for that matter, to any person in need of help, nothing is more important than the kind of relationships he has with people around him. Patients are people in trouble, usually serious trouble, when they come under the care of the nurse, and they are seeking safety, security, and comfort. The nurse provides that in her therapeutic relationship with them, using both verbal and nonverbal methods of communication. In any interaction, the nurse either helps a patient meet his needs and increases his sense of well-being, or she interferes with his satisfaction and increases his discomfort—there is no neutral position.

COMMUNICATING WITH PATIENTS

Sometimes the nurse feels uneasy or uncomfortable or at a loss as to how to communicate with a patient. This may also be true in social situations with healthy people. Probably the most difficult is the initial meeting—"getting acquainted"—with someone new. Sometimes it helps to remember that the patient is probably as uneasy as the nurse is, maybe even more so.

First of all, it is important for the nurse to convey to the patient that he is important and that she wants to help him. For the nurse, tell the patient who you are, that you are there to help him, and that you'd like to get to know him better: ask him if you can visit for a little while. Sometimes patients have difficulty expressing themselves in words, so the nurse might suggest doing something together—a game or a walk, for instance. Often, when you are doing something with another person, the discomfort decreases and communication comes easier. If the patient cannot express himself verbally, then the nurse must learn to communicate with him nonverbally and at the same time encourage him to put his thoughts and feelings into words. In other situations, it is possible for the nurse to talk to the patient in such a way that concern and interest are communicated without expecting a response. For example, the nurse may say something like, "You look uncomfortable. Is there some way I can help you?" Or the nurse might say, "I'm here to help you, and when you feel able to talk, I'll be here to listen." With other patients, the nurse might show them pictures out of a magazine and help them to identify things in the pictures. Sometimes just to sit with a patient and not talk at all is therapeutic—the feeling is conveyed that the nurse is interested enough to spend time with him regardless of his inability to talk.

Second, it is important for the nurse to convey to the patient that she is honest and trustworthy. For the nurse, don't overwhelm him with questions of a personal nature that might be embarrassing to answer until you have established a relationship. If the nurse must ask the patient personal questions for treatment purposes, explain why and don't overdo it—keep it short and matter-of-fact. Avoid such clichés as "You'll feel better soon" or "Everything's going to be all right." Tell him instead, if he is frightened, that you are here to see that nothing untoward happens to him. Explaining events and surroundings in a quiet, matter-of-fact way helps the patient to trust the nurse. For the nurse, be sure you follow through with what you say. Don't say you'll be back in ten minutes if you don't plan to be. If you are late, explain why. Despite what we think sometimes, patients are most often very capable of understanding explanations or forgiving our mistakes if given the opportunity. For the nurse, if you make a mistake, tell the patient so and ask him to forgive you. Don't say things you don't mean or can't carry out. Don't make promises that can't be kept. The patient's ability to communicate with the nurse depends upon the trust level the nurse is able to establish. The patient's communications should be treated with respect and confidentiality, only to be recorded or reported as treatment goals require and with his knowledge.

Third, it is important for the nurse to communicate with each patient as an individual. That means the nurse has to get to know the patient in order to understand what he is saying and how to help him. The best way to do this is by listening. For the nurse, try to put yourself in the patient's place and see the world through his eyes. If you don't understand what the patient is trying to communicate, tell him so and ask him to explain it to you so that you can understand. Check with the patient to validate your conclusions to make sure you have understood him correctly. You can ask him "Is this what you are saying?" or "This is what I understand you to be saying; is it correct?" or simply repeat in question form the last part of his statement.

Fourth, it is important for the nurse to accept and respect the patient despite the symptoms of his illness. For the nurse, with a delusional patient, avoid arguing with him about the reality of his perceptions. Try to point out reality to him as you see it, and help him accept the fact that he may not be able to see it that way at this particular time because of his illness. Do not agree with delusions or hallucinations either, but find ways to accept how the patient might feel without rejecting him or putting him down. The nurse might say, "I can understand how you might feel that way, but this is the way I see it." With some patients it may be necessary to object to certain kinds of behavior, and this should be done in a firm and matter-of-fact way, laying out alternatives if possible. The nurse might say, "I don't like that kind of behavior and suggest that if we are going to continue our discussions you will have to do this or that. What do you think is the best for you?" With elderly people, it is well for the nurse to remember they may have many interests and it is the nurse's responsibility to find out what they are and use them to draw the other person out. The conversation may be family related or job related: what the patient used to do for fun and work. Or it may be related to current events—elderly people are often more knowledgeable and perceptive than we realize. With angry or depressed patients, often the best thing for the nurse to do is listen, and let the patient get his feelings out in the open. Just talking about how you feel helps to relieve the feeling. After the patient has expressed his feelings, then it is often possible to help him find solutions or alternate ways of behaving that will make him feel better.

There is no way to provide a ready-made conversation or specific way of communicating with patients. Each nurse has to find ways that are most effective for the people and circumstances concerned. But if the nurse tries to be herself, expresses care and concern for the patient, uses the therapeutic methods outlined, and makes corrections as they are needed, the communication process between nurse and patient is apt to be effective.

REFERENCES

Almore, Mary G.: "Dyadic communication," *American Journal of Nursing, 79* (June, 1979) pp. 1076–1078.

Angelini, Diane J.: "Non-verbal communication in labor," *American Journal of Nursing, 78* (July, 1978) pp. 1220–1222.

Berne, Eric: *Games People Play,* Ballantine Books, New York, 1978.

Harris, Thomas: *I'm OK–You're OK,* Avon Books, New York, 1976.

Holm, Carol S.: "Deafness: common misunderstandings," *American Journal of Nursing, 78* (November, 1978) pp. 1910–1912.

Kalkman, Marion, and Anne Davis: *New Dimensions in Mental Health—Psychiatric Nursing,* 5th Edition, McGraw-Hill, New York, 1979.

Mitchell, Ann Chappell: "Barrier to therapeutic communication with black clients," *Nursing Outlook, 78* (February, 1978) pp. 109–112.

Moritz, Derry Ann: "Understanding anger," *American Journal of Nursing, 78* (January, 1978) pp. 81–83.

Murphy, Joan C.: "Communicating with the dying patient," *American Journal of Nursing, 79* (June, 1979) p. 1084.

Noble, Mary Ann: "Communication in the ICU: therapeutic or disturbing?" *Nursing Outlook, 79* (March, 1979) pp. 195–198.

Powell, John: *Why Am I Afraid To Tell You Who I Am?,* Argus Communications, Niles, Illinois, 1969.

Ramaekers, Sister Mary James: "Communication blocks revisited," *American Journal of Nursing, 79* (June, 1979) pp. 1079–1081.

Reik, Theodor: *Listening with the Third Ear,* B. J. Publishing Group, New York, 1977.

Zimmerman, Beverly M.: "Human questions vs. human hurry," *American Journal of Nursing, 80* (April, 1980) p. 719.

Chapter 4

Human Growth, Development, and Function

We have discussed basic human needs, communication, and human relations in an attempt to understand ourselves and others better and thus to improve our care of patients. Let us now investigate what makes people different from one another, how they get to be the kind of people they become, and why they behave as they do. We might have called this chapter "What Makes People Tick," or "What Makes Sammy Run."

Human growth and development is an interwoven, interrelated, dynamic process affecting the whole person. It is a process of becoming what one potentially is. It includes all aspects of the person—physical, emotional, and social. It is learning what one is expected to know, and becoming what one is expected to be. It is the accumulation of all the experiences a person has, which in turn determines how he functions, how he thinks and feels and acts as a human being. It is a lifelong process that begins in this world before birth and ends with death.

Each person comes into this world as a unique individual, unlike all others. He is endowed with a wide range of possibilities and a variety of needs. Through his interactions with his environment, he must learn how to maintain survival and attain security. He must learn how to satisfy his needs in acceptable ways. He must learn how to live in harmony with others and at peace with himself. What he learns as a child determines the kind of person he becomes as an adult. For each person life is made up of the perception of certain goals that he wishes to obtain, and the fulfillment of at least some of these.

A great deal of controversy has raged in the past over whether heredity or environment plays the greatest role in influencing human growth, development, and function. Likewise, there are disagreements over whether a person is born with certain kinds of behavior (instinctual) or whether he acquires them after birth (learned behaviors). At any rate, it is generally agreed that both heredity and environment play essential roles in each person's growth, development, and function as a human being. It is further generally believed that everyone is biologically equipped with certain kinds of responses, which can be elicited only by certain stimuli from the environment. Our discussion will follow along these lines of general agreement.

FACTORS WHICH INFLUENCE GROWTH AND DEVELOPMENT

There are many specific factors which influence the future of every human being and determine the general pattern of his functioning as a person. These factors may be divided into two groups—those we come into the world with, and those we acquire after we get here. Genes, maturation, and intellectual and physical capacity and characteristics fit into the first group. Learning opportunities, significant other people, interpersonal relationships, satisfaction of basic needs, and experiences with illness fit into the second group.

Hereditary Factors

Genes. Genes account for physical characteristics, such as body build, complexion, features, hair and eye color, and sex. From our parents we inherit our physical makeup—the systems, organs, and parts of the body and how they are put together. For example, if a person inherits a defective heart valve which limits his activities in life, this influences the kind of person he becomes. We inherit also our intellectual and physical abilities and capacities.

An individual's hereditary endowment is determined by what the germ cells (the egg cell of the mother and the sperm cell of the father) bring to the union. Each of these germ cells contains half (23) of the number of chromosomes found in other cells in the body. When the two germ cells, the egg and the sperm, unite, the new cell, the zygote, has the required number (46) of chromosomes, and thus the new human being begins. The chromosomes contain the genes which are the bearers of a person's heredity. Each gene is a giant molecule and consists mainly of deoxyribonucleic acid (DNA), which governs the formation of other protein molecules from which the new cells come. The chromosomes from the male and female germ cells unite in different combinations, and hence different children inherit different combinations of genes from the same parents. This accounts for the similarities and the differences between a child and his brothers, sisters, parents, and grandparents. Only identical twins have identical chromosomes and genes.

Maturation. Because he is a member of the human race, as well as the product of two particular human beings, each new person comes into the world equipped with a certain developmental pattern called maturation. Maturation can be defined as the sequence in which biological structures appear and new functions develop. Although each individual has his own variations, his physical and mental growth patterns resemble those of the same age, sex, and culture. For example, the developmental direction proceeds from his head to his extremities. The infant learns to hold up his head before he sits. He sits before he stands. He stands before he walks. Development also proceeds from the general to the specific, from large muscle to small muscle control and coordination. He learns to grab before he can grasp. He learns to walk before he can run.

The degree of neuromuscular development determines to some extent what the child accomplishes and when. For example, he cannot be toilet trained until the muscles which form the sphincters for the digestive and urinary tracts can be controlled. He cannot walk until muscle coordination is possible. He cannot pick things up until the small muscles have developed. Development moves from the whole to the part, from the random to the orderly, from the general to the specific.

Intellectual and Physical Capacity. A child's mental development begins long before he is able to think. His mastery of the intellectual functions involved in the cognitive process—sensation, perception, attention, memory, association, and thought—is related to his emotional and social development. For example, he cannot learn to read unless he has inherited sufficient physical and intellectual capacity to do so. Nor can he learn to read until his nervous and muscular coordination has reached a sufficient level of development. Further, he cannot learn to read unless he has the opportunity, stimulus, and encouragement to do so. The laws of growth and development apply to the total person. His physical, neuromuscular, and intellectual development influence and are influenced by his emotional, social, and spiritual development.

We all come into the world with the same basic needs—food, clothing, shelter, activity. However, they occur at different times, and in different combinations, and with different priorities. We come equipped with biological or instinctual drives that are designed to help us survive. These drives propel us in the direction of the satisfaction of our basic needs.

The inherited potential of any individual either develops or does not, depending upon certain factors in his environment. Our major focus will be, then, upon the factors that influence what and how an individual learns in interaction with his environment.

Environmental Factors

Learning Opportunities. First of all, what the person learns and how he learns it will be determined by the kinds of learning opportunities the environment provides him. For example, the child may learn incorrectly from his parents that blacks are inferior to whites. Unless he has some opportunity to learn differently, he will grow up with that prejudice and behave accordingly as an adult. It is obvious that the kind of environment which provides a wide variety of learning opportunities will better prepare the person for living. If he grows up in a family where reading is discouraged or even ridiculed, he may never experience the pleasure or value of literature, and he is not likely to hold reading or literature in very high regard, nor the people who enjoy such pursuits. If he grows up in a family which provides him with limited opportunities, he may go outside his family to find other opportunities, and his behavior may then be different from other members of the family. He may have inherited great intellectual capacity, but unless he has the opportunity to develop his potential through formal and informal education, he will not become an intelligent person. The converse is also true. He may have inherited low intellectual ability, but if he is given many opportunities to develop his full potential, he may be better off intellectually than someone more highly endowed.

He needs to learn not only what he must know and how he must behave, but how to continue learning. All of his abilities are relative to the one inclusive ability—his ability to learn. To stop learning is to stop growing, and to stop growing is to die.

Significant Others. The second important influence of the environment upon the individual is the kind of significant people with whom he comes in contact. The child learns to be the kind of adult he becomes from the adults around him—the models he has to imitate or identify with. For example, if a little boy is surrounded only by female figures as he grows up, his speech, gestures, his way of walking, even the way he combs his hair or dresses may resemble what we call typically female behavior. Such effeminate behavior is likely to provoke criticism from his peers, teachers, neighbors, and others. However, unless he has an opportunity to learn different behavior from someone significant to him, like the scoutmaster or teacher or coach, he is not likely to change. In fact, he may suffer from trauma and stress sufficient to cause further disturbances in his behavior.

If a child grows up in a family where the significant members do not trust one another or anyone outside the family, the chances are that he will not trust others either. If he grows up with people who are loving, trusting, honest in their relationships with themselves and with others, he is likely to have similar attitudes towards others.

Interpersonal Relationships. The kinds of interpersonal relationships a child has with significant people in his environment will influence the kinds of relationships he is able to establish with others. He learns how to communicate with other people from those who are significant to him. By such communication he attempts to satisfy his basic needs and the basic needs of others, thus forming the basis of successful human relations. What he learns from his experiences with others guides the intra-personal part of his communication system. What he perceives, how he evaluates it, what he decides about it, and how he signals others are all affected by his experiences in life. For example, if he has learned from his experiences that mothers are cold, rejecting, unloving people, his communication and relationships with mother figures, such as nurses, will be so affected.

Satisfaction of Basic Needs. Another environmental factor that influences the kind of person an individual becomes is the satisfaction of his basic needs. How, by whom, and how well his needs are satisfied will affect the way he sees himself and others and the world he lives in. If he is well cared for by his parents, then he is likely to develop the ability to relate successfully with others, to reach out for further learning experiences, and to tolerate the inevitable failures that learning brings.

Illness. Another environmental factor which influences the development of a person is the kind of experiences he has with illness. A person's state of health (physical, emotional, social) depends upon the physical endowments with which he was born, the kinds of illness he has been subjected to in his life, and the ways he has learned to cope with the enemies of health. The enemies of health can be listed as injury, infection, malformation or malfunction, and stress. Some people list stress as the primary enemy of health, with injury, infection, malformation, and malfunction named as the aides or complications or results of stress. For example, two different children in the same family may inherit diabetes and yet develop into very different kinds of people because of it. The response will depend upon the severity of the illness and the child's reaction to it. It will also depend upon the attitude of the parents toward the illness, the love and acceptance the child receives, the successes or failures he has in school, and so on. One child may turn out to be dependent, controlling, and backward because of his illness. Another child may turn out to be independent, spontaneous, alert despite his illness. For example, a young man who was born with defective vision became an outstanding professional football player, because he learned how to accept the deficit and compensate for it so that it did not become a handicap. If a person can be described as mentally alert, emotionally stable, and socially acceptable, then his organs and systems can be judged to be performing well.

STAGES IN THE LIFE CYCLE

Each person proceeds through a series of stages in life—infancy, childhood, adolescence, and adulthood. In each state the individual is faced with certain problems which he must master if he is to proceed to the next stage with vigor and confidence. These problems are called developmental tasks; the individual must accomplish these if he is to be judged by himself and others as a reasonably happy, successful person. Successful achievement of these developmental tasks as they occur leads to happiness and success with later tasks and will influence his future development. Failure leads to unhappiness, disapproval by society, and difficulty with later tasks. If the problem is well solved at the time it appears, the person's progress to the next stage is assured, and he acquires a degree of sturdiness for the future. What he learns in each stage forms either a firm or a shaky foundation for healthy adjustment.

At each stage there are evidences of earlier stages and hints of further development. Growth and development is a succession of spurts and plateaus, rather than a smooth, even progress. An individual's maturity can be measured at any stage of development; in other words, at any age it can be measured in terms of how well he has mastered the developmental tasks which he has faced, and thus how he feels about himself, other people, and the world in which he lives.

Developmental tasks arise from a combination of factors acting together—physical growth, pressures from society, and the needs of the emerging personality. If a child has received the necessary love, encouragement, and guidance, his individual rate of development can be trusted. Each person has his own timetable, although there is a certain consistency about the growth pattern. Children in different societies learn early which responses are favored and which are frowned upon. They also learn that different responses are expected of them at different stages. For example, what was right at age two is no longer all right at age four. A person's adjustment at any age depends upon the appropriateness of his physical, emotional, and social responses, and his ability to cope with life's challenges.

To master the developmental tasks, the child must have mature, giving adults to guide him. It is important to provide the child with suitable opportunities to practice the desired activities. Otherwise, he may try to provide his own, or resort to undesirable responses. Teaching is essential to his survival, security, and healthy adjustment. As different needs emerge, he attempts to satisfy them through whatever channels are available to him. He must also be provided with opportunities and safety valves to relieve the pent-up feelings that accumulate in response to frustration.

Customarily we think of growth and development as being limited to childhood, but the struggle to grow and develop is a part of our behavior throughout life. To deny ourselves and others the opportunity for growth is to jeopardize human health and happiness. We are all familiar with the person who shuts out life by closing the door to the acquisition of new knowledge and new behavior, who is satisfied with "the good old days." The impulse to learn is an innate tendency, and the fact that the impulse survives at all is evidence of its strength. Children find out early that learning is dangerous and is sometimes even discouraged. The first word the infant learns is not "Mommy" or "Daddy" but "no." If you have ever watched children playing, you have seen the little girl, pretending to be the mother, who shakes her finger at the pretend child and says, "No, no, no, no, no!" It is not too unusual for the child to go through his own stage of saying, "No, no, no, no, no!" to his mother. To grow or learn or to succeed in life, a person must have the kinds of human relationships which sustain him and give him the strength to conquer new heights.

The stages of life are described in different ways by different authorities. They are called the stages of psychosexual, or psychosocial, or personality development. Our discussion will follow that pattern set by Erikson in his book, *Childhood and Society* (see Fig. 5). He calls these stages the eight ages of man, in each of which a person faces certain crises in his psychosocial development. We will divide the stages into infancy, early childhood, play age, school age, adolescence, adulthood, the middle years, and later life. In each stage, the person is faced with different problems to be mastered, different sources of stress, different expectations for his behavior. There are no sharp lines which distinguish the stages, nor hard and fast norms which establish a given age for a particular stage. However, we will assign approximate ages for each stage, so that when we talk about

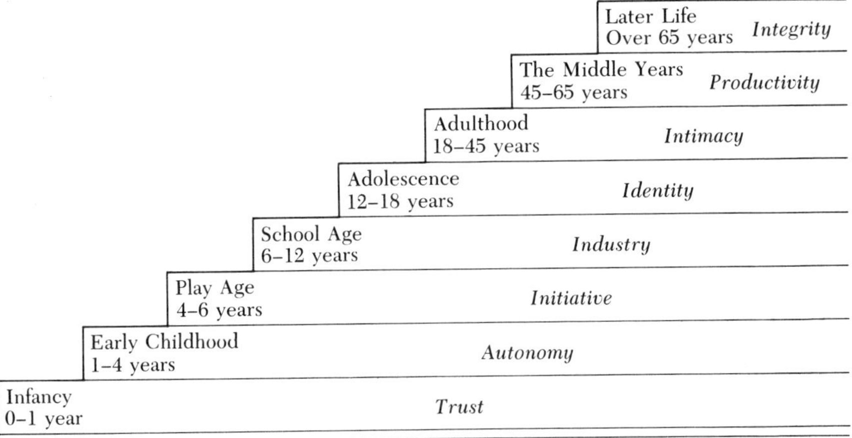

Figure 5. Stages in the life cycle. (Adapted from "Eight Ages of Man," in Erik H. Erikson, *Childhood and Society,* 2nd Edition. W. W. Norton & Company, New York, 1963, page 273.)

a particular stage, we have some general idea about the age period as well.

Infancy. In the first year of life, the individual must learn many kinds of things pertaining to himself, the people around him, and the world he lives in. Furthermore, what he learns sets the stage for all his future learning. Infancy is often called the oral period because it is with his mouth that the infant learns about himself and the world. He gets his food by sucking. He explores his fingers and toes and objects from his environment by putting them all into his mouth. He gains pleasure from cooing, crying, and gurgling. In order for him to have good feelings about himself and others, it is necessary for him to experience satisfaction. His satisfaction centers around the meeting of his physical needs, including how he is held, spoken to, and looked at, when he is fed, whether he is kept clean, dry, and comfortably warm, and whether he is allowed freedom of expression and movement. All of these interactions convey to him whether or not he is loved and determine whether or not he experiences the necessary feelings of worth and belonging. The degree to which his needs are met gently and with respect will determine the degree to which he develops the *sense of trust,* the first essential step toward achieving successful relationships with others. He learns to trust others by the way he is treated. He learns to trust himself through his rapidly developing ability to eat, grasp objects, sit, stand, walk, and so on. He develops a certain basic faith in himself and the people around him.

Early Childhood (1 to 4 Years). As he increases in size, coordination, and ability, the child begins to assert his individuality.

It is necessary for him to experience feelings of self-reliance and adequacy in order to develop the second essential, the *sense of autonomy*. He learns how to coordinate his own actions so as to manipulate objects in his environment. All the while he is learning that he is a separate person in his own right. He has difficulty understanding what is tolerated, what is forbidden, and what is approved. Since he learns these things through experimentation, frustration is inevitable and he needs patient understanding from an adult to help him accept the necessary restrictions. He also needs opportunities to get rid of the steam that builds up inside him in response to failure and frustration and restrictions. There are so many obstacles to freedom of action that he does not know where he stands, and easily doubts his own strength and ability. He must have many opportunities and encouragement to exercise his independence by being allowed to make choices he is ready and able to make and by having his feelings and wishes respected.

Play Age (4 to 6 Years). Having established himself as an individual, the child begins to develop the *sense of initiative*. He gets satisfaction from trying out his own powers of action and imagination. He is curious about everything—his own body, the relationships of people around him, the nature of things and how they affect him—which accounts for the terribly trying period of "Why?" He watches what adults do, and then tries to do what he has seen himself. Many parents have been sobered by seeing themselves reflected in their child's behavior during play, like the little girl scolding an imaginary child, or the little boy smoking an imitation cigarette. The child needs many outlets for his creativity, with only enough curbing to help him achieve the necessary social acceptability. Unnecessary, arbitrary, or roughly-applied restrictions may curtail his sense of initiative or make him resentful.

School Age (6 to 12 Years). At about six, imitation and imagination are not enough—the youngster wants to be doing the real thing. The little boy wants to use the real saw and cut up the board. The little girl wants to make cookies out of real flour and bake them in the oven. Thus the person develops the *sense of industry*. This is usually a period of calm, steady growth, in which the child learns to play and work productively with others outside the family. His experiences provide him with the basis for responsible citizenship, cooperative effort, and adult productivity. It is the age of keen competition, group activities, great enthusiasm and energy, and rapid growth in every direction. He wavers between the baby and the responsible person, so that on the one hand he is independent and reasonable, and on the other, he is helpless and demanding. He develops a keen interest in relationships outside of the family, develops "crushes," and may even transfer his allegiance to others. He begins the struggle to achieve maturity, and may rebel against established routines and parental standards.

Adolescence (12 to 18 Years). Perhaps no stage in life is so full of stress and conflict for all people concerned as this period of transition from childhood to adulthood. It is full of pitfalls and dangers, confusion and instability, progress and regression, socially unacceptable and successful behavior. It is the age in which the person is trying to establish his *sense of identity* as a person, as an adult, as a man or woman. Everything that ever was a problem for him plagues him now. Heavy demands are placed upon him, but he is not told how to meet them. He is leaving the comfortable, familiar role of the child for something new, different, frightening, and he is not sure he wants any part of it.

He is treated on the one hand like a child, and on the other, like an adult. He is given the family car to drive for the evening, but told to be in at 10 P.M. He has great sensitivity and little emotional control. It is an age of experimentation and investigation and rebellion. He is not sure who he is or what he is or what he wants to be. He needs adult guidance, but he has trouble accepting it, let alone asking for it. He does not trust his innermost secrets, feelings, or ideas with adults, because he might be misunderstood or perhaps ridiculed.

Group experience and security with his peers are of primary importance. He can accept the controls of his friends more easily than he can his parents'. Characteristic of the group influence is the game of chicken. One must do whatever the group dictates or be called chicken, and almost every adolescent would rather be dead than be chicken. His need to belong and his search for identity govern his actions.

It is also a time for rapid physical change, including sexual changes. His need for food increases, and he has a voracious appetite. He can eat the whole platter of meat prepared for the family meal and still be hungry. The awakening of sexual drives and urges confuses and surprises him and sometimes makes him feel guilty. The development of his sexual organs and the appearance of secondary sexual characteristics fluster and embarrass him.

He questions and challenges the whole universe, social standards, basic attitudes toward life, accepted ways of behaving, ethical and moral values. He demands a part in society, even though he often does not know what to do with it. He wants "to be where the action is," as sometimes expressed in slang. He is very sensitive to dishonesty, dislikes it intensely, and suspects most adults of practicing it deliberately. Again, slang reflects this feeling and is responsible for the cry from the youth of the country to "tell it like it is."

He is difficult for most adults to understand, relate successfully with, or even tolerate, but he needs all the help they can give him. To develop the sense of identity, he needs healthy social experiences with his own group. He needs help in accepting and understanding his sexual drives and urges and finding acceptable ways of expressing these. He needs help in learning the masculine and feminine roles in life. He needs encouragement, especially by example, to develop his own code of ethics or values. He needs respect and assistance in choosing the kind of preparation best suited to develop his physical, intellectual, and social potentialities. He needs fun, adventure, success—and lots of love!

Young Adulthood (18 to 45 Years). If the individual has developed the necessary social sense of trust, autonomy, initiative, industry, and identity, he is well prepared to acquire the sense of intimacy, productivity, and integrity associated with maturity. As an adult he is expected to be primarily independent, giving, and cooperative in contrast to the characteristics he had as an infant—dependent, receiving, demanding. In Freud's words, the healthy adult should be able "to love and to work." In early adulthood he faces first the problem of independence, responsibility for himself. He must be able to satisfy his own needs in socially acceptable ways. He is generally expected to support himself, establish his own home, and begin his own family life. If he has a healthy perception of himself and others and the necessary strength to tolerate stress, he is ready to grow further. He develops the *sense of intimacy* through his interactions in marriage and parenthood. To be a giving, loving, cooperative parent he must have received the necessary love, because a person cannot give from a vacuum, but must give from a surplus.

The Middle Years (45 to 65 Years). To develop the *sense of productivity,* an individual must have gained sufficient appreciation of himself. He must have attained a certain degree of self-satisfaction, and believe that what he has produced has been worthwhile. Then he can move from the kind of self-centered life, in which his major responsibility has been his own family, to a broader concern and involvement with society and all mankind. One of the major problems he faces is the change in his own physical appearance and ability. Gray hair and sagging muscles require that an individual revise his picture of himself, his body image, and that is no easy thing to do. Beauty parlors, health resorts, gymnasiums, and country clubs are crowded with middle-aged people trying to recapture something of their youth. For the woman, the problem culminates in the loss of reproductive function, the menopause. If she is satisfied with her life, it may pose no great problem to her, but if she is unhappy with the way things have gone up to that time, she may experience great stress. Menopause is a symbolic event.

Later Life. Again, if one has lived successfully through the other stages, it is not too difficult to enter the last stage in one's life with the *sense of integrity.* It is the feeling that one has done what he had to do and done it not too badly, the feeling of having come full circle, that gives comfort and peace in later life. The ultimate achievement in life is self-fulfillment—the acceptance by each person of what he is, what he has done, and what he has become as a unique, exciting, rewarding experience for which he is grateful. With such achievement death loses its sting. As Erikson says, "Trust means the assured reliance on another's integrity . . . Healthy children will not fear life if their elders do not fear death."

An individual faces a number of problems in later life, and he needs all the strength and assistance he can muster. He faces a steady decrease in status and ability. Forced retirement and a decline in physical and intellectual ability catch many people unprepared. A man loses many formerly enjoyed sources of satisfaction—family, friends, marriage partner, job, activities. He finds himself in family and financial situations in the role of a dependent—and many times unwanted. Often he faces the end of his life in loneliness and despair.

In each stage of development, a person is expected to master certain kinds of behavior and achieve certain basic attitudes toward himself and others. In each stage, as well, he faces particular sources of stress to which he reacts with anxiety (Table 1). How well he succeeds in each stage in acquiring the kind of thinking,

TABLE 1. BEHAVIOR, ATTITUDES, STRESSES TO BE MASTERED IN EACH STAGE OF THE LIFE CYCLE

Stage of Life	Age	Major Behavior to be Learned	Basic Attitudes to be Acquired	Major Stresses to be Mastered
Infancy	–1	Eating Sitting Standing Grasping	Trust	Weaning
Childhood	1–12	Walking Continence Coordination Cooperation	Autonomy Initiative Industry	Toilet training Restrictions
Adolescence	12–18	Sexual role Group interaction Preparation for life work	Identity	Sexuality Dependence vs. independence Authority
Adulthood	18–65	Independence Responsibility for self, family Giving Loving Working	Intimacy Productivity	Leaving home Getting a job Marriage Parenthood Changes in body image
Later Life	65 and over	Responsibility for group, society	Integrity	Decrease in status and ability Loss of sources of satisfaction Death

feeling, and doing that leads to the satisfaction of his basic needs in socially acceptable ways is a measure of his adjustment, maturity, and mental health.

REFERENCES

Axline, Virginia: *Dibs: In Search of Self,* Ballantine Books, New York, 1976.

Dresen, Sheila E.: "Autonomy: a continuing developmental task," *American Journal of Nursing, 78* (August, 1978) pp. 1344–1346.

Dyer, Wayne W.: *Pulling Your Own Strings,* Thomas Y. Crowell Co., New York, 1978.

Erikson, Erik: *Childhood and Society,* W. W. Norton & Co., New York, 1964.

Hogan, Rosemarie: *Human Sexuality: A Nursing Perspective,* Appleton-Century-Crofts, New York, 1980.

Knowles, Ruth Dailey: "Dealing with feelings: disputing irrational thoughts," *American Journal of Nursing, 81* (April, 1981) p. 735.

Kubler-Ross, Elizabeth, ed.: *Death: The Final Stage of Growth,* Prentice-Hall, Englewood Cliffs, New Jersey, 1975.

Masters, William H., et al.: *The Pleasure Bond,* Little, Brown, New York, 1975.

McCullers, Carson: *The Member of the Wedding,* Bantam Books, New York, 1966.

McKeel, Nancy Lynn: "Child abuse can be prevented," *American Journal of Nursing, 78* (September, 1978) pp. 1478–1482.

Randolph, Bonnie Moore, and Clydene Ross Valliere: "Consciousness raising groups," *American Journal of Nursing,* 79 (May, 1979) pp. 922–924.

Redl, Fritz: *When We Deal With Children,* Free Press, New York, 1966.

Satir, Virginia: *Peoplemaking,* Science and Behavior Books, Palo Alto, California, 1972.

Webster-Stratton, Carolyn, and Kate Kogan: "Helping parents parent," *American Journal of Nursing, 80* (February, 1980) pp. 240–244.

Chapter 5

Healthy Adjustment

The way a person learns to function, the kind of person he becomes, can be further understood in terms of the development of his personality in interaction with his environment. We hear comments like, "He has lots of personality" or "He is a well-adjusted person," referring to a person's popularity and how well-liked he may be. However, when we use those terms in psychiatry, they have a slightly different meaning. Personality means the sum total of the behavior patterns of the individual. Adjustment means the relationship between an individual and his environment, as measured by the degree of satisfaction of his basic needs and the acceptability of his behavior. A person comes into the world as one kind of person—the infant—dependent, demanding, receiving. He is expected to become the opposite kind of person—the adult—independent, cooperative, giving. How well he accomplishes this change depends upon the development of his personality.

PERSONALITY DEVELOPMENT

Needs. The infant comes into the world and interacts with those in his environment as a bundle of needs, the first stage of his personality. He sees himself as the center of the universe, in fact, as the universe itself. He controls the world around him—one is never so powerful as when he is an infant. Think of the way in which the family interacts with a new baby. The whole household is turned upside down, and even the lives of the people around him are rearranged so as to provide for his every comfort. For example, the common habits of sleeping may be completely changed following his arrival. Father may have to sleep in a different part of the house in order to get sufficient rest. An older child may have to give up the privacy of his room in order to accommodate the crib. Mother's sleeping pattern may change drastically to fit the infant's feeding schedule.

The infant occupies the center of the stage so that his every demand can be met. If he wants something, he lets everyone around him know it. He does not understand or tolerate postponement; when he wants something, he wants it now. There is no question in the minds of people around him that he wants something, although there may be some question as to what it is he wants. Is he hungry, or wet, or is there a pin sticking him, or is he just exercising? Parents learn to distinguish one demand from another. The cry is different when he is hungry from that when he is exercising his lungs. At any rate, the people around him respond to his demands and see that his needs are met, so that he is comfortable and happy again.

Everything comes to the infant. He is always on the receiving end—he gives nothing of himself. It is true that his parents derive pleasure from him, but he does not give that to them. They get it from the satisfaction and pleasure they feel in producing such a delightful creature. For that matter, he is in no position to give—he has to receive something before he can give anything. He has to receive satisfaction, comfort, security, and care from those around him, before he is able to give those same things to others.

Self. Personality-wise, the infant is described as dependent, demanding, and receiving. However, he has to learn to be the opposite kind of person, the adult, whose personality is described as independent, cooperative, and giving. His lessons, therefore, start early and very soon the infant begins to learn that if he is to get what he wants, he must behave in certain ways. He learns that if he turns his mouth up in what mother interprets as a smile he gets certain rewards.

As he begins to appreciate the distinction between himself and his environment, we see the emergence of the second part of his personality, the self. It is the job of the self to find ways of filling his needs, of keeping him in peace and harmony. The function of the self is determined by the perception one has of himself and others. It is that part of the personality which evaluates what is going on inside the individual, what the situation is in his environment, and what he must do in order to meet his needs. It is that part of the personality which is oriented not only toward his inner needs, but toward reality as well—toward the goal of satisfying one's needs in interaction with significant others.

Conscience. It is not long after the emergence of self, that the child begins to learn that there are rights and wrongs, do's and don'ts, good and bad behavior. For the one he is rewarded, for the other he is punished. What was accepted once, now is no longer permitted. He is prevented from putting things into his mouth for investigation both by physical restraint and by verbal and nonverbal admonition, "No, no, no, no, no!" Thus he begins to incorporate the standards, values, and mores which guide the behavior of people in his society. He begins to develop that third part of his personality we call conscience. A person doesn't come into the world knowing right from wrong, and what he learns as right and wrong depends upon the standards of the people around him and what he is able to incorporate. His parents and significant other people around him are his models, and he learns his set of rules and regulations in interactions with them. It is not so much what they say that determines what he learns as what they do. He learns to treat others as he himself is treated. For example, if he is treated with honesty and respect, he tends to think of himself and others with respect, and he incorporates honesty in his behavior as a guide. If, on the other hand, he learns from those around him to take what he wants without regard for honesty and respect, he tends to acquire different values and behaves accordingly. For a person to be mentally healthy the parts of the personality must fit together in a balanced, integrated, proportionate fashion. He must be able to maintain peace within himself and harmony between himself and others if he is to function in a well-adjusted manner.

The thoughts, wishes and actions of an individual are tempered by the society or culture in which he grows up, specifically by the environment provided by his parents. In other words, the thinking, feeling, and doing of the person is adapted to the physical and social environment of which he is a product. If that environment is healthy, he has a better chance of being healthy; if it is unhealthy, he is more likely to be sick. The National Association for Mental Health states that people with good mental health have the following characteristics:

1. They feel comfortable about themselves.
2. They feel right about others.
3. They are able to meet the demands of life.

EMOTIONAL MATURITY

The individual comes equipped with certain physiological responses to stress (adaptation) and acquires certain other psychological methods of defense (adjustment), both of which become automatic, unconscious, habitual behavior. The purpose of his behavior, whether physical or emotional in origin, is to protect the life and security of the individual. The success of his behavior is measured by how effective it is in satisfying his basic needs in socially acceptable ways.

No other creature spends so much time preparing for life under the guidance of parents. Parents not only endow the person with his potentialities, but they also provide for the development of those potentialities as well. That is why parental influence is so important in determining an individual's healthy adjustment, and why great stress is placed upon the patient's growth and development in psychiatric treatment.

If a person's personality is properly proportioned and balanced, he is better prepared for meeting the demands of life, developing healthy attitudes toward himself and others, and enjoying succeeding stages of the life cycle. He is likely to become a competent, successful, well-adjusted, mentally-healthy, emotionally-mature adult, whom Saul, in his book, *Emotional Maturity,* describes as follows:

1. Predominantly independent and responsible, with little need to regress.
2. Giving and productive but still able to relax and receive.
3. Cooperative rather than egotistical and competitive.
4. In relative harmony with conscience, integrated with mature feelings and behavior.
5. Sexually free, integrated with mating and responsible productivity, sexual and social.
6. Hostility toward himself and others minimal, but available for defense and constructive use.
7. Grasp on reality clear and unimpaired by childhood distortions.
8. Discriminating and highly adaptable, free from childhood patterns.

Adjustment

All organisms have or acquire methods of adapting or adjusting to life conditions in their environments. It is a simple matter of survival—adjust or perish. The possum plays dead, for example, in the hope that the enemy will pass him by and thus spare his life. The chameleon changes his color to match that of his immediate surroundings, so that the enemy, not being able to detect him, will not attack him. The gazelle develops his long legs so that he can outrun his enemies. The lion develops his teeth, claws, and muscular strength to conquer his enemies and satisfy his basic need for food as well.

Man is no exception. The individual finds himself almost from the beginning of life in opposition to the demands made upon him by the society of which he is a product. He adapts to society's demands by the physical and neuro-muscular growth changes taking place in him, and he adjusts to these demands by his emotional and social development. For example, the infant is perfectly happy with the method of eating which comes naturally to him—nursing. However, his society, in the specific form of his mother, does not allow him to continue using this method past a certain age, usually sometime within the first year of life. He is expected to learn a completely new method of eating, as well as a new menu. Since he is unfamiliar with both and happy with his old ways, he is not eager to change. In fact, he may strenuously resist his mother's attempt to feed him puréed beets with a spoon. However, his own physical and neuro-muscular growth requires that he change from milk to solid foods, and, in addition, his emotional and social development require him to change what and how he eats in order to master the expectations and meet with the approval of his mother. So, as a matter of survival and security, he adapts and adjusts to the new behavior that is expected of him.

The whole process of growth and development is a progressive series of such adaptations and adjustments. It is, therefore, essential that the resulting conflicts be resolved if a person is to move through the various stages of life with health and vigor. If he is to survive and feel secure, he must learn ways of handling the conflict and ways of behaving which not only protect and defend him, but at the same time promote the satisfaction of his basic needs.

ANXIETY

Anything that poses a threat to the survival and security of the individual calls forth a reaction which we call anxiety. Anxiety can be defined as an unpleasant subjective response to a perceived physical or psychological threat composed of fear and tension. Conflict, ambivalence, stress, trauma, and frustration are all life experiences which contain a source of threat to the survival and security of the individual. The danger can be real or potential, internal or external, but always it represents a threat to the survival or security of the person. Anxiety can be useful and productive when it motivates the individual to action. It is a warning, a cue to danger, an alarm which says to the person, "Look out, you're in danger, do something to protect yourself or you will perish." The person responds by trying to protect himself from harm—and as a result we see fight, flight, or paradoxical behavior. Anxiety can also be harmful and destructive when it overwhelms the person. It may be more than he can handle, or the way he has learned to combat it may be ineffective, or his life situation may prohibit its relief. Then we see disturbances in his behavior.

Anxiety is composed of a feeling response, fear; a physiological response, tension; and an action response, fight or flight. In periods of anxiety, a person may experience feelings of apprehension, uneasiness, discomfort, anticipation, or a sense of impending doom or disaster. The physiological reaction to anxiety may increase, decrease, or distort the function of any part of the body. For example, the individual may experience dry mouth, nausea, rapid pulse, increased respiration, or vomiting, diarrhea, urination, perspiration, and headache. In behavioral reactions we may observe irritability, restlessness, sleeplessness, preoccupation, anorexia, nail biting, and excessive eating, drinking or smoking.

Anxiety is a fact of life, and the individual experiences it almost from the beginning. Some people believe, for example, that birth itself is an anxiety-provoking situation for the newborn. At any rate, the infant's initial relationship with the world is full of anxiety-provoking situations. Mother turns out to be not only the source of satisfaction, but the source of frustration as well. The infant experiences feelings of comfort and security when his needs are satisfied, and feelings of anxiety and insecurity when they are not. How mother interacts with him, the feelings she has about him, the way she treats him, how she cares for him, all help to determine whether she increases or allays the anxiety he is bound to experience.

In interaction with his mother and the world, then, the infant experiences anxiety in response to the conflict, ambivalence, stress, trauma, and frustration that he encounters. How he learns to handle this feeling of anxiety in interaction with his mother sets the stage for his way of behaving with the rest of the world for the rest of his life. Since it is not possible (or even desirable) to eliminate the sources of anxiety, it is essential for him to learn ways of successfully adapting and adjusting to it. It is necessary to avoid, disguise, deny, or in some way relieve the physiological and psychological responses to anxiety, and we see the results of the individual's attempts to do just that in his behavioral response.

The Physiological Response

To better understand the reactions we will see to stress, as well as some of the somatic forms of psychiatric treatment, let us first look at the physiological response to anxiety. Anxiety stimulates the nervous system as a whole, which, in coordination with the suprarenal glands, is responsible for equilibrium or homeostasis in the body.

The Central Nervous System. The central nervous system (CNS), made up of the brain and spinal cord, directs and coordinates all of the other body systems. The autonomic nervous system (ANS) is governed by the hypothalamus of the brain, in close relationship with the pituitary gland. The pituitary gland is the master gland which directs and controls the functions of all the rest of the glands in the endocrine system. One of the functions of the hypothalamus is to relay the sensory stimulation, emotions, and basic impulses to other parts of the brain. It accomplishes this function in cooperation with the reticular-activating and limbic systems which carry the impulses from all parts of the body up the brain stem, and on to the cortex and brain centers.

The Autonomic Nervous System. The autonomic nervous system helps to regulate essential body functions such as heart rate, blood pressure, and digestive and excretory functions which occur automatically and are not under our voluntary control. The system is responsible for preparing a person for action in time of stress, either fight or flight. It is made up of two parts, the sympathetic and the parasympathetic systems, which, with their antagonistic actions, provide the necessary checks and balances to maintain equilibrium or homeostasis. The sympathetic system, for example, takes charge in an emergency; it dilates the pupil of the eye to provide a wider range of vision and dilates the bronchial tubes to provide for a greater intake of air. It quickens and strengthens heart action and constricts blood vessels to increase the circulation. It lessens peristalsis and constricts sphincters to inhibit bowel and bladder functions. It decreases glandular secretion and contractions to cut down on nonemergency functions. The parasympathetic system is in charge of the nonemergency functions of the body, and does just the opposite of the sympathetic system. It constricts the pupil and the bronchial tubes, slows and weakens heart action, dilates blood vessels, increases digestive processes, relaxes sphincters, and increases glandular secretion and contractions.

General Adaptation Syndrome (GAS). When faced by a threat, the body is automatically prepared for the emergency by the sympathetic system. Since the discomfort of preparation cannot be tolerated for very long, the parasympathetic system goes into action to relieve the situation, to restore law and order and permit normal functioning. If the parasympathetic system for some reason is unable to restore equilibrium, or if the stress situation continues over a prolonged period of time, the organ, system, or person affected may wear out under the strain. For example, in response to prolonged anxiety, an individual might first blanch, then blush, then faint.

Hans Selye (see References) describes this physiological response to threat as the general adaptation syndrome (GAS). The three stages of the physiological response he calls alarm or emergency, resistance, and exhaustion.

The Psychological Response

We like to think of our behavior as governed largely by our rational logical thinking, and it is not easy for us to see that emotions underlie all our behavior. A person thinks and does in accord with how he feels, especially about himself and other people. Less of our behavior is under our control or direction than we generally like to believe. Man's behavior may be compared to the iceberg—one-third is above the surface or under our conscious control, and two-thirds is submerged, under the control of our pre- or sub- or unconscious.

The ways or methods that the individual learns of defending himself psychologically are just as essential to his self-protection, survival, and security as the physiological response. These ways or methods are called mental mechanisms, defense mechanisms, or coping methods. They are learned in interaction with significant other people in the environment and they become unconscious, automatic processes which underlie all behavior and help to shape a person's life style.

The coping methods are used in a variety of combinations by both healthy and unhealthy people. The methods in themselves are neither healthy nor unhealthy, but the way in which a person uses them or the results which they produce in behavior may be judged to be healthy or unhealthy. They tend to confirm the person's perception of himself and the world he lives in. The healthy use of the coping methods is determined by how successful they are in relieving anxiety and promoting the satisfaction of basic needs in socially acceptable ways.

The Coping Methods

Repression. In reaction to stress, the first line of psychological defense is that of repression. In repression an individual excludes from his awareness unpleasant or unwanted experiences, emotions, or ideas. None of us could bear to see ourselves constantly exposed with all our faults showing, so we learn to keep out of our awareness those things about ourselves and our lives that we find unbearable. A person could not survive the constant bombardment of sensory stimuli surrounding him, so he simply excludes part of it, and lets through what he can tolerate. He does this automatically and unconsciously. For example, a person may not be able to remember the name of another individual about whom he has strong negative feelings.

Conversion. In conversion an individual attempts to deny or relieve his emotions by changing them into physical symptoms. Most of us have experienced physical symptoms in response to the wear and tear of ordinary living. For example, if a person has many frustrations on the job, he may react with a headache at the end of the day rather than with feelings of anger or despair. A nurse may react to an unrewarding assignment with chronic low-back pain, which she attributes to being on her feet all day rather than to the lack of fulfillment. Even physical illness can be seen as an attempt to adapt to the stresses of life.

Introjection. In introjection a person incorporates the ideas, objects, and persons of his environment into his own personality. When he experiences frustration, his emotional response is directed inward toward himself rather than outward toward his environment. For example, if a nurse fails to get sufficient satisfaction in her job, instead of blaming her supervisors or her co-workers, she may feel she is inadequate, or may suffer from blue spells. A person reacts to the death of someone he loves (a major frustration) not with anger but with overwhelming grief or despair.

Displacement. In displacement a person transfers the emotions associated with one idea, object, or person to another. For example, a mother lessens her feelings of failure as a parent by worrying about her son's reputation rather than about the unhappiness which has caused him to turn to drugs. Sometimes nurses are overly concerned about performing relatively unimportant tasks away from the bedside in order to avoid facing the inadequacy of their relationships with patients.

Projection. In projection a person attributes his own thoughts, feelings, and actions to the external environment. It is the opposite of introjection because the person turns his feelings outward upon the environment and the people in it rather than inward upon himself. For example, the student may explain his failure in a course by stating that the teacher didn't like him. A nurse may try to explain away her own inadequacy by blaming her failures upon the supervisor, the patient, or her co-workers.

Fantasy. In fantasy a person substitutes a more pleasant, satisfying, or rewarding situation of his own creation for the real one. Daydreaming is a common example, in which we substitute a more complimentary ending to situations that have not turned out well for us during the day. In order to protect our self-esteem, we imagine "I should have said" situations. As in dreams, one may think, feel, and do in fantasy what would not be possible in reality. In nursing, we may encounter patients who alleviate the pain of their existence by thinking of themselves as more successful or important than they actually are.

Dissociation. In dissociation a person detaches himself, his emotional investment, or certain aspects of himself from interactions with his environment. He observes rather than experiences life, as if it were, indeed, a stage, and the individual merely acting. Automatic behavior, like sleep walking, is an example of dissociation. A person may not allow himself to become involved in a serious relationship because of his fear of being hurt. A patient may give the appearance of being unconcerned about a life-threatening illness such as cancer in an attempt to control his overwhelming fear.

Regression. In regression a person returns to earlier, more comforting but less mature ways of behaving. For example, a person may eat to alleviate his dissatisfaction with life. He may fall asleep when the going gets too rough. He may break into tears whenever he is faced with possible failure. In nursing, we may care for physically ill patients who demonstrate regression by behaving in ways more characteristic of the infant than of the adult—dependent, demanding, receiving.

Fixation. In fixation an individual stops at a particular stage of development as a result of too much or too little satisfaction of basic needs. It's as though he stops growing at a particular time in his life and is stunted as a result. For example, a man continues to behave like the high school athlete he once was because he got so many rewards in that period of his life that he has never been able to move on to more mature successes. A nurse may behave in immature ways because she was never allowed to be dependent as a child.

Identification. In identification an individual thinks, feels, or acts like another person or group of people who are significant or important to him. A person may be more comfortable where there are fewer conflicts of interests, so he becomes more like the others from whom he gets his satisfaction. If a person is to be successful, he must make some identification with those around him. Often there is a similarity even in the appearance of the people who are closely identified—husband and wife, brother and sister, or members of the same group, such as nurses. For example, to the adolescent, identifying with his own group is of primary importance, and it accounts for the rigid adherence of many young people to the current fashions in dress and hair styles. Many patients need approval so badly that they try to be "the good patient" even when it is contrary to their own best interests.

Rationalization. In rationalization a person finds a more plausible reason for his behavior than the real one. Usually the result is a partial truth, rather than a whole truth. It is an attempt to make our behavior more acceptable to ourselves and others. For example, a woman may try to justify her shopping spree by saying she really needed some new clothes when her closet is full of perfectly adequate, though not new, clothing. A frequent excuse which nurses use for not being more effective or successful is to say they didn't have time to do something, when they have eight hours every day.

Compensation. In compensation a person makes up for his deficits or inadequacies in one area by excelling in another—he does something he can do well instead of something he does poorly. If a person wants to do something very much, but he finds that he cannot, he makes up for his disappointment by excelling at something else. For example, the young boy who wants desperately to play football but cannot because he is too small makes up for the deficit and alleviates the hurt by becoming an honor student. A nurse who is not good at technical work may devote more time and energy to her relationships with patients.

Reaction Formation. In reaction formation a person denies certain unacceptable aspects of his behavior by developing the extreme opposite kind of behavior. An example is the sweet, overly-polite way of behaving which some people develop in order to deny unacceptable angry feelings. It is not uncommon that the "good Christian" is also the town gossip. Nurses may feel that it is not professional to have tender feelings so they deny those feelings by developing a rough, gruff manner.

Restitution. In restitution an individual atones for his unacceptable ideas or feelings or actions. It is a kind of undoing to make up for something thought or felt or done that is not acceptable to one's self or others. For example, the successful businessman may attempt to atone for his questionable sales practices by giving to charity. In nursing, we may care for patients who try to make up for some of their symptoms or ways of behaving by buying our forgiveness or approval with gifts.

Sublimation. In sublimation a person directs his unacceptable impulses into constructive channels. For example, a professional football player directs his aggressive impulses into ferocious blocks and tackles and is handsomely rewarded for it. If a nurse experiences frustrations in her work, she may take up gardening. In this way she relieves her pent-up feelings of hostility and satisfies needs as well, since she gets praise and recognition for her gardening efforts.

Substitution. In substitution a person replaces unacceptable ideas, objects, or persons with more acceptable ones. We take our hostile feelings out on those people whom we trust, respect, and love because they are safer than the people who provoked the feelings in the first place. For example, a man or woman may look for the kind of mate (or boss) who can be a father or mother substitute. People who have no children often substitute pets, dogs or cats, as objects of their love. A nurse may have a frustrating day with a disagreeable physician, but rather than express her feelings to him, she goes home and gets into an argument with her husband.

All of these coping methods are used in an attempt on the part of the person to adjust to reality, to relieve anxiety, to restore equilibrium, to keep peace within himself, and to promote harmony between himself and others. The more methods an individual has at his disposal, and the more successful he is at using them appropriately, the better his preparation for meeting the stresses he will encounter during his life. It is difficult to separate the coping methods into definite concrete entities because they work together in determining behavior. Thus, any particular act or way of behaving may result from the fusion of several coping methods in an individual's attempt to protect himself, respond to the demands of life and meet his needs.

To qualify for healthy adjustment, the person must have achieved certain goals. He must have:

1. Changed from a dependent, demanding, receiving infant to an independent, cooperative, giving adult.
2. Developed a healthy personality with needs, self, conscience in proportion and balance.
3. Inherited and developed an efficient nervous system.
4. Learned the necessary coping methods and a degree of success in using them appropriately.
5. Acquired the characteristics of emotional maturity and mental health.

Failure to achieve any of these goals will result in disturbances in a person's adjustment and productive functioning.

REFERENCES

Falk, Gerhard, and Ursula Falk: "Sexuality and the aged," *Nursing Outlook, 80* (January, 1980) pp. 51–55.

Glasser, William: *Mental Health or Mental Illness,* Harper & Row, New York, 1970.

Jourard, Sidney, and Ted Landsman: *Healthy Personality: An Approach From the Viewpoint of Humanistic Psychology.* 4th Edition, Macmillan Publishing Company, New York, 1980.

Jungman, Lynne B.: "When your feelings get in the way," *American Journal of Nursing, 79* (June, 1979) pp. 1074–1075.

Knowles, Ruth Daily: "Dealing with feelings: managing anxiety," *American Journal of Nursing, 81* (January, 1981) pp. 110–111.

Kovar, Lillian: *Wasted Lives,* Gardner Press, New York, 1979.

McConnell, James V.: *Understanding Human Behavior,* Holt, Rinehart & Winston, New York, 1974.

Meltzer, Herbert L.: *The Chemistry of Human Behavior,* Nelson-Hall, Chicago, 1979.

Memmler, Ruth, and Dena Wood: *The Human Body in Health and Disease,* 4th Edition, J. B. Lippincott Company, Philadelphia, 1977.

Richter, Judith M., and Rebecca Sloan: "The relaxation technique," *American Journal of Nursing,* 79 (November, 1979) pp. 1960–1963.

Rubin, Theodore Isaac: *Inner Peace in an Age of Anxiety,* Viking Press, New York, 1980.

Salinger, J. D.: *Catcher in the Rye,* Bantam Books, New York, 1977.

Saul, Leon: *The Childhood Emotional Pattern and Maturity,* Van Nostrand Reinhold Company, New York, 1979.

Schatzinger, Lynn H., et al.: "Spinal fusion: emotional stress and adjustment," *American Journal of Nursing,* 79 (September, 1979) pp. 1608–1612.

Selye, Hans: *The Stress of Life,* McGraw-Hill, New York, 1975.

Chapter 6

Reactions to Stress

We have defined stress as physical or psychological force that, when applied to a system, is sufficient to cause strain or distortion in the system, or when very great, to alter the system. Let us concentrate on the psychological force that affects people in their efforts to live successfully, and investigate the reactions that result in certain kinds of behavior, healthy and unhealthy.

A person experiences stress when he is confronted with situations in life which require him to take some action in order to resolve the crisis. For example, anything which interferes with the satisfaction of his basic needs (frustration) threatens his survival or security, gives rise to anxiety, and calls for action. What the person has learned in interaction with his environment about himself and the world he lives in shapes his reaction to stress into a pattern of behavior or particular life style. Sometimes people are described in terms of the way they learn to live. For example, a person who reacts characteristically to stress with fight behavior may be described as a "fighter" with "spunk" or "guts" or "courage." If the person reacts with flight behavior, he may be described as "flighty," "detached," "a cool customer," or "a brain." If a person reacts with paradoxical behavior, he may be described as a "a weak sister," "sickly," "paranoid," or "neurotic."

Patterns of behavior or life styles as reactions to stress are in themselves neither healthy nor unhealthy, as we shall see in the following examples. The degree of healthy adjustment is determined by the success of a person's behavior in meeting his needs and resolving the situational crisis. When his action fails to do this, we see the emergence of unhealthy behavior patterns and the symptoms characteristic of certain kinds of mental illness.

For example, the eccentric millionaire who believes his heirs are just waiting for him to die so they can get their hands on his money is not usually regarded as behaving inappropriately. However, an individual who is not rich and believes the same thing is likely to be looked at with some question. If he goes several steps further and calls the police repeatedly to complain about people trying to break into his house and steal his money, he is likely to be considered mentally ill. If he protects himself by barricading himself in his house, arming himself with a gun and threatening to shoot anyone who approaches, he is likely to be apprehended and taken off to the mental hospital.

The more versatile or flexible a person is, the more adaptable, better adjusted, more appropriate or realistic is his behavior, the better prepared he is to meet and master the stress of different life experiences. Also, the more likely he is to be able to learn new methods, new competencies, new ways of behaving that help him accommodate himself to the changes in expectations that accompany the various stages in the life cycle.

SOURCES OF STRESS

Stress may arise as a result of frustration, conflict, ambivalence, or trauma. The crisis may be within the individual himself in the form of a struggle between his desires and his conscience. It may result from a confrontation between the individual and the people around him, such as whose needs are going to be met first. It may be primarily environmental, such as changes in expectations for a person in a particular period of the life cycle or in cases of national emergency such as war.

Frustration. Any interference in the satisfaction of a person's basic needs is a source of stress. The interference may be a result of delay or postponement, which the individual must learn to tolerate in the process of growing up. It may be the result of failure —a person tries to obtain satisfaction and fails. It may be the result of a loss of the source of satisfaction, such as in the separation of infant and mother. Whatever the cause, the individual must learn to handle the resulting inner feelings of anger, despair, guilt, or anxiety in ways which are socially acceptable and at the same time give him relief, if he is to remain healthy.

One youngster may fly into a rage when satisfaction is denied him. Another may cry as if his heart were broken. Another may take his good coat and run away from home. Another may become silent, sullen, unresponsive. Another may become physically ill. How he responds depends upon what he has learned about himself and life. Whether or not he changes his behavior depends upon his ability to change and the opportunities he has had to learn other ways of responding than those he has already experienced.

Conflict. A fundamental source of stress is the struggle in each of us between our innate desires and the restrictions placed upon us by our society, internalized by us in the form of conscience. One example of this is the personal struggle everyone experiences between the desire to be cared for and the desire to care for one's self and others. We come into the world as dependent creatures and we are expected, in the process of growth and development, to become independent creatures. The learning process involved is always stressful and not always successful. Frequently the youngster wishes to be more independent than his parents allow him to be, while the adult often wishes to be more dependent than either he or his life situation allows him to be.

Sometimes society places demands upon the individual that cause severe stress—for example, war. War represents, especially in this nuclear age, a threat to the survival of mankind. Not only does a young man have to face death, but he must not show his rage, his terror, or his revulsion to the whole situation. He is required to go under penalty of law, whether he wants to or not—and very often he has nothing to say about it. Characteristic of conflict is the fact that it is not easily or simply resolved. If he defies the requirements, he is apt to find himself at odds with his friends, parents, society, even himself.

Ambivalence. Opposing feelings within the individual which originate in the mother-infant relationship are often a source of stress. When the infant finds mother to be both the source of satisfaction and the source of frustration in his life, he experiences the condition known as ambivalence. When she satisfies his needs and he experiences comfort, pleasure, security, his feelings toward her are positive, and this is experienced as love. When the demands she places upon him cause frustration, he experiences discomfort, pain, anxiety; his feelings toward her are negative and are experienced as hate. This primary relationship sets the pattern for others, so that any meaningful relationship which serves as a source of both satisfaction and frustration arouses feelings of ambivalence in us. We experience the greatest pleasure and the greatest pain in relationships with those we love most deeply. The Mills brothers used to sing an old song that some of you may have heard, "You always hurt the one you love, the one you shouldn't hurt at all." People who are important to us are often a source of frustration because they do not always behave as we would like them to.

Often a person cannot tolerate the degree of discomfort that accompanies ambivalence, so he tends to get rid of one aspect of the dual feeling, either the love or the hate, by using whatever coping methods he has learned. In most circumstances the unacceptable feeling is that of hate, because most of us learn early that a person shouldn't hate other people, especially mothers. It is not safe because it is necessary to have mother's love and approval, and if we hate, we run the risk of losing that love. Hate generates stress because the rules and regulations of society say that we should love our mothers.

Trauma. Psychological injury is apt to be more painful and lasting than physical injury. A child experiences trauma when he suffers rejection, overprotection, or inconsistency on the part of his parents. If a person has heard all his life that he has been the cause of his mother's death because she died in the act of bringing him into thc world, he is apt to experience extreme stress. In order to survive, he must find some way of relieving the intolerable pain. If a girl repeatedly is made aware of the disappointment her parents feel because she is not a boy, she will find some way to behave that will alter their feelings toward her and thus relieve her own.

On the other hand, a child who is not allowed to learn and do things for himself will be just as severely crippled as if he did not have healthy legs to stand on. If he is not allowed to fall, he will never learn to walk or run or jump for joy. If he is protected from life and its hardships he will be completely unprepared for living, and his first real conflict is likely to defeat him.

Perhaps the most serious injury is done to the child who is confused by the inconsistent erratic behavior of his parents. He has great difficulty figuring out how to behave when he does not know whether he will be accepted or rejected. It is impossible for him to learn to trust himself and others if he is rewarded sometimes and punished at other times for the same behavior, or if there is a contradiction between what his parents say and what they mean, between the content and the intent of their communication.

SEVERITY OF STRESS

Duration. The severity of the stress that a person experiences depends upon a number of factors in his life situation. The first one is the length of time the person finds himself subjected to the stress. If the stress is sufficiently prolonged, just the physiological response alone may lead to exhaustion. The old saying, "You can get used to hanging if you hang long enough" isn't true; the longer you hang the harder it is to maintain life, psychologically speaking. It is true that in order to survive an individual must find some way of adapting to his circumstances; otherwise he may die. If the stress is short-lived, an individual has a better chance of mustering his strength and withstanding the force because, for one thing, it does not destroy his faith in himself or the future. If it goes on and on, a person loses his morale, undermining his strength and hope and lessening his ability to withstand the force.

Intensity. If the issues at stake are important to the individual's survival or security, the severity of the stress is greater. If a young man finds that his life is threatened, as it is in time of war, he may experience severe stress. If an adolescent finds that his peer group's sense of decency is in direct conflict with his own, severe stress may result. If a man has strong negative feelings toward his job, which must serve as his major source of satisfaction, he too may undergo severe stress.

When a person finds himself in a situation in life which is entirely unfamiliar to him, he will suffer greater stress than when he is faced with familiar problems. Also, if the stress situation appears suddenly or unexpectedly and he has no time to prepare for it, the severity of the stress will be greater. If a person is used to being treated with love and respect, he may experience great stress when he finds himself surrounded by cold, rejecting people. On the other hand, if he is a person who has been kicked around all his life, he may feel severe stress when he finds himself suddenly surrounded by warm, accepting people.

Individual Factors. Not only does the degree of stress depend upon the kind of stress, its quality and quantity, but it also depends upon the affected individual and how he looks at himself and the world around him. For example, if the individual has *not* developed the initial sense of trust, whenever he meets with criticism from others his security may be severely threatened, and he may react inappropriately in an attempt to defend himself. If a person whom he doesn't trust offers him a suggestion for improvement, he may interpret that as an attack and react with hostility. We call that defensiveness. If, on the other hand, a person *has* developed a sense of trust, the other individual may be very critical of him without his feeling threatened and throwing up barriers, and he may therefore be able to profit from the criticism.

The degree of stress depends, as well, upon the competence of the individual in handling it. If he has been exposed to different kinds of stress, has learned a variety of effective coping methods, and has had a sufficient degree of success in life, he is pretty well equipped to meet and deal with stress situations. If, on the other hand, his environment has been limiting and his success minimal, he will have little tolerance for stress, let alone an ability to meet and deal productively with it. The kind of stress a person experiences at any one time in his life is directly proportionate to the degree of interference in the satisfaction of his basic needs and to his ability to master the stress.

LIFE STYLES AS REACTIONS TO STRESS

We have already discussed in Chapter 4 the major stresses that face the individual during infancy, childhood, adolescence, adulthood, and later life. How a person masters the stress of each period in his life is a measure of how successful he will be in mastering the particular stress in succeeding periods of his life. However, an individual may experience stress at any time in his life for which he is unprepared, and he may succumb to it, be crippled by it, or adjust to it.

Not only does each stage in the life cycle have its peculiar kind of stress, but in addition the individual may at any time be attacked by the other enemies of health—injury, infection, malfunction, or malformation. A disfiguring injury is a source of severe stress at any age in life, but to one person it may be such a severe blow that his behavior and outlook on life are changed, while another person suffers no maladjustment. An infection can leave one person severely handicapped emotionally, while another takes it in stride. One individual may accept a physical or intellectual handicap from birth, while to another it is a constant source of severe stress. Cancer is a stress situation for patient and family alike because of the threat to life, its sudden appearance, unknown quality, and lack of predictable cure. However, every individual afflicted with illness experiences and reacts to it differently, depending upon how it affects him and how capable he is of adjusting to the stress.

Aggressive Behavior. The basis of the aggressive pattern of behavior is the fight response to stress or anxiety—the fight to satisfy one's needs, to protect one's self, to succeed, the fight for survival and security. Early in life the person with aggressive behavior acquires a peculiar sensitivity to situations in which he experiences inadequacy, a strong sense of rejection, and in which he expects punishment. As a child, the frustration of his physical, emotional, and social needs provoked strong feelings of ambivalence, and subsequent life experiences that produce self-doubt touch off the sequence of inadequacy, rejection, and hostility which is a natural response to the accompanying threat. The core of his behavior pattern centers around how he handles the feelings of hostility and aggression.

If the individual develops an oversized conscience, he is likely to turn the hostility and aggression inward upon himself, using the method of introjection. He learns from his experiences with the people around him that hostility and aggression are intolerable or unacceptable. He feels sure that he will be punished for feeling the way he does about his mother or father because he thinks he is bad to feel as he does. To rid himself of the feeling of guilt and to atone for his bad feelings, he punishes himself. He feels sad or hurt or disappointed in reaction to the frustrations he experiences in his life.

If the individual develops an undersized conscience, along with the distorted picture of himself, he is likely to turn his hostility and aggression outward upon the environment, using the coping method of projection. From experiences with the people around him, he learns that the way to get what he wants is to take it. He learns to protect himself by hitting the other fellow first. He fails to incorporate the rules that govern social interaction. He feels angry, hostile, or aggressive in reaction to the frustrations he experiences in life.

If the individual develops a fairly well-balanced personality, he may direct the hostility inward, then outward, using the coping methods of substitution or sublimation. From experiences with the people around him, he learns acceptable outlets for his feelings of aggression and hostility. As a child, he learns to substitute his toys for people. He learns to bat a ball or play pingpong or hunt. He learns to rake or hoe or mow the lawn. He learns to compete and win the prize. He may feel angry or guilty or anxious, but he handles it differently, he controls and expresses his feelings in productive ways.

Passive Behavior. The passive pattern of behavior or life style is related to the basic response of flight—avoid the conflict, run away from trouble, get out of the situation. The person with passive behavior learns early in life that feelings, one's own as well as other people's, are not to be trusted. He experiences a series of grave disappointments or betrayals in his interactions with people. He develops a sensitivity to contradictions or inconsistencies between the content and the intent of communication from other people. His attitude toward himself is self-depreciatory, and he experiences marked insecurity in his relationships with other people. The core of his behavior pattern is his failure to externalize his emotional attachment and relate successfully.

His early experiences with significant people in his environment lead him to develop an attitude of indifference or aloofness. He refuses to invest his emotional energy in the environment or attach any enduring emotional interest to persons or objects outside himself. Feelings which he cannot accept or express are separated from himself, using the coping method of dissociation. The natural human tendency to interact with others is inhibited, the regular channels of communication are cut off, and the accompanying energy or emotional capacity is transferred to himself. Narcissism or self-love becomes a major source of satisfaction when the individual invests his emotional energy in himself.

The resultant feelings of loneliness can be handled in a variety of ways. One rather common way of getting compensation as well as social approval is by intellectual achievement—the quiet, studious, well-behaved, successful individual we call the introvert.

The person's unusual difficulty in socialization may be combined with daydreaming, using the coping method of fantasy. He may never grow up, or in periods of stress, he may return to earlier ways of behaving more characteristic of the infant, using the coping method of regression. His behavior pattern may be that of the dependent person, who remains on the receiving level rather than becoming predominantly giving. It may be difficult for him to postpone his own satisfaction in order to provide for the security and survival of another person. His behavior may be described as immature, irresponsible, or infantile.

Paradoxical Behavior. Paradoxical behavior is a response to stress in which an individual reacts in a way that looks inconsistent with or contrary to his best interests or the demands of the situation. Rather than dealing with the threat in a direct way by fight or avoiding it by flight, the individual distorts or disguises it so that the accompanying anxiety is reduced and some sort of adjustment is made. His early experiences with significant people in his environment may be similar to either or both of the previous behavior patterns. The way he looks at himself and other people may also be similar. The difference lies in the coping methods upon which he relies and the kind of behavior which results.

Suspiciousness or active distrust is a combination of aggressive and passive behavior patterns. The individual's early experiences are similar to those of the person who develops the pattern of introversion. He learns from his experiences not to trust himself and others, particularly when it comes to feelings. He develops a sensitivity to situations which make him feel inadequate and inferior, often related to too high demands being placed upon him by his parents. He is extremely sensitive to the opinions of others, without sufficient self-confidence or interpersonal skill to evaluate those opinions objectively. He does not adequately develop the sense of trust or autonomy, and the result is often a person with chronic insecurity, sensitivity, pride, and suspiciousness. His behavior makes it extremely difficult for him and others to develop social or interpersonal effectiveness. As in introversion, he separates from himself unacceptable feelings or desires, but he goes one step further—he projects these faults or failures upon others. His behavior, then, serves to relieve his anxiety by getting rid of his intolerable feelings, maintains his self-esteem by making him superior to others, and provides a ready explanation for any failure or inadequacy on his part.

The individual who uses physical symptoms as a major method of adjustment is also using a combination of aggressive and passive behavior patterns. He learns from his environment that feelings of hostility and aggression are unacceptable or unsafe. However, in reaction to stress, he learns to disguise and express such feelings in physical symptoms, using the coping method of conversion. His behavior serves to relieve his anxiety by getting rid of intolerable feelings, atone for them by his physical suffering, and provide for meeting his dependent needs by being taken care of as well.

DIMENSIONS OF HEALTH AND ILLNESS

The degree of mental health or the extent of mental illness is measured by the individual's success in meeting the demands of life, in weathering the storm. Reactions to stress are on a continuum, ranging from the most effective to the most ineffective, from healthy to psychotic (see Fig. 6). There are no sharp distinctions between normal and abnormal, or between the categories of abnormal behavior. Mental illness is primarily a disruption in the individual's ability to relate successfully with others and stems from his lack of preparation for successful living, the nature of the stress that he faces at a particular time in his life, or the loss of personal or environmental resources. Mental illness may be broadly defined as an unsuccessful attempt on the part of the person to adjust to life, to restore equilibrium, to relieve anxiety, or more simply, to satisfy his basic needs in socially acceptable ways.

The Healthy State. The healthy person enjoys a large degree of self-fulfillment and is coping successfully with life's problems. Physically, his body organs and systems perform well. He satisfies most of his needs in fairly acceptable ways. He is at relative peace

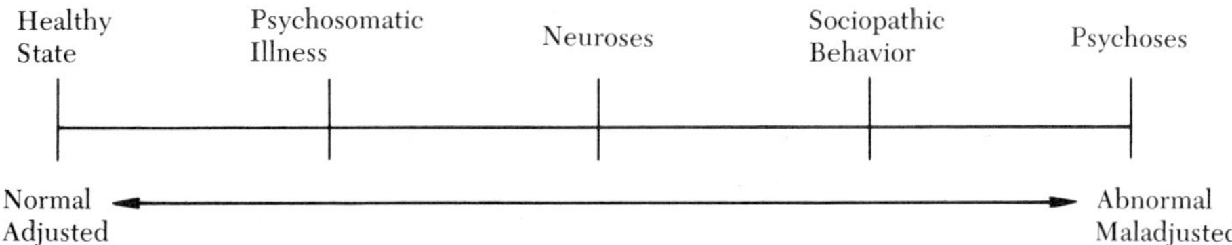

Figure 6. Continuum of behavioral reactions to stress. Healthy and sick behaviors have similarities as well as differences. They tend to shade into one another rather than existing as distinct categories. The closer the behavior is to being socially acceptable and meeting the needs of an individual, the greater the degree of health and vice versa. Thus the sickest way of reacting to stress is psychotic behavior because it is the least acceptable and offers the least satisfaction.

within himself and in general harmony with his environment. His needs, self, and conscience are in proportion and proper balance for healthy functioning. He is characteristically independent, cooperative, and giving.

Psychosomatic Illness. In psychosomatic illness, the individual suffers from some physical disease resulting from prolonged stress and chronic anxiety. There is an interruption of his satisfaction, but his ways of getting it remain generally acceptable. His external self is often the direct opposite of his inner self and in conflict, so he tries to protect himself by denying his unacceptable feelings. He is overly independent, cooperative, and giving in an attempt to counterbalance his inner dependent, demanding, and receiving strivings. The individual suffering from psychosomatic conditions is generally treated medically in the general hospital and occasionally receives psychiatric treatment on an outpatient basis. We will discuss some of the more common psychosomatic conditions related to the body systems which they affect in Chapter 16. (See also Appendix B, Classification of Mental Disorders, "Somatoform Disorders" and "Psychological Factors Affecting Physical Condition.")

Neuroses. In neuroses, the individual experiences overwhelming anxiety from which physical and psychological symptoms result. He gets some satisfaction but not sufficient, and his behavior loses some of its acceptability. He lacks self-acceptance and uses repression too much so that his satisfaction is inhibited and his hostility increased. He is generally described as a dependent, inadequate, hostile person. He resorts to substitutive and symbolic methods to relieve his anxiety, but is not quite successful and this results in the neurotic conflict. He is unable to give up his way of behaving (even though it leaves him dissatisfied) for healthier methods which are foreign to him—like the old saying, "A bird in the hand is worth two in the bush." He is generally treated in the doctor's office, frequently changing doctors, or in the general hospital, and sometimes he receives psychiatric treatment on an outpatient basis. We will discuss the common neuroses in Chapter 15. (See also Appendix B, "Anxiety Disorders," "Somatoform Disorders," and "Dissociative Disorders.")

Sociopathic Behavior. In sociopathic behavior, the individual often discharges his pent-up physical and psychic energy upon the environment in antisocial attacks. His behavior nets him little satisfaction, and his methods are socially unacceptable. His lack of control and rejection of authority are demonstrated in hostile, aggressive acting out against society. He has developed little self or conscience, so that his basic needs and impulses are expressed directly in the dependent, demanding, receiving ways characteristic of the infant. He is unable to postpone his satisfaction and he has few coping methods at his disposal. This individual is generally in difficulty with the law and is often incarcerated in jail, prison, or some other correctional institution, seldom receiving psychiatric treatment. We will discuss sociopathic reactions in Chapter 14. (See also "Personality Disorders" in Appendix B.)

Psychoses. In psychoses, the individual's behavior shows severe interference with effective functioning, involving his thinking, feeling, and doing. His behavior does not gain him the satisfaction he needs, and it is not acceptable to himself and others. He either is ill-prepared for the task of living, or experiences too much stress for him to master, or a combination of these. There are characteristic disturbances in his behavior corresponding to the different forms the illness takes.

Organic mental disorders are those in which we see behavioral or psychological disturbances due to transient or permanent dysfunction of the brain. They include (1) primary degenerative dementia, senile onset, with delirium, delusions, or depression or uncomplicated; (2) primary degenerative dementia, presenile onset; (3) multi-infarct dementia; and (4) substance-induced, including those caused by alcohol and drugs (see Appendix B).

The resulting symptoms are of two kinds—those due directly to the CNS dysfunction and those due to the individual's psychological reaction to the additional stress. For example, the aging process is likely to be stressful for most people; most adjust to it, but some develop the physical and psychological symptoms of senile dementia—loss of intellectual ability, impairment of judgment and memory, and symptoms of depression or schizophrenia. These individuals may be treated medically and psychiatrically in general or psychiatric hospitals, nursing homes, and doctors' offices or other outpatient facilities.

The functional psychoses are those of psychogenic origin or without clearly defined physical disease or structural change in the brain. The nonorganic mental disorders include schizophrenic and affective disorders, in which there is no clearly defined physical disease or structural change in the brain. In the emotional and psychological reactions to the stress of living we see the most severe disturbances in the individual's functioning. The person, as a result, has distortions in thinking, disturbances in mood, and increased or decreased motor activity. There is serious disruption in his personality organization, his ability to correctly evaluate external reality, and his behavior toward his environment and other people (see Appendix B). The patient may be treated medically and psychiatrically in a general or psychiatric hospital or doctor's office or other outpatient facility. We will discuss the three most prevalent psychotic disorders—schizophrenia (Chapter 11), depression (Chapter 12), and psychoses associated with the aging process (Chapter 13).

All kinds of behavior patterns and life styles are considered healthy so long as they serve the function for which they are intended—the satisfaction of basic needs in socially acceptable ways. The behavior pattern or life style of the individual depends upon what he inherits, what he acquires from his environment, and what kind of stress he experiences in life. The development of healthy reactions, or the opposite, mental illness, is rather like building a house. In building a sturdy structure, it is important to use good material to start with, mix the materials together in proper balance and proportions, and use the best tools possible in the building process. Such a house is likely to withstand the customary storms and various seasons of the environment. However, no matter what the degree of sturdiness or how well built it is, if a storm of sufficient severity occurs, the house will not be able to withstand it. Similarly, abnormalities or maladjustment or mental illness occur when the structure is not too sturdy to start with and the first big wind that comes along shakes it apart. When the storm is sufficiently intense or prolonged or widespread, even the sturdy structure is not able to withstand it and it succumbs to the pressure. Some individuals weather the storm or adjust; others develop physical disease or symptoms which incapacitate them; others act out their conflicts in antisocial attacks and get into trouble with the law; others develop severe disturbances in thinking, feeling, and doing which disrupt their inner peace and their harmony with others and make it impossible for them to cope with the demands of life.

REFERENCES

Baruch, Dorothy: *One Little Boy,* Dell Publishing Company, New York, 1964.

Billings, Carolyn Veronica: "Emotional first aid," *American Journal of Nursing, 80* (November, 1980) pp. 2006–2009.

Buckalew, M.W.: *Learning to Control Stress,* Rosen Press, New York, 1979.

Finesilver, Cynthia: "Reducing stress for cardiac catheterization patients," *American Journal of Nursing, 80* (October, 1980) pp. 1805–1807.

Grubb, Davis: *Night of the Hunter,* Penguin Books, New York, 1977.

Harris, Merril: "Understanding the autistic child," *American Journal of Nursing, 78* (October, 1978) pp. 1682–1685.

Hoff, Lee Ann: *People In Crisis,* Addison-Wesley, Reading, Mass., 1978.

Lynch, James J.: *The Broken Heart,* Basic Books, New York, 1977.

Maugham, Somerset: *Of Human Bondage,* Penguin Books, New York, 1978.

Schulberg, Bud: *What Makes Sammy Run?* Penguin Books, New York, 1978.

Smith, Marcy J. T., and Hans Selye: "Reducing the negative effects of stress," *American Journal of Nursing, 79* (November, 1979) pp. 1953–1955.

Wendt, Roselyn L.: "Good morning, world. I'm glad to be back," *American Journal of Nursing, 1979* (May, 1979) p. 949.

Wilson, Ronald W., and Bonnie J. Elmassian: "Endorphins," *American Journal of Nursing, 81* (April, 1981) pp. 722–725.

Chapter 7

Treatment of Mental Illness

As our knowledge and understanding of mental illness have increased, the treatment of psychiatric patients has changed accordingly. When the causes of illness were not obvious, primitive man attributed them to malignant forces either human or superhuman. He then treated the illness by *magical* or religious means—incantations, rituals, exorcism, prayer, and penance. If the illness was caused by evil spirits, one had to get rid of them, and this was done primarily by inflicting punishment upon the sick person or banishing him from the group in atonement for his sins.

Then came the ages of reason and enlightenment, and man's ailments were described in terms of biology, physiology, and anatomy. The explanation of illness and the approach to treatment were based upon the natural sciences and were largely *organic.* There was also an emphasis upon social reform and a more humane treatment of all unfortunate people, including the mentally ill. Vincenzo Chiarugi (1759–1820) in Italy, Philippe Pinel (1745–1826) in France, and Benjamin Rush (1745–1813) in the U.S. helped to release the mentally ill from their chains and dungeons and change society's attitudes toward them so that they could be considered as sick human beings deserving of treatment. At the beginning of the modern era the organic approach to mental illness was enhanced by Emil Kraepelin (1856–1926), a German neuropsychiatrist, who spent years evolving a system which is still used today to describe and classify disorders in behavior (see Appendix B).

Over a period of years, improvements were made in the methods employed in the observation and classification of mental illness, and people began to be more compassionate in their attitudes toward the mentally ill. Likewise, the aura of fear and magic surrounding mental illness began to subside, although there is still some residue of it today. Psychiatry began to deal with the patient as a whole person, and the *psychological* approach to psychiatric treatment came into being.

Sigmund Freud (1856–1939), an Austrian neuropsychiatrist, made significant contributions to psychiatry, society, and man's understanding of himself. He established psychology as a valid method of systematically observing and explaining man's behavior. He developed a method of treatment, *psychoanalysis*, based upon his theories regarding personality development and structure, which he supported with rigorous scientific research and voluminous clinical data. Freud and his followers made many valuable contributions to the understanding and treatment of mental illness and had great influence on modern psychiatric treatment. Some of Freud's colleagues disagreed with him and modified the psychoanalytic approach or established other schools of thought, among them Eugene Bleuler, Carl Jung, Otto Rank, Mortimer Adler, William Alanson White, and Adolf Meyer. Contributions from a host of others form the nucleus for modern psychiatric theory and practice in the United States. Prominent among these are Franz Alexander, Erich Fromm, Harry Stack Sullivan, Karen Horney, Frieda Fromm Reichman, Erik Erikson, Carl Rogers, Maxwell Jones, Bruno Bettelheim, Leon Saul, Karl and William Menninger and many others.

Modern psychiatric treatment uses a multi-disciplinary, multilateral approach. The sick person today is likely to be treated with everything and by everybody in his environment, hopefully with one person, usually the psychiatrist-physician, directing or coordinating the joint effort. Psychiatric treatment incorporates recent advances in biochemistry, microbiology, genetics, and pharmacology, along with refinements in psychology, sociology, criminology, economics and learning theory. Let us look first at the physical, organic, or somatic forms of treatment in current use.

SOMATIC TREATMENT

Shock Therapy. The first kind of shock treatment to be used was that induced by insulin. In 1933, Sakel reported that insulin used in a high enough dosage to produce coma reduced overactivity in excited patients, particularly those suffering from schizophrenia. Some schizophrenic patients, particularly young acutely ill patients, did seem to benefit from insulin shock therapy. However, the treatment procedure was time-consuming, expensive and hazardous, requiring especially skilled physicians and nursing staff. Since treatment results were not particularly positive, this form of treatment has largely disappeared. Other shock-producing drugs, for example metrazol, were tried with similar results.

In 1938 Cerletti and Bini introduced electroshock treatment, which replaced shock-producing drugs. It is sometimes called electro-convulsive therapy (ECT) to distinguish it from other forms of electrical stimulation. Treatments are usually given three times a week for a six-week period, or a series of eighteen. However, they are tailored to the individual needs and response of the patient. They may be given in varying frequency, from several in one day to one treatment a month. For a particular patient, a total of three or four treatments may be sufficient to restore optimum function, while for another patient, it may require more than one series. Because of the introduction of psychoactive drugs, particularly antidepressants, ECT is seldom used anymore, and is even prohibited in certain states. It may be used in very severe cases, especially if the patient does not respond positively to drug therapy.

Drug Therapy. Drugs have been used for many centuries to reduce man's tension in reaction to stress. The use of alcohol and opium go back to ancient times, and even the primitive medicine man or witch doctor used roots and herbs in many of his magico-religious rituals and ceremonies. The use of drugs has been considerably refined and has become much more scientific in modern medicine, particularly in psychiatric treatment.

1. TREATING PHYSICAL CONDITIONS. Drugs are used in different ways and for different purposes in psychiatric treatment. First of all, they may be used to treat the physical condition of the patient. In relieving the physical symptoms, the patient's stress and anxiety with their accompanying psychological symptoms are also relieved. For example, a patient with a high fever may experience the psychotic symptom of hallucinations. When the infection is treated with antibiotics, such as penicillin, the physical and psychotic symptoms disappear. A patient with CAS may have attacks of vertigo which seriously interfere with his functioning and make him increasingly irritable and suspicious. When the attacks are relieved with medication such as Antivert, the disturbances in his behavior likewise disappear. A patient may become severely depressed as a result of endocrine dysfunction during menopause. With the administration of a hormone such as Premarin, both the physical discomfort and the depression are alleviated. Patients with rheumatoid arthritis may be relieved of physical and psychological symptoms with the administration of corticosteroids. Cortisone diminishes the inflammatory process, thus reducing pain, and at the same time increases the patient's sense of well-being.

2. USE OF PLACEBO. A whole variety of drugs are used because they are the favorite remedies of the patient or physician.

These drugs might well fit into the placebo category because their success is primarily dependent upon the faith they invoke in the patient rather than upon their chemical properties. For example, many people take aspirin, an analgesic, to relieve tension and help them sleep, even though it has no sedative action. Many people take over-the-counter medicines to relieve gastric distress, even though they have no specific antacid or smooth muscle action.

Doctors often prescribe nonspecific remedies for patients whose physical symptoms have an emotional basis. If the remedy works, and it often does, it is because of the patient's faith in the helping ability of the physician, or because of the belief that medicine of any kind helps relieve distress. Studies have been done which demonstrate the relationship between the therapeutic effectiveness of the medications being given and the attitudes held by the nursing staff giving them and the patients receiving them. When the attitudes indicate a belief in the medication's helpfulness, improvement tends to take place in the patient's behavior, even though the drug may be a placebo. Whereas when both staff and patients feel the medication will not help, no improvement or further disturbance may take place in the patient's behavior, regardless of the chemical properties of the drug.

3. SEDATIVES AND STIMULANTS. Another group of drugs are those used to sedate or stimulate the patient's functioning, particularly his activity. For example, chloral hydrate is often used as a sedative to produce sleep in patients who are restless, agitated, tense, and anxious. Sometimes barbiturates, such as Amytal Sodium, are used to quiet very excited, aggressive patients. However, barbiturates, like bromides, must be used with extreme caution because they may excite the patient further rather than sedate him. Stimulants, such as caffeine and Adrenalin, may be used in certain illnesses involving circulatory difficulty. Amphetamine derivatives, such as Benzedrine and Dexedrine, may be used to treat patients with depression, usually in conjunction with other drugs.

4. PSYCHOACTIVE DRUGS (see following list). The most common group of drugs used to relieve reactions to stress are the psychoactive drugs, sometimes referred to as ataractic, psychotropic, psychophysiological, psychopharmacological, or pharmacotherapeutic. These drugs account for some of the major changes in psychiatric treatment, and in addition, they do not have the many undesirable side effects of the sedatives and stimulants mentioned above. They have reduced the violence of mental illness, made it possible for patients to be treated more easily at home or in the community, reduced the length of the hospital stay, and made it possible for very agitated and regressed patients to participate more readily in other forms of treatment. There are three kinds of psychoactive drugs used to relieve anxiety and counteract

its manifestations—antipsychotic, antianxiety, and antidepressant. The fourth kind, antiparkinsonism drugs, relieves side effects of phenothiazines. Although the action of these drugs is not fully understood, in general they seem to inhibit the function of the subcortical areas of the brain—the hypothalamus, limbic system, and reticular activating system—and thus lessen the effect of anxiety on the autonomic nervous system (see pages 60–61).

CLASSIFICATION OF COMMON PSYCHOACTIVE DRUGS*

I. The Antipsychotic Drugs (major tranquilizers)
  A. Butyrophenone—Haldol
  B. Rauwolfia
    1. Reserpine—Serpasil
    2. Deserpidine—Harmonyl
  C. Phenothiazines
    1. Dimethylamine—Thorazine
    2. Piperazine—Compazine, Prolixin, Stelazine, Trilafon, Triavil
    3. Piperidyl—Mellaril
    4. Piperacetazine—Quide
    5. Acetophenazine—Tindal
    6. Triflupromazine—Vesprin
    7. Mesoridazine—Serentil
  D. Thioxanthenes (phenothiazene-like)
    1. Chlorprothixene—Taractan
    2. Thiothixene—Navane
  E. Lithium carbonate—Eskalith, Lithane, Lithonate
  F. Dihydroindolone—Moban
  G. Dibenzoxazepine—Loxitane
II. The Antianxiety Drugs (minor tranquilizers)
  A. Meprobamate
    1. Miltown
    2. Equanil
  B. Hydroxyzine
    1. Atarax
    2. Vistaril
  C. Chlordiazepoxide—Librium
  D. Diazepam—Valium
  E. Clorazepate—Azene
  F. Lorazepam—Ativan
  G. Oxepam—Serax
  H. Prazepam—Verstran

*More detailed information may be found in Appendix C.

III. The Antidepressant Drugs (psychic energizers; psychostimulants)
  A. Monoamine oxidase inhibitors (MAOI)
    1. Hydrazines—Marsilid, Marplan, Nardil, Niamid
    2. Nonhydrazines—Parnate, Eutonyl
  B. Nonenzyme inhibitors
    1. Imipramine—Tofranil, Imavate
    2. Amitriptyline—Elavil
    3. Desipramine—Pertofrane, Norpramin
    4. Nortriptyline—Aventyl, Pamelor
    5. Protriptyline—Vivactil
    6. Doxepin—Adapin, Sinequan
    7. Amoxapin—Asendin
    8. Maprotiline—Ludiomil
    9. Trimipramine—Surmontil

IV. The Antiparkinsonism Drugs (anticholinergic; antimuscarinic)
  A. Procyclidine HCl—Kemadrin
  B. Benztropine mesylate—Cogentin
  C. Biperiden HCl—Akineton
  D. Trihexyphenidyl HCl—Artane

Tranquilizers are used to relieve reactions to stress manifested by distorted thinking, hyperactivity, and disrupted interpersonal relationships. They calm a person and make him feel more comfortable and relaxed without impairing his conscious awareness or intellectual functioning. Tranquilizers may be divided into two groups—the antipsychotic and the antianxiety drugs, also called major and minor tranquilizers. The antipsychotic drugs are used for major disturbances in the person's adjustment, and the medications most commonly prescribed are of the phenothiazine group and include such trade names as Stelazine, Thorazine, Compazine, Mellaril, and Taractan. The antianxiety drugs are used for less severe emotional disturbances, and the medications most commonly prescribed are meprobamate, hydroxyzine, chlordiazepoxide, and diazepam and include Miltown, Equanil, Atarax, Vistaril, Librium, and Valium. (See preceding list and also Appendix C.)

Antidepressant drugs may also be divided into two groups—the monoamine oxidase inhibitors (MAOI), sometimes referred to as psychic energizers, and the nonenzyme inhibitors, sometimes referred to as psychostimulants. Since the MAOI drugs were found to produce many undesirable side effects, they are seldom used and many are no longer on the market. The most commonly prescribed medications include Tofranil, Elavil, and Aventyl. Antidepressants relieve reactions to stress manifested by melancholy, retardation, and tension. Unfortunately, the response to antidepressant drugs may not be so dramatic or positive, so that often the severely depressed patient receives a combination of antidepressant and tranquilizing drugs, and sometimes ECT as well. They are used to elevate the patient's mood, stimulate his activity, and give him hope again.

Another group of drugs, the *antiparkinsonism agents,* are often used in conjunction with phenothiazine tranquilizers to counteract their side effects. Large doses of tranquilizers may produce various kinds of extrapyramidal symptoms—akinesia or muscle weakness and fatigue, dyskinesia or involuntary muscle movements, akathisia or motor restlessness, and pseudoparkinsonism. The most commonly prescribed medications include Kemadrin, Cogentin, Akineton, and Artane.

There has been some investigative and experimental use of hallucinogenic drugs in psychiatric treatment. However, since neither their action nor their therapeutic value has been clearly established, their use is not extensive and has even been outlawed in some states. The two most common drugs in this group are mescaline, which comes from the buttons of the peyote cactus, and lysergic acid diethylamide (LSD), which comes from ergot, a fungus growth that causes rye cereal to rot. They are sometimes referred to as "mind-expanding" drugs and are used therapeutically to help the patient recall and, hopefully, resolve some of the unpleasant experiences or conflicts that he has pushed down into his unconscious mind, using the coping method of repression.

There is no question as to the value of somatic treatments or even the necessity, especially with severely disturbed patients or those who have been ill for a long time. However, they do not combat the cause of the anxiety or change the person's basic reaction to it. They offer temporary relief to the person who is so overcome by the stress in his life situation that his fear, tension, and anxiety hamper his ability to function. They are emergency measures to maintain the patient's life. They can help the patient face and deal more realistically with internal and external problems if they are used appropriately. If they are misused, they can compound the patient's problems and make matters worse rather than better for him.

PSYCHOLOGICAL TREATMENT

It seems obvious that the best approach to treatment is one that uses a combination of physical, psychological, and social factors. A man falls ill as a person—not as a nervous system, nor as a personality, nor as an isolated creature. The patient has a right to expect not only survival, but security and health when he comes to us for help. We can best help the maladjusted, emotionally disturbed, mentally ill person by assisting him in his search for greater satisfaction of his needs and better ways of going about it. The only way he can end that search is through some kind of corrective emotional experience with people, which will help him change his perception of himself and the world he lives in.

Psychoanalysis. One of the primary forms of psychological therapy, psychoanalysis, has changed little since its conception by Freud over fifty years ago. Although it is based upon very complex psychodynamic principles, we will try to describe the treatment process briefly. The treatment usually consists of fifty-minute sessions, as many as four or five times a week, over an extended period of time, which may mean years. Traditionally, the patient lies on a couch and the therapist sits out of sight so as not to distract him, though this practice is often modified. The patient is instructed to talk as freely as he can about anything he wishes, and this is called *free association.*

During the course of treatment, the patient's unconscious repressed desires are brought out into the open so that they may be examined and modified. In this way, the internal conflict which forms the basis of his disturbed adjustment is resolved. This is accomplished by the therapist's interpretation of the patient's free associations and dreams. Sooner or later the patient projects his attitudes about others upon the therapist, and acts out with him the conflicts he has had with his parents. This is called *transference.* The therapist interacts with him in such a way as to correct his misinterpretations about others, and thus resolves the external conflict. The patient comes to see himself and others more realistically in the mirror which the therapist holds up to him; that is, he gains *insight.*

Many people have departed from the orthodox psychoanalytic method of treatment, which can be used only with a limited number of selected individuals. It is expensive, time-consuming, and requires special training. For example, to become a psychoanalyst, the therapist, already a psychiatrist or psychologist, must undergo further training in a psychoanalytic institute, including personal analysis. However, the principles upon which psychoanalysis is based are used in many of the other forms of psychological and social treatment.

Psychotherapy. Psychotherapy may be defined as a planned psychological procedure undertaken by a specially trained professional person to restore a patient to mental health. Although many things we do with patients are therapeutic, they don't all fit in the category of psychotherapy. There are various kinds of psychotherapy, and the kind used with a particular patient depends upon the training and preference of the therapist and the needs and abilities of the patient. *Psychoanalytically oriented* psychotherapy means dealing with repressed, unconscious material in an effort to produce insight and change. *Supportive* psychotherapy means allowing the patient to be dependent upon the therapist while the therapist is reenforcing the positive attitudes the patient has toward himself and others. *Reality-oriented* psychotherapy means dealing with the here-and-now problems in an effort to help the patient face up to his responsibility for his own behavior.

The treatment may be conducted in a one-to-one situation, with therapist and patient, called *individual* psychotherapy, or it may be conducted with a group of patients and one or two therapists, that is, *group* psychotherapy. Sometimes a patient participates in both kinds of therapy. There are advantages to both, and again the selection of the type of therapy is determined by the therapist and the patient. Group therapy has been used to great advantage in large hospitals for the mentally ill, such as state and federal hospitals, because so many more patients can be treated.

To become a psychotherapist, the person must have special training, including supervised practice in the clinical field, whether he be a psychiatrist, physician, psychologist, social worker, or registered nurse. Individual treatment usually consists of fifty-minute sessions at least once a week, over a relatively short period of time (six months to a year). Patient and therapist face each other and discuss aspects of the patient's problems.

Special forms of psychotherapy include play therapy, family therapy, and counseling. Although some therapists hold to the classic psychoanalytic approach in the treatment of children, many advocate other techniques, particularly *play therapy.* The emotionally disturbed child is encouraged to express his feelings freely in a warm, permissive atmosphere with an accepting, supportive adult. In the play sessions, the child acts out his problems, particularly concerning his parents, by using such avenues of expression as toys, molding clay, puppets, and finger painting. The emotionally disturbed child has great difficulty communicating at all, but when he does it reflects the degree and kind of problems he is faced with. The therapist using play therapy can help the child to relieve his pent-up feelings, learn how to handle his feelings more constructively, experience a correction in his perceptions of himself and his parents, or compensate in part for some of the deprivation, isolation, or suffering in his life.

Like play therapy, *family therapy* is a special form of psychotherapy. Many therapists treat more than one member of the family because very often the illness lies in the disturbed family relationships rather than in just one member of the group, particularly in the case of disturbed children. Family-centered therapy is a fairly recent development in psychiatry, and the whole family is treated together at the same time by one or more therapists. It is a kind of select form of group psychotherapy, with the family as the group members. This form of therapy provides a rare opportunity for the therapist to help correct defects in the communication process within the family, particularly in the case of schizophrenic children. A great deal of work has been done in this field, and you will find some reading references which report on this kind of treatment (see Caplan, 1964).

Another development in psychiatric treatment is a special kind of psychotherapy called *counseling.* Counseling is usually directed toward a specific problem area of a client's life, rather than toward attempts to change him or his style of living. For example, vocational counselors help a person with problems pertaining to work, such as preparing for a certain job, or selecting a job suitable to the individual. Marriage counselors help people resolve serious problems in their marriage which they cannot handle by themselves. Spiritual counselors help a person with problems pertaining to his spiritual life or religious belief. School counselors help students with problems pertaining to school, such as the choice of curriculum, or relationships with other students and teachers, or how to study. All are directed toward helping the counselee, client, or patient function more effectively by using guidance, advisory, and sometimes healing techniques.

There are many different kinds of groups, including therapy, recreational, educational, and growth groups. These are variously referred to as encounter groups, sensitivity training, Gestalt groups, TA groups, psychodrama, Reality Therapy, nonverbal therapy, and so on. These groups generally give the patient an opportunity to seek validation, give and receive feedback, and test new ways of behaving that may bring him greater success in living. There has been a great increase in self-awareness and consciousness-raising groups that focus on self-healing practices, discovery of the real self, body-mind integration, and responsibility for self and life.

Crisis Intervention. Although crisis intervention is more of a process than a specific treatment method, it should be mentioned here. It will be discussed further as it relates to community mental health nursing in Chapter 17.

The term "crisis" may be defined in different ways, but one way we are already familiar with is related to medical conditions. For example, we refer to the crisis of a high fever, in which the fever reaches a peak and then breaks and drops suddenly to a normal temperature or below. There are emotional and social crises as well as physical ones. As we have seen in Chapter 4, Erikson refers to developmental crises in each of the stages of a person's life cycle. He sees a crisis as a turning point in one's life that presents the opportunity for growth and self-realization. As a person masters the crisis, he emerges "with an increased sense of inner unity, with an increase of judgment, and an increase in the capacity 'to do well' according to his own standards and to the standards of those who are significant to him" (Erikson, 1968, p. 92). Caplan, too, emphasizes the growth potential for the individual as an outcome of crisis, rather than seeing it as a catastrophe that results in pathological behavior. He explains crisis as occurring "when a person faces an obstacle to important life goals that is for a time unsurmountable through the utilization of customary methods of problem solving. A period of disorganization ensues; a period of upset during which many abortive attempts at solution are made" (Caplan, 1964, p. 18).

Life crises can be equated with particularly stressful periods in one's life that urgently require a resolution. They represent a severe threat to the satisfaction of basic needs and result in a state of disequilibrium from which the person must extricate himself in order to survive. Thus, it is a period of increased vulnerability as well as increased potential for growth. At the time of the crisis, the person is overwhelmed—he is in serious trouble, the old methods of solving problems don't work for him, and he may need assistance in weathering the storm. That assistance, when given by a professional, is called crisis intervention.

The assistance may take different forms—physical, emotional, or social—depending upon the needs of the individual and the circumstances surrounding him in the crisis situation. For example, he may need intensive tranquilization to lessen the extreme tension and give him some rest and comfort. He may need supportive psychotherapy in order to find new solutions among his own resources. Temporary removal from the social situation that has provoked the crisis might be necessary. He may need all three of these or something entirely different.

The form, then, that crisis intervention takes depends upon the needs of the individual involved, the resources that he has within himself, and the ability of the therapist and others around him to help. The focus is upon the here and now, rather than what has happened to him in the past or why. The assistance is aimed toward giving him immediate relief in an intolerably painful situation. It requires an astute assessment of the individual and his social situation, an immediate decision about a course of action, a resolution of the existing crisis, and assistance in making realistic plans for the future. It is a preventive as well as a treatment measure to help the stricken individual avoid disastrous consequences.

The Nurse-Patient Relationship. Nurses have a unique opportunity to form a therapeutic or helping relationship with patients because they "live" with them. They are where the action is. They are key figures in determining the effectiveness of the treatment program or individual care plan. They are the filters through which all communication flows to and from the patient. They interpret and implement hospital and clinical policy. They control the rewards and punishments for patients. They are the treatment models for patients. Whether the patient lives or dies, whether he feels secure or anxious, whether he returns to health or remains sick (especially for the hospitalized patient) depends in large measure upon how skilled the nursing staff are in observing, analyzing, and responding to the patient's needs in interaction with him.

The nurse uses her own healthy personality to help the patient correct the distorted perceptions he has of himself and the world he lives in. She provides for the satisfaction of his needs, directly when he is unable to help himself, and indirectly by helping him utilize the resources within himself and his environment. In her verbal and nonverbal communication with him, she provides continuous, nonevaluative, corrective feedback that helps him improve his own ability to communicate effectively. In her interactions with him, she helps him learn how to go about getting more satisfaction of his needs in more acceptable ways.

The nurse is not only a therapeutic agent for the patient, she is also a social agent. She creates the environment necessary for the patient to get well. She guides his social participation, teaches him new social skills, or helps him regain those he has lost. She provides the opportunity for him to practice new ways of behaving. She is often in the position of family counselor, advising the family what to bring, how often to come, what to do and say, how to help the patient. She encourages the patient to form mutually helpful relationships with those in his immediate environment and then go on to new relationships and new environments without her.

And she does this not just for one patient, but for a ward full of patients in the hospital, or a number of individuals and families in the community, for her particular clients if she is a counselor, her students if she is a teacher, or her staff if she is a supervisor.

SOCIAL TREATMENT

Recent emphasis has been placed upon the treatment of the patient as a member of a group—the family, the society, the world—rather than a single, isolated individual. This emphasis has led to greater use of social approaches in treatment, based upon certain factors. First, psychiatric illness is primarily a disruption of the patient's ability to relate successfully with others. Second, the patient must learn, or relearn, how to assume responsibility for the welfare of himself and others. Third, members of the patient group, as well as members of the staff, often become therapists or treatment models for other patients. Fourth, any group of people who are allowed to govern themselves or participate in decisions that affect their lives will hold greater possibilities for each member's growth toward self-fulfillment, interdependence, individual and social responsibility than one which is subject to authoritarian control. Fifth, what happens in patient groups is similar to what happens in families, and therefore, experiences in the patient group offer unique possibilities for correcting a patient's distorted perceptions of himself and others.

Environmental. The kind of climate or environment which surrounds a person directly affects his state of health or well-being. This is true of the healthy person as well as the sick, but it is a particularly crucial factor in the treatment of the mentally ill. This may be because the mentally ill person is peculiarly handicapped in his ability to interact effectively with his environment, or perhaps because he has never had the kind of healthy environment that is required in order to learn how to function successfully. To a patient in a psychiatric hospital, or for that matter, to any person in need of help, nothing is more important than the kind of people he comes in contact with. Therefore, of particular significance to the sick person is the psychological environment, which is in part determined by the kind of physical environment provided.

Various organized efforts are used to surround the patient with the kind of supportive environment conducive to learning new or more successful methods of living. Such environmental approaches are called by various names, such as milieu therapy, attitude therapy, therapeutic community, or social psychiatry. At the Menninger Psychiatric Hospital in Topeka, Kansas, a set of attitudes was developed which could then be prescribed for the staff to follow with individual patients. For example, the attitude of "kind firmness" might be prescribed for a patient with a severe depression. He would then be treated by everyone in a kind manner but with extreme firmness, an attitude designed to help him externalize his hostility and thereby alleviate his self-punishment. Often, such a patient is assigned menial tasks, which are meant to provoke him into expressing his anger. It is important for the staff to follow through with the attitude prescribed, and be prepared to accept the hostile outbursts from the patient toward the nurse, doctor, or hospital. The student will find some reading references in this kind of treatment.

The therapeutic community approach is attributed largely to Dr. Maxwell Jones, who instituted several programs in Great Britain and the United States. Such programs generally follow the same design. All of the activities in which a particular patient participates are integrated in such a way that they provide a therapeutic program for him. Staff and patients alike participate in the decision-making. Often patients are provided with paid jobs, either within the hospital community or in the larger outside community.

Many hospitals, both general and psychiatric, utilize the basic principles of attitude therapy and the therapeutic community. Patients may participate in regular policy-making sessions directed toward solving the problems of group living. These sessions are sometimes called ward government or ward management, or patient-staff meetings. They may discuss such problems as what to do about the patient down the hall who makes so much noise at night that the rest of the patients have trouble sleeping, or whether or not a particular patient should be given permission to go home for the weekend, or where to go on their next shopping trip to town.

Behavior Modification. Traditional forms of psychiatric treatment are based upon the belief that a patient's symptoms or problems or behavior stem from internal causes. Traditional psychotherapy, therefore, is aimed toward the relief of internal conflict, which in turn relieves the symptoms. On the other hand, behavioral psychology is based upon the belief that symptoms or problems or behavior are a result of environmental influences. Behavioral therapy, therefore, is aimed toward changing the behavior directly, rather than indirectly, by altering the patient's way of responding to environmental stimuli. Rather than paying attention to what the patient is (e.g., sad or happy), behavioral therapy pays attention to what the patient does (e.g., he cries or laughs). In either case, the therapeutic goal is the same—to help the patient find better ways of satisfying his needs; it is the approach that is different. Behavior modification may be defined, then, as a method of treatment that utilizes planned changes in the environment to assist the patient in learning new, adaptive ways of behaving.

What constitutes a behavior problem or problem behavior is a matter of social judgment based upon cultural standards. Behavior in itself is usually neither good nor bad, except for specifically condemned activities such as incest, but it becomes so for most of society, including the nurse and the patient, under different sets of environmental circumstances. For example, taking another person's life is generally condemned, but doing so in defense of one's self or one's country is not only acceptable, it is even regarded as honorable. Or the behavior itself may be generally acceptable, but how and when it occurs may be the problem. For example, laughing at a funeral is generally unacceptable, and laughing excessively anywhere or anytime becomes a problem. On the other hand, not laughing when it is called for, such as at humorous events in life, is also likely to result in social problems. We might say, then, that there are three kinds of problem behavior: (1) condemned behavior, regardless of how rare, such as incest; (2) excessive behavior, such as laughing or talking incessantly or inappropriately; and (3) deficient behavior, such as not laughing or responding when it is called for.

Treatment approaches for behavior modification consist of classic or respondent conditioning, and operant conditioning or learning theory. Most people have read about Pavlov's experiments, in which he was able to get dogs to salivate by ringing a bell. This was accomplished by presenting food and the ringing of a bell simultaneously enough times so that the weaker stimulus (ringing bell) could elicit the same response as the stronger stimulus (food). The focus in respondent conditioning is the manipulation of *stimuli* as they affect *involuntary* activities. However, the most commonly used approach in behavior modification is operant conditioning or learning theory, established by B. F. Skinner. The focus here is upon the *consequences* of behavioral response rather than the stimuli, and *voluntary* activities rather than involuntary. A continuous schedule of reinforcement is set up so that for every desirable response a positive consequence occurs. As long as the therapist controls reinforcement, he can accelerate (increase) or decelerate (decrease) target behaviors. However, extinction of the desired behavior may occur if the response is not followed long enough by a positive consequence.

Positive reinforcers (or rewards) are important in helping patients change their behavior and are a common part of our social system; for example, we get paid for doing a certain job. It is important, therefore, to determine what represents a positive reinforcer for each patient. A reward for one person is not necessarily a reward for another; therefore, the treatment plan must meet the needs of the individual patient. For example, with regressed, retarded, or socially deprived patients, the most potent reinforcer may be food or treats, whereas, for another patient, it may be pleasurable activities, such as favorite games or TV shows. For still another patient, the most potent reinforcer may be the verbal approval of nursing staff or other patients.

Behavior modification is a process for dealing with social problems of human beings. It consists of (1) assessment—defining, observing, and recording behavior and the circumstances in which it occurs; (2) intervention—application of specific treatment techniques; and (3) evaluation—observing and recording the patient's reaction to the treatment, testing the accuracy of the assessment, identifying the relationship of change to techniques used, and measuring how long the improvement lasts.

Usually a behavioral agreement or contract is made with the patient, so that he knows exactly what activities are to be performed and what rewards are to be delivered. The terms must be clearly specified, so that the occasion is set for the desired effect. Therefore, the stimuli preceding the desired behavior should indicate when, where, and under what conditions the response is to occur, and the response should be followed by a specific positive reinforcement. The more powerful the consequences, the greater the likelihood that the behavior will be accelerated. One of the most potent reinforcers is social agreement or the approval of significant others in one's environment, such as the nursing staff. The nursing staff, as we have said before, have direct, frequent, and prolonged contact with patients, particularly hospitalized patients. They are often in control of the reward system and determine (consciously or unconsciously) who gets rewards and who does not. The nursing staff are of primary importance in any behavior modification treatment program for patients in either the hospital or the community, where they control the consequences of a patient's actions.

Shaping, or handshaping, occurs when each step the patient takes in the direction of the desired or target behavior is positively reinforced. It begins with activities the individual is capable of performing and ends with the behavior to be produced. The reinforcement should be potent, consistent, and delivered immediately after the desired behavior occurs. However, too much reinforcement reduces the likelihood of the next step occurring. Progress depends upon the patient's mastering each step, one at a time, until the final result is reached. The requirements for reinforcement are raised slowly but surely for each step, always within the capabilities of the individual patient. Some patients, for example those who are mentally retarded, socially deprived, or severely withdrawn, have lost or never developed certain social behaviors. With these patients it may be necessary to demonstrate and imitate, or physically guide the patient through the required steps to the goal behavior. Let's say the behavior one hopes to produce is the patient's taking care of his own personal hygiene. The nurse may set up a series of achievable steps, such as washing his hands, washing his face, combing his hair, brushing his teeth, taking a bath, putting on his underwear, putting on his shirt, putting on his socks, putting on his shoes, and tying his shoes. Each of these activities would be rewarded repeatedly until the patient is able to do them on his own. The end result is his ability to care for himself, but he accomplishes this one step at a time, with each step being rewarded until it can be done without reward.

To obtain desirable changes in patient behavior, then, desired response is reinforced continuously until it is established. After the behavior is taking place frequently, the reinforcers can gradually become more intermittent. As social reinforcers, such as verbal approval, gradually replace material reinforcers, such as food, other desirable behaviors begin to occur in addition to the ones specifically accelerated. The real test of the effectiveness of the treatment is fourfold: (1) changes in behavior last; (2) the changes in one situation can be transferred to others; (3) the patient can behave more competently; and (4) the patient can change and control his own behavior.

Activity Therapy. An important part of the environment includes the kinds of activities in which the patients participate. Most hospitals have some kind of planned program in occupational therapy (O.T.), recreational therapy (R.T.), and industrial therapy (I.T.). Activity therapy offers patients an opportunity to dissipate excess energy in a productive way, practice social skills and problem solving in a protected environment, learn more creative ways of self-expression, become more independent and responsible, and find greater satisfaction of basic needs in more socially acceptable ways.

In occupational therapy, a patient accomplishes these goals primarily by producing something with his hands. It may be building a bedside stand for himself, or making a crib for his youngster. It may include fancy work, ceramics, leather work, cooking, and handicrafts of all kinds. It may result in the patient's contributions to art, drama, music, dance, and literature.

In recreational therapy a patient accomplishes the goals primarily by playing some game or participating in some kind of fun activity. It may include sports, like basketball or softball; social activities, like dancing or playing cards, or going to movies; or individual pleasure, like reading or listening to music.

In industrial therapy, a patient accomplishes the goals primarily by learning to do a particular job that contributes to the welfare of himself and others. It may be a job on the ward for a patient who cannot yet go out on his own, or a job on the paint crew of the hospital. It may be a job in the community doing housework or gardening.

Whatever the activity, it should be chosen with the particular patient in mind, and should not be used just to pass the time or just to keep patients active and busy. It should be directed toward the fulfillment of the specific needs of the patient for whom it is prescribed or recommended so as to aid in the restoration of the patient's health. The following guidelines should be used in selecting activities: (1) the activity should fit with the patient's particular life style; (2) it should be one which holds real interest and purpose for him; (3) it should capitalize upon his assets and abilities; (4) it should be short enough for him to attain the sense of accomplishment; (5) it should give him some new experiences; (6) the patient should be allowed as much freedom of choice as possible; (7) he should be given only the amount of help that he needs; and (8) the activity should be his, not the hospital's or the staff's.

Educational Therapy. Most educational efforts are directed toward promoting the patient's self-esteem, his ability to care for himself and others, and his participation in the community as a contributing member. Classes may be offered in such personal subjects as hygiene, grooming, homemaking, and cooking. The classes may be directed toward preparing the patient for some occupation, like carpentry, small motors repair, nursing, typing, sewing; or the classes may be primarily for self-expression or pleasure, like art, music lessons, modern dance, and ceramics. An individual patient may be assigned a tutor to help him learn to read and write English, or to help him keep up with his class at school, or to help him prepare for entrance exams at college. Patients may attend special classes at schools in the community, or continue to go to school during the day and return to the hospital at night, or they may attend regular school classes at the hospital.

Any treatment program or individual patient care plan, to be effective, must be aimed at meeting the needs of the individuals for whom it is intended. Those needs include physical, emotional, and social needs, so the program must include physical, emotional, and social treatment. Treatment is aimed toward the whole person, not parts of him, and not him in isolation, but as a member of a group. Successful and comprehensive treatment has as its goal helping the patient maintain survival, attain security, and return to optimum functioning. It utilizes all of the people, physical facilities, activities, supplies and equipment that surround the patient and form his environment or world.

REFERENCES

Amdur, Mark, and Marcia Cohen: "Medication groups for psychiatric patients," *American Journal of Nursing, 81* (February, 1981) pp. 343–345.

Caplan, Gerald: *Principles of Preventive Psychiatry,* Basic Books, New York, 1964.

DeGennaro, Marion D., et al.: "Antidepressant drug therapy," *American Journal of Nursing, 81* (July, 1981) pp. 1304–1310.

Erikson, Erik: *Identity and the Life Cycle,* W. W. Norton & Co., New York, 1980.

Erikson, Erik: *Identity: Youth and Crisis,* W. W. Norton & Co., New York, 1968.

Fink, Max: *Convulsive Therapy,* Raven Press, New York, 1979.

Harris, Elizabeth: "Lithium," *American Journal of Nursing, 81* (July, 1981) pp. 1310–1315.

Harris, Elizabeth: "Anti-psychotic medications," *American Journal of Nursing, 81* (July, 1981) pp. 1316–1323.

Hollister, Leo: *Clinical Pharmacology of Psychotherapeutic Drugs,* Churchill Livingstone, New York, 1978.

Kazdin, Alan E.: *Behavior Modification in Applied Settings,* Dorsey Press, Homewood, Ill., 1975.
Klein, Donald F., et al.: *Diagnosis and Drug Therapy of Psychiatric Disorders,* 2nd Edition, Williams & Wilkins, Baltimore, 1980.
Krause, Marie, and L. Kathleen Mahan: *Food, Nutrition and Diet Therapy,* 6th Edition, W. B. Saunders, Philadelphia, 1979.
Linder, Robert: *The Fifty Minute Hour,* Bantam Books, New York, 1976.
McAfee, Heidi Ann: "Tardive dyskinesia," *American Journal of Nursing, 78* (March, 1978) pp. 395–397.
Misner, Susan J.: "Using art therapy techniques in staff and patient education," *Nursing Outlook, 79* (August, 1979) pp. 536–539.
Neuman, Frederic: *The Seclusion Room,* Viking Press, New York, 1978.
Perry, Samuel W., and George Heidrich: "Placebo response: myth and matter," *American Journal of Nursing, 81* (April, 1981) pp. 720–725.
Roberts, Mary Jo, and Marcia Canfield: "Behavior modification with a mentally retarded child," *American Journal of Nursing, 80* (April, 1980) p. 679.
Rogers, Carl: *Encounter Groups,* Harper & Row, New York, 1973.

Chapter 8

The Nurse-Patient Relationship

It is easy to see at this point that it is difficult to define exactly what the psychiatric nurse does that is different from any other kind of clinical treatment and nursing practice. Furthermore, because the nursing functions overlap and fuse with those of other members of the treatment team—psychiatrist, physician, psychologist, social worker, activity therapist—it is not always possible to separate and designate what is specifically nursing.

There is not only some confusion as to what constitutes psychiatric nursing, but there is some controversy as well. Some people identify psychiatric nursing according to where it is done. Thus, all nursing care given in a psychiatric unit or mental hospital would be called psychiatric nursing, while all nursing care given somewhere else would not. Still another way of identifying psychiatric nursing is on the basis of the kind of patients who receive the care. Thus, if patients for whom the nurse cares are designated as psychiatric patients or diagnosed as mentally ill, then what she does would be called psychiatric nursing; if the patients are not so designated, then what she does is something else. Still another way of identifying psychiatric nursing is on the basis of the kind of preparation, education, and experience the nurse has had. Thus, if she has had special classes or clinical experience in the care of psychiatric patients, she would be called a psychiatric nurse; if she has not had such special preparation, she would not be so called. Still another way to identify psychiatric nursing, or at least the psychiatric nurse, is on the basis of the kind of person giving the care. The personal qualities of the psychiatric nurse are listed as alert, mature, intelligent, neat, orderly, stable, flexible, cheerful, sympathetic, objective, patient, and so forth and so on. If she is none of these, then, apparently, she is not giving psychiatric nursing care no matter what she does, where she does it, or who the recipient is.

Obviously, all of these attempts to identify or describe psychiatric nursing leave something to be desired. They fail to identify and define what psychiatric nursing is on the basis of what the nurse does and how she does it in the course of giving comprehensive care to sick people.

Psychiatric nursing is not determined by the place where it is given—nursing care of psychiatric patients may take place in general hospitals, community centers, or private homes as well as specific hospitals designated as psychiatric. It is not determined by the diagnosis of the patient—psychiatric nursing is an important part of the care of physically ill as well as mentally ill patients. Many of the basic elements of effective psychiatric nursing apply, generally, to any person-to-person relationship, any field of nursing, or any kind of human endeavor.

The heart of nursing, indeed the very art of nursing itself, lies in the relationship between the nurse and the patient. The nurse has a primary role in the treatment of the patient, particularly the psychiatric patient. The nurse's therapy consists of ongoing, corrective feedback in the communication process which we discussed in Chapter 3. The purpose of the nurse-patient relationship is to help the patient satisfy his needs in more acceptable ways. This is accomplished by helping the patient learn new methods of functioning from his interactions with the nurse. The nurse either helps the patient through her relationship with him, which adds to his comfort and security, or she does not, which adds to his discomfort and anxiety. The effectiveness of the nurse's therapy depends upon her ability to correctly observe, evaluate, and respond to the patient's needs, and that ability is, in turn, directly dependent upon her knowledge, understanding, and skill in interpersonal relations.

All of these statements about psychiatric nursing imply the nurse's therapeutic use of herself in her relationship with the patient. The nurse uses her own healthy personality and the various methods of communication as treatment tools to help the patient make the necessary corrections in his own faulty communication process. She helps him learn not only from her relationship with him, but also from his experiences in everyday life.

Let us, therefore, draw the following conclusions: psychiatric nursing means that kind of nursing practice which provides the therapeutic relationships and environment necessary in order to help patients meet their needs, and at the same time, correct the unhealthy aspects of their behavior. The nurse carries out the traditional nursing functions—observation, communication, care—in the accomplishment of this therapeutic goal. The person who, through her nursing actions, provides the therapeutic relationship and environment, no matter where it takes place or who the patient is, is giving psychiatric nursing care. Any member of the nursing staff, regardless of education or experience, participates to some degree in giving such care.

BASIS FOR NURSING ACTION

The overall objective in nursing is to increase the patient's sense of well-being. This requires the accomplishment of the threefold goal of helping the patient (1) maintain survival by relieving his suffering; (2) attain security by meeting his needs; (3) restore health by combating his disease. Any one nursing action may accomplish all three aspects of the goal, or it may take more than one nursing action to meet each aspect of the goal. For example, the nursing action of giving the ulcer patient his between-meal snack may help to relieve the pain, satisfy his needs for food, love, and belonging, and reduce the irritation to the lining of his stomach. On the other hand, with a patient who is brought to the emergency room with a severe laceration, the nurse's first action may be to stop the bleeding. Her second action may be to meet his needs by comforting him. Her third action may be to put him to bed so as to help him recover from the trauma.

The nurse accomplishes this threefold goal through the traditional nursing functions of observation, communication, and comprehensive care. She sees what the situation is, discusses this with her co-workers and the patient, and does whatever is required and appropriate in order for the patient's needs to be met. What she observes and what she learns from others helps to determine what she does, so that observation and communication are crucial steps in effective nursing. If she relies only upon her own observations, the resulting action may be inappropriate, incomplete, or incorrect. If she relies only upon her own observations and those of her co-workers, the resulting action again may be inappropriate, incomplete, or incorrect. If she relies upon her observations, those of her co-workers, and those of her patient, the resulting action is more likely to effectively fulfill the threefold nursing goal.

For effective nursing, the nurse's actions must be based upon certain facts. First of all, patients are people in trouble, usually in serious trouble, when they come under the care of the nurse. Second, to effect a cure, the patient's treatment takes into consideration the particular sick person and his circumstances, not just his disease or his symptoms. Third, the nurse-patient relationship is a primary form of treatment which provides the patient with the opportunity to satisfy his needs.

For effective nursing, the fundamental attitude of brotherly love must underlie all nursing actions. Erich Fromm defines "brotherly love" as "that desire to further another human being's life," which has the characteristics of concern, respect, knowledge, and responsibility (see references in Chapter 2). The nurse must have care or concern for all people; in other words, she must care about the welfare of others. She must have respect for each individual, not just because he is a patient, but because he is a person worthy of her respect. In order to help him, she must learn all she can about him and his needs, about herself and her impact upon others, and about people in general and the reasons behind behavior. She must have that sense of responsibility which enables her to help others satisfy their needs, postponing her own satisfaction so that the patient's needs take precedence.

For effective nursing, the nurse's relationship with the patient must be a therapeutic or helpful one. Carl Rogers has expressed the philosophy of a helping relationship with great simplicity, "If I can provide a certain type of relationship, the other person will discover within himself the capacity to use that relationship for growth, and change and personal development will occur" (see references, Chapter 1). The characteristics of such a relationship are, as he says, acceptance, honesty, understanding, and faith. The nurse must believe that the patient has a right to be exactly as he is. She must be able to accept the patient as a person of essential worth and dignity, regardless of his appearance, behavior, or station in life. The second characteristic is a scrupulous, and often painful, kind of honesty. The nurse must be what she professes to be, mean what she says, and act in accord with her beliefs. (In communication terms, the content and intent of her message or response must be in harmony.) What she does must be in accord with what she thinks and feels; there is no room for phoniness if she is to be helpful to the patient. Third, the nurse must have the kind of understanding that enables her to see and accept the patient's private world through his eyes. She must have the empathy that helps her understand, not how *she* might feel in the situation, but how the *patient* feels in the situation. And last, she must have faith that she and the patient will discover within themselves the resources necessary to help him move toward health. Even though a person's capacity to learn or grow or change may be buried under layers of defenses or hidden behind elaborate facades, it awaits only the proper conditions to be released and expressed and fulfilled. The effectiveness of the nurse can be measured by how successful she is in providing those conditions. Each of us has within himself the seed, the soil, the climate for establishing many helping relationships. All that remains is the cultivation and that work is the essence of nursing.

Certain fundamental concepts form the guidelines for effective nursing: (1) to establish a working relationship, the nurse must accept the patient exactly as he is; (2) the only successful nursing care is based upon the whole person, not the symptom or the disease; (3) people tend to behave in accord with what is expected of them; (4) effective nursing action is related to correct identification of the problem; (5) any single nursing action either decreases or increases the patient's sense of well-being; (6) the effectiveness of the action is based upon the technical and interpersonal competence of the nurse.

COMMON NURSING PROBLEMS

In carrying out patient care, the nurse is faced with many problems which can seriously interfere with her effectiveness. These problems seem to group themselves into common areas with each nurse, each patient, and each circumstance varying to some degree. To be successful, the nurse must be able to effectively solve or handle problems as they arise in her care of patients. The common problem areas include the nurse herself, the patient's behavior, other staff, the patient's family, the physical difficulties, and the community where the care is given.

The Nurse Herself. It is always more comfortable to explore, and sometimes put the finger on, the other fellow's problems or sore spots rather than one's own. However, if the nurse is to be really competent in her relationships with others, she must be able to look at, accept, and assume responsibility for her own behavior. Her effectiveness as a nurse is directly dependent upon her attitudes toward herself and others. Our attitudes are a result of the knowledge we have acquired and the experiences we have had with people and life. Attitudes can only be changed by gathering further knowledge from new experiences. The more knowledgeable the nurse is about human behavior, including her own, the better her chances for success in helping others. The more positive and realistic her experiences in life, the more likely she is to be seen by others as helpful. The nurse's attitudes will color her perception, her judgment, her behavior, and thus, will influence her whole communication process.

I believe successful, effective nurses become so only after considerable personal effort and sometimes struggle. I don't believe "good" nurses are born or are made; I think they make themselves. Obviously, it helps if a nurse's life experiences have led her to two basic attitudes—acceptance of herself, and compassion toward others. I do not think there is any one kind of person who makes the "good" nurse, nor any one set of attributes or qualities that such a nurse should possess. In fact, I do not even believe that a nurse must necessarily be "good" or "kind" or "successful" in her own life in order to be effective in nursing. However, I do believe that there are certain characteristics that are fundamental to the achievement of the necessary interpersonal competence in nursing.

First, the nurse must be both physically and emotionally healthy. If she is to be the patient's sending and receiving set, her own communication or transmission must be in first-rate condition. The nurse is not only the eyes and ears of the physician and other members of the treatment team, but she is often the interpreter and spokesman for the patient, doctor, hospital, family, and sometimes community. How she interprets and responds to the patient's message will determine whether she increases or decreases his sense of well-being. How she interprets the patient to those around him will determine whether or not he is treated with acceptance, honesty, understanding, and faith by other important people in his environment, including his family, other patients, and other staff.

Second, the nurse must be secure enough within herself to be flexible. She must have the ability, willingness, and desire to change, to improve, to learn. As soon as she becomes satisfied with herself, her performance, her convictions, she is in danger of closing off her mind and herself to further learning. To be successful in human relations, one must always be receptive to new possibilities. That means that the nurse must always be in a position of being less than sure of herself and the correctness or rightness of her actions. She must always be in the position of questioning her actions, as well as the actions of others, in order for improvement to take place. She must be able to tolerate, accept, and redirect the anxiety that is associated with not knowing all of the answers, the fear that accompanies the recognition of possible failure, the tension that is required to produce action, and the hostility that results from frustation.

Third, the nurse must be emotionally mature enough to be able to postpone the satisfaction of her own needs. She must be able to allow the patient's needs to take precedence over her own. It takes great strength and self-control on the part of the nurse not to indulge her own needs, impulses, and feelings rather than those of the patient. A willingness to invest and give of one's self comes from an inner reservoir of strength and courage. It must be accompanied by the knowledge that giving is more rewarding than receiving, and that the act of giving replenishes, rather than depletes, one's supply. A willingness to give is preceded by the fact that a person must have received before he can give, he must have been cared for before he can care for others, and he must have been helped before he can be helpful. There are some people who simply cannot give or care for others or be helpful because they themselves have not received enough from others to have the necessary surplus. They are still striving to get, to be cared for, to be helped, so that their needs come first.

Fourth, the nurse must be able to accept, allow, and even foster the patient's independence. I think one of the most difficult things in any successful relationship is to recognize the other fellow's right to be himself instead of the person you want him to be. We all have the tendency to try to make the other fellow over into a reflection of ourselves, or our ideal, rather than to help him develop his individual potential. One of the hardest things for a teacher to accept is the time when the student is able to accomplish things for himself, even though that is the goal for which both teacher and student have been struggling. The student may no longer need the teacher, in fact, he may have surpassed her or grown beyond her. I am sure there is a similar problem for parents with their children—to let them grow up into their own selves must be very difficult. I know it is the same for nurses, particularly with psychiatric patients for whom the nurse has become a treatment model, and in whom she has invested a great deal of herself. The tendency is to hang on to the patient, to continue or even foster his dependence upon her, for the satisfaction of her own needs rather than his.

Fifth, the nurse must be able to accept, understand, and modify her impact upon others. She must be able to assume responsibility for her own behavior so that she does not need to be defensive about it. If she sees that the other person, particularly the patient, has taken offense at her action, then it is up to her to change her behavior accordingly. It is not up to the other person to accept her or change his behavior. If the nurse can be responsible for her own behavior, then she does not need to worry about the other fellow—he will respond to the best of his ability and competence. Because of the nature of her work, she often has knowledge of the most intimate aspects and inner faults of an individual's life and person, including patients, families, co-workers. She stands in a privileged position with personal information that does not belong to her. How she uses that position and that information measures her stature as a nurse—and a person.

The nurse is not expected to be either a saint or an expert in human relations, although it may sound like it; but she is expected to be an honest, responsible, competent human being if she is to be successful in helping others. She must be able to deal effectively with fear, failure, and frustration, her own as well as those of others. She must be able to figure out what is required in the way of help, and then provide that in her relationship with the patient. She must be genuine in her desire to help because she will not be successful without it. She is required to use both skill and intuition in identifying and providing what is needed. Her knowledge and experience are both important so long as they contribute to her ability to help the patient. She should not be expected to be on duty twenty-four hours a day, seven days a week. She needs time for herself when her needs and desire to be cared for take precedence over everything else. She also must be able to be cared for and get sufficient help in her personal life or off-duty time, that she is not tempted or driven to do so in her relationships with patients. Successful relationships with patients are an important part of the nurse's job, and as such, must be learned and worked at. Such an important part of her job cannot be ignored, left to chance, or left for someone else to perform.

The Patient's Behavior. Certain symptoms in the patient's illness may pose greater problems to the nursing staff than others. These include manipulative, combative, self-destructive, complaining, and regressed behavior, physical pain, suffering, and approaching death. Sometimes a patient displays more than one of these kinds of behavior problems, and such a patient is apt to be the center of controversy, the eye of the storm, in a psychiatric ward or hospital. He often brings out conflicts that exist within individual nurses, conflicts between members of the nursing staff, and conflicts between the nursing staff and other people.

Manipulative Behavior generally refers to a person's attempts to use others to his advantage, or change the environment to suit his purposes. We all use one another to satisfy our needs, and we attempt to change our environment and other people in it to more nearly suit our purposes. If the person is skillful in managing his environment to better satisfy his needs, he is often considered well-adjusted or successful by others. However, if he is not skillful, as is often the case with the patient, he is apt to evoke strong negative feelings in others, including the nurse. The nurse's reactions may be those of anger, dislike, rejection, retaliation, and punishment. Often such a patient is labelled a "manipulator," which is like waving a red flag in front of most members of the nursing staff. They tend to build up negative attitudes toward such a patient, sometimes without even seeing him or having any interaction with him. Such preset attitudes are apt to insure negative behavior on the part of the nurse and the patient simply because people tend to behave in accord with expectations.

It is important for the nurse to accept and understand that the behavior is a symptom of the patient's illness and must be dealt with as such if the patient is to be helped. The reason for such behavior is very often the patient's underlying feelings of inadequacy, inferiority, and unworthiness. He does not like himself, and therefore he finds it hard to believe that anyone else can like him. He behaves in such a way as to corroborate his belief that other people do not really like him, and this results in repeated testing to see if people really mean what they say. Indeed, the patient with this kind of behavior is difficult to like, and is sometimes heartily disliked by those who interact most often with him—the nursing staff. Thus, inadvertently, they participate in the symptoms of his illness.

To interact successfully with the manipulative patient, the nurse must be firm, matter-of-fact, and realistic in her approach to the patient. She must be able to set the limits that he cannot set for himself without rejecting or punishing him. She must be able to set realistic goals for him which he can reach, so as to overcome his pattern of failure and frustration. She must be able to anticipate and accept his need to repeatedly test her honesty. She must be able to recognize, control, and redirect her anger and disappointment when he fails, as everyone sometimes does, so as not to retaliate. Only through such positive interaction can she help him build a healthier concept of himself, and thus make a fundamental contribution toward changing his behavior. In addition, the entire nursing staff must work closely together so as to provide continuity and consistency in the care of the patient.

Self-destructive Behavior often accompanies manipulative behavior and further complicates the nursing problems. The reason for such behavior, again, is the patient's underlying feelings of inadequacy, inferiority and unworthiness. Because of these, his needs are frequently not met, and he turns his reaction to such frustration (anger) inward upon himself in a destructive way, hurting himself. By so doing he hurts all of those around him, particularly those who care about him. The ultimate in self-destructive behavior is the act of suicide which punishes not only the victim but society as a whole and his friends and family in particular.

The nurse's response to a patient's threatened suicide, suicidal attempt, or successful suicidal act is often one of mixed feelings of responsibility, guilt, and anger. When a patient inflicts wounds upon himself, even minor ones, the nurse's reaction is often one of anger. Sometimes the nursing interaction with the patient becomes so focused upon the symptom of self-destruction that the patient as a person is neglected. Nurses have said to the oncoming shift, "Well, we got him through our shift, now it's up to you."

Self-destructive behavior is threatening to the nurse because it interferes with the satisfaction of her needs. Her frustration may lead to feelings of helplessness and hopelessness. If a patient is bent on self-destruction, it seems almost impossible to deter him—he seems to manage to hurt himself somehow. When he succeeds in hurting himself, he insures the nurse's sense of failure because she feels responsible for maintaining his survival, helping him attain security and relieving his suffering, not the opposite.

Sometimes the nurse attempts to defend herself by reducing the seriousness of the situation, particularly if the self-destructive behavior is accompanied by manipulative behavior, as it often is. The nurse may say, "He's just trying to get attention," or "You have to ignore him when he acts like that." As a result, the patient may be driven in his frustration and sick behavior to more serious and more inappropriate acts of self-destruction, and sometimes even to death.

To interact successfully with the self-destructive patient, the nurse must help to turn his reaction to failure and frustration outward. In so doing, she must be prepared to accept his hostile outbursts, and channel them into acceptable or constructive outlets. The best deterrent to self-destructive behavior is the nurse's presence, so she needs to spend as much time as possible with the patient. This closeness can also be used to convey to the patient that he is an important person to the nurse, and thus help to correct some of his feelings about himself. It is very important for the nurse to help the patient control his impulses, and this may be done by establishing definite limits or restrictions for him. Whatever is done should make clear to him that every effort will be made to prevent him from hurting himself.

Combative Behavior includes threatening, assaultive, destructive, impulsive acts which the patient directs toward the environment or the people in it. Such behavior often strikes fear in the hearts of the nursing staff and seriously interferes with their effectiveness. Fear has a certain contagious quality about it, and if one nurse is afraid of the patient, other nurses frequently get caught up in the feeling. As President Roosevelt reminded the American people in time of great threat to the national security, "The only thing we have to fear is fear itself." If the patient senses that the staff are afraid of him, it makes him all the more insecure and promotes his aggressive behavior.

Often the nurse feels that the behavior is personally directed. For some reason the patient doesn't like her—when she is trying to do everything she can for him. Her tendency is to counterattack or defend herself by attacking the patient first. For example, if the patient gets the least bit upset or irritable or agitated, the nursing staff may descend upon him to sedate him or seclude him or give him treatment. The patient, already apprehensive and angry, may fight for his very life until he is finally subdued.

To interact successfully with the combative patient, the nurse must first of all possess sufficient physical courage to be able to withstand the threat of assault. Secondly, as with self-destructive behavior, the patient should be controlled in such a way as to prevent him harming others. It is never helpful for the patient to express his feelings in harmful ways. Such behavior only increases his apprehension, anger, and destructive behavior because it means he is out of control. Third, the nursing action taken to control the behavior should be instituted calmly, swiftly, and decisively. Fourth, as soon as the patient is able to control his behavior himself, the restrictions should be lifted so that he is not punished for doing something which he cannot help.

Complaining Behavior includes critical, sarcastic, demanding behavior. Often the basis of the behavior is the patient's underlying sense of fear, failure, and frustration. The nurse may defend herself with rejection of the patient. When the patient is met with a negative reaction from the nurse, instead of helping him correct his behavior, the interaction serves to increase or enhance it because he suffers even more from the sense of failure.

For some patients the behavior is a way of getting rid of pent-up feelings, or letting off steam, and should simply be acknowledged as such. For other patients, it is behaving as a patient is expected to behave—he isn't supposed to be happy in the hospital. For other patients it is a way of displacing the anxiety they feel about their illness, separation from their families, or general dissatisfaction with their lives. For still other patients it is a legitimate criticism of their treatment programs and the people serving them.

To interact successfully with the complaining patient, the nurse must be able to listen to what the patient is saying. She must try to determine what lies behind his behavior and interact with him accordingly. She must be able to accept the behavior as a symptom of his illness from which he will recover with her help. She may need only to listen and acknowledge what he is saying. She may need to agree with him that he has a right to complain because he feels bad. She may need to make necessary corrections in his care so as to relieve his anxiety or discontent. She may need to stay with him for longer periods in order to lessen his feelings of apprehension, loneliness, and isolation. She may need to anticipate his requests and supply them before he becomes demanding, sarcastic, critical or complaining.

Regressed Behavior includes incontinence, poor personal hygiene, poor eating and toilet habits, and excessive dependence upon the nursing staff. The nurse sometimes reacts to the patient's regressed behavior with ridicule or rejection. Such a negative reaction from the nurse may re-enforce, prolong, or exacerbate the behavior because the more anxious and insecure the patient feels, the more regressed and infantile he becomes.

Sometimes the regression is a result of profound stress in the adult patient's life which he tries to handle by returning to earlier forms of behavior that once brought him safety and comfort. This kind of regressed behavior usually accompanies severe mental or physical illness which disrupts the patient's life and seriously interferes with his functioning. Sometimes the regression is a result of severe deprivation in the adult patient's early life from which he never recovers and beyond which he does not advance. This kind of regressed behavior usually accompanies severe mental retardation or physical handicaps. In either case, the adult patient displays various behaviors that are characteristic of infancy or early childhood, and are inappropriate and unacceptable in the adult.

While some dependency on the nurse may be necessary and even rewarding for the nurse, she may become fatigued and irritable if the patient relies too heavily upon her. If she finds the patient always underfoot, demanding her attention and services, she may not be able to tolerate this drain upon her resources, and she may react by forcibly pushing the patient away from her. Continued excessive dependency on the part of the patient often represents a failure to the nurse in her efforts to help him move in the direction of healthier methods of adjustment.

There is a difference between dependency and the need for support. All of us need to feel the support of those people in our lives who are important to us. In stress situations that confront the patient, he particularly needs to feel the support of the nursing staff. In such situations, the nurse may do for him what he is capable of doing for himself in order to demonstrate that she really cares for him and understands how he feels. However, for the nurse to promote a patient's dependency upon her by not allowing or not encouraging or not teaching him how to do for himself is to deny him self-esteem, self-worth, and self-identity. It is sometimes easier for the nurse to go ahead and take care of the patient rather than encouraging him to take care of himself, but in the long run, it always interferes with his recovery, optimum functioning, and sense of well-being.

To interact successfully with the regressed patient, the nurse must be able to accept infantile behavior in the adult. She must be able to help the patient learn more appropriate behavior, step by step, in much the same fashion as the child does. She must be satisfied with small gains and able to lead the patient out of his regression one step at a time. She must be prepared for the patient's temporary lapses and occasional hangups in the slow process of training or retraining for social effectiveness. She must be able to give generously of herself, especially in terms of time, interest, patience, and praise.

Physical Pain, Suffering, and Approaching Death (see Kubler-Ross, 1974) of the patient often pose special problems for the nursing staff. A great deal of the nurse's effectiveness depends upon her own attitude toward life and death. If she is generally apprehensive, fearful of being hurt, or afraid of dying, she is likely to have greater difficulty dealing therapeutically with the patient who has a serious, life-threatening, or terminal illness.

In an attempt to make the suffering patient and herself feel better, she may assume an attitude of false optimism and utter empty reassurances such as "You're going to be all right" or "Don't you worry about a thing." Such nursing action is an affront to the comprehending patient because it denies the reality of his situation and symptoms as if they did not exist. Further, such action does not allow him to talk about whatever is bothering him, including his suffering, and it only increases his feelings of isolation, apprehension, and loneliness. The nurse may try to get the patient to "buck up" and "face it like a man." This may be more than he can manage which will add to his feelings of discomfort and misery.

Pain and suffering, death and dying are facts of life that must be dealt with realistically and compassionately. The nurse needs to spend enough time with the patient so that he may talk if he wishes. If she is always in a hurry, or is abrupt and disinterested in her manner, or brushes him off, he may not take a chance on being rejected. However, if the nurse stays with him and devotes her full attention to him and his concerns, he may feel free enough to talk to her. He may need an opportunity to express his feelings and sort out his thoughts so that he can accept what must be with as much integrity, dignity, and courage as he can muster. The nurse needs to listen to what he has to say. It may not require any comment from her at all, or only sufficient prompting for him to get it out of his system. He may not want to talk, or be able to talk, in which case the nurse may care for him in silence, but that silence can convey her concern for him and her interest in him. Her presence alone may be of comfort to the patient, and give him the courage and strength he needs to meet the situation. It will be a help if he knows he is not alone or abandoned, and that someone really does care about him. Pain, suffering, and even death can be tolerated better if the patient knows somebody cares about him. He may need to cry, and this is sometimes a good way for him to relieve tension. The nurse should accept and comfort him, not try to make him stop by cutting him off with such admonitions as "You shouldn't be crying; it isn't good for you," or "There's nothing to cry about." He needs as much comforting as the hurt child. However, it is important that the nurse not move to the opposite extreme and overdo it. She can make him feel worse by causing him to feel sorry for himself, more apprehensive about his chances of recovery, or smothered or overwhelmed by her over-concern.

Other Staff. The nurse's problems with her co-workers often revolve around her feelings of loyalty, respect, trust, and responsibility toward other people and her job. Honest disagreement and criticism of one another can be a necessary and helpful exchange among the nursing staff. However, gossiping about another worker, undercutting what he is trying to accomplish, or saying "yes" when she means "no" can seriously interfere with the nurse's effectiveness. You may have heard the comment, "She's a good nurse, but she can't get along with people." Well, that's a contradictory statement and an impossibility to achieve. The relationships between staff directly affect patient care because they either promote or interfere with the nursing staff's relationships with patients and the provision of a therapeutic environment.

Sometimes the nurse is misguided by her loyalty toward fellow workers and deliberately overlooks or does not report mistakes that they make. In so doing, she not only does the patient—to whom she has a primary responsibility—a disservice, but she also does the individual for whom she covers up and her other fellow workers a disservice. If a mistake is called to the individual's attention, or is reported to someone else, it can be corrected. Otherwise, it cannot. The nurse also has a legal and ethical, as well as moral, obligation to see that patients get the best care possible, which means that errors should be eliminated as far as possible, and certainly, corrected when they are made.

The nursing staff share a common goal—the patient's well-being—and their effectiveness in achieving that goal is determined in part by how well they work as a team or unit. All of their actions should be directed toward that common goal; anything that they do which interferes with the accomplishment of that goal interferes with their effectiveness. Social or personal relationships or exchanges between staff members can seriously interfere with the care of the patients if they take priority or are carried on to the exclusion of the patient's needs.

A common problem, particularly in a hospital where there are students, is the orientation, education, supervision, and evaluation of new staff members. Older, senior, or permanent nursing staff are usually the real instructors and supervisors for students of all kinds. New staff members generally do what they see others doing, not what they are told to do in class or conference or somewhere else. A new person tends to fit himself into the ongoing pattern of activity if he wishes to become a member of the group. Only if he does not care what others think of him, or if he is particularly brave, foolhardy, or aggressive, will he face off in disagreement with older, more secure, wiser people than he. What the new staff member learns, how he feels about his job, what things he sees as significant and important, what attitudes he holds toward patients, are all directly dependent upon how he is treated and what he is taught by members of the nursing staff.

Nurses often object to the role of instructor or supervisor, and sometimes voice their objection with such comments as, "I came here to work with patients, not nursing staff." Certainly patient care, present and future, depends directly upon what students learn from members of the nursing staff, particularly those who set attitudes on the ward. If a nurse is really interested in caring for patients, she cannot ignore her responsibility of teaching others what she herself is fortunate enough to know already. That includes accurate and helpful performance evaluations of nursing students or new staff or staff members in junior positions.

Another common problem among nursing staff is the lack of continuity of care from one shift to another. Most nurses describe this problem as "poor communication," but it is usually more than just a lack of passing information back and forth between shifts. It usually involves a serious difference of opinion as to how patients should be cared for, and what actions the nurse should take in carrying out that care. If one shift feels that patients should have a voice in their own treatment by making decisions which concern them, and another shift feels that patients should be told what to do, there is not likely to be much continuity of care no matter how much information is passed back and forth. Such discrepancies in care serve to confuse the patients, and often make them more anxious and unsure of themselves. If a particular plan of care or approach has been decided upon for a particular patient, or group of patients, then it should be carried out by all personnel who deal with that patient or group of patients. Whether a member of the nursing staff disagrees with the plan or not is not the issue. Any plan that provides for consistency in the patient's care is apt to be better than none, or better than two or three different plans put into effect by different shifts or individual nurses. That is not to say that differences of opinion or disagreements as to approach are not healthy or legitimate, but they should be expressed and explored before decisions are made, not afterward. Changes may be instituted, but they should be discussed and incorporated as modifications of the plan so that everyone may follow them. It is like the family situation—if mother and father approach problems in life from entirely different or opposite points of view, the children under their care are apt to grow up with a great deal of ambivalence and confusion about themselves and life. There must be some compromises in treatment programs and individual care plans for patients, and all staff members should care for the patients within that framework. Otherwise, each one is pulling the patient in a different direction, and he cannot help but suffer further damage.

Sometimes rivalry or jealousy develops between members of the nursing staff or between shifts, interfering with communication and comprehensive patient care. Often the day shift is involved in the direct planning for patients, and the other shifts, particularly the night shift, may not have a chance to participate in important decisions about patient care and ward policy. To avoid negative reactions which may actually prevent continuity of care, all staff members should be encouraged to participate as fully as possible in making decisions which they are expected to carry out. If individual staff members have difficulty carrying out certain approaches, they should be helped to see how important it is to the patient that he know what to expect, and thus predict, in relationship to his environment and the people in it. There are usually many different and equally legitimate forms of treatment for any individual patient, but it is essential to the patient's sense of well-being that efforts be made by the whole staff to carry out whatever form of treatment has been decided upon.

Nursing staff on the various shifts sometimes experience feelings of divided loyalty and responsibility. They may have to make a choice between carrying out what is expected of them by their shift charge or supervisor, or carrying out what is expected of them according to the selected treatment program for the patients. Again, to avoid such conflict, it is wise to include key nursing personnel in the overall planning conferences whenever possible, and when not possible, to consult with them individually. Most nursing staff understand and accept problems and decisions that are presented from the point of view of the patient's welfare rather than the wisdom of the plan or those who designed it.

Authority Figures. Authority figures include medical and nursing supervisors, instructors, chiefs of service, and administrators. A major problem for nursing staff occurs when there is a conflict of interests, expectations, status, orders, therapeutic approach, or authority among these people. Probably one of the most common problems occurs when the physician and nursing supervisor are not in accord, and the nursing staff get conflicting orders. In such cases, if the nursing staff are not sure which way to act, they may split into two groups, one going one way and one another, with the patient left somewhere in the middle.

The traditional relationship between nurse and doctor is a very complex and contradictory one, but the success of it seems to depend upon each of the participants playing his role correctly, or according to the game rules. The nurse often knows the individual patient, the overall treatment program, the hospital rules and regulations, and what course of action is most likely to succeed much better than the doctor, particularly if he is new on the scene or relieving somebody else. It is important that she suggest a course of action that is in the best interests of the patient. It is up to her to do this in such a way that it is accepted by the doctor. The doctor on his part must solicit the advice of the nurse in such a way as to make the interests of the patient the priority.

A problem which sometimes occurs is related to the focus of nursing service and the assignment of priorities. If the authority figure takes precedence over patients' needs, then the nursing staff are likely to drop whatever they are doing to serve the supervisor. It used to be common practice in large mental hospitals and in general hospitals as well, that when the supervisor came on the ward everyone stood at attention much as in the military service, and the visiting dignitary was escorted around the facility, doors being opened for him as the procession advanced. These days it is more usual for the supervisor to be treated like the human being he is, worthy of respect but not the entire attention and service of the nursing staff. It may be, however, that some supervisors or some nursing staff are unable to give up the old "spit and polish" way of doing things, and the relationship between supervisor and staff takes precedence over the relationship between patient and staff.

In many hospitals, the nursing staff functions as an extension of the administrative staff, particularly on the afternoon and night shifts, when the regular administrators are not on duty. In such a situation, it is not uncommon for the nurse on duty to be in a position of objecting to a doctor's order which runs counter to hospital policy. This may cause some conflict, particularly when the relationship or communication between nurse and doctor is not very good to start with, or when it involves the question of therapy.

Another problem, which seems to be a product of modern times, is that the decisions, plans, and programs made at the administrative level are not always the same as those actually carried out in practice at the ward level. Treatment programs described by administrative and professional staff in various scientific journals may be completely foreign to the nursing staff supposedly carrying them out. Sometimes the nursing staff who have not been included in the planning do not realize that what they are doing even fits into an overall treatment program. Sometimes they do not understand the treatment program so they are hardly in a position to carry it out. Sometimes the treatment program described exists only in the minds of the planners, or in the words they use to describe it. John Kenneth Galbraith, Harvard economist, called this practice the "wordfact," and he goes on to say, "The wordfact makes words a precise substitute for reality. This is an enormous convenience. It means that to say that something exists is a substitute for its existence. And to say that something will happen is as good as having it happen. The saving in energy is nearly total."

Sometimes, in large hospitals in particular, there are problems in the relationships between the various departments which serve the patients. If there are not clear lines of authority and responsibility and communication, there may even be a vying among departments for their fair share of the money, staff, patient's time, and recognition available in the institution, which they believe they deserve.

The Family. The nursing staff often have serious problems relating successfully with the patient's family. In the past (and perhaps it still exists to some extent) it has been traditional for the nursing staff not to give any information about the patient to his family, relatives, visitors, and callers. When someone asks how a patient is getting along, the nurse's standard answer is "as well as can be expected," which contains no information at all. Sometimes when the family is persistent in trying to find out how the patient is, the nurse will advise them to talk to the doctor or social worker. Actually, there are situations which may demand more knowledge and skill than the nurse possesses, or situations which might better be handled by the physician or social worker or someone else who is slightly removed from the direct care of the patient. However, very often the family is asking for some word of comfort from the nurse, in order to relieve their own tremendous anxiety, guilt, or concern regarding the patient. The nurse, in order to relate successfully with the family, should give an answer to the question, not refer them to someone else or give no answer at all, both of which only serve to increase their feeling of frustration. Sometimes all it takes from the nurse is a simple statement of fact regarding the patient's condition, such as, "He slept better last night," or "He seems kind of restless today," or "His appetite has improved." The answer does not usually require a detailed description of his medical condition, which the nurse is not in a position to give and which the family does not expect anyway.

Another problem with families centers around ways in which they express their anxiety, guilt, or concern for the patient, ways which may be difficult for the nursing staff to handle. Some families are demanding and critical of the service or care the patient is receiving. Some are suspicious and distrustful of the staff who are caring for the patient. Others are rejecting, neglectful, or even abusive toward the patient.

If the nurse takes the family's behavior personally, she will be hurt and angry, and this will interfere with her relationship with them. If she tries to change their behavior by argument or criticism, she will probably make things worse instead of better. If she cuts them off, ignores them, orders them about, or tries to keep them from seeing the patient, their anxiety is likely to increase, and their behavior will follow suit.

To be successful, the nurse must try to allay the family's anxiety, and thus help them understand the situation the patient is in. It may be helpful to explain what is being done for the patient and elicit their cooperation. It may be helpful to acknowledge the fact that they must be worried or alarmed about the patient. It may help to allow them to participate in the patient's care by showing them how to do things for the patient or how to help the patient do things for himself. It may help to include them in the admission, treatment, and rehabilitation plans and procedures involving the patient and his care.

The Physical Facilities. The physical facilities themselves may lack the proper therapeutic atmosphere. Some hospital buildings presently in use were built in another era when the treatment philosophy was focused upon incarceration, isolation, and custodial care of the mentally ill. It is difficult to make such forbidding, barren housing into therapeutic surroundings for patients. Bathing, toilet, and sleeping facilities are often insufficient and arranged for maximum observation and safety precautions, and for minimum privacy and comfort. Remodelling may be done in order to create individual cubicles to protect the patient's sense of modesty and decency. Nothing is more degrading or injurious to self-esteem than to have to expose one's self and one's most intimate functioning to strangers. The patient, already low in self-esteem and high in sensitivity, needs all of the privacy that can be managed.

The furnishings need not be elaborate but should be as homelike as possible. State mental hospital furniture is noted for its prison-like appearance—heavy, dark, and usually in poor repair. Paint, bright cushions, drapes, curtains, and plants or flowers do a lot to change a drab and depressing atmosphere to a cheerful and liveable one. The arrangement of furniture should encourage one-to-one and small-group interaction. A huge day room with the chairs lined up all around the wall can be one of the most desolate, uninviting sights in a psychiatric hospital. Bedside stands for cosmetics and other personal belongings and individual closets or lockers for clothing add to the personal touch as well as promote the independent functioning of the patient. It is important to the patient's sense of well-being that he have as many of his personal belongings as possible. Personal belongings are an extension of the person, and as such, have great significance to the individual. His own clothing is of particular significance. If it is necessary to provide clothing for him it should be tailored to his needs and marked for him.

It is important that the patient be involved in maintaining his own and the group's living area as well as his personal belongings. He should be included in making decisions about what should be done when and how and by whom, much as he would at home. The arranging, cleaning, and decorating of a ward, which used to be done by the nursing staff, particularly in large mental hospitals, now may be done by patients using their patient-staff or ward government meetings to make the necessary plans. This is an important way of helping the patient learn how to assume responsibility for himself and others, establish his independence, interact in a socially acceptable way, become involved with reality, and build his sense of personal worth and ability so that he can cope adequately with his environment. If the nurse denies him the opportunity to participate in this way, she overlooks an excellent way of helping him reach optimum functioning.

Supplies and equipment can be as outmoded, and as obsolete as the physical facilities, particularly if no effort has been made to keep them up to date. The patients' survival and security may be directly related to the kinds of provisions that are made in this area. Outdated supplies and equipment can endanger the patient's safety, health, and sense of well-being. For example, it may be safer (and incidentally cheaper in the long run) to provide disposable equipment for the giving of medications, syringes and cups, than to risk possible transmission of infection and misuse of equipment, or expend the amount of nursing time necessary to wash and sterilize such equipment. Because of their experience of shortages in the past, nursing staff often have a tendency to hoard supplies such as linen, cleaning solutions, and disinfectants. Such practices may be changed if the nurses are provided with supplies in sufficient amounts to give adequate care to patients over a prolonged period of time, or by asking nursing staff to assist with the planning and provision of supplies on a hospital-wide basis.

The Community. The establishment of effective psychiatric treatment programs depends directly upon attitudes of the people in the surrounding community. In the first place, the nursing staff caring for patients are products and residents of the community. If they are rejected, looked down upon, or criticized for their work with mentally ill patients, they may react with bitterness, resentment, or embarrassment which will, undoubtedly, interfere with their effectiveness in relating to patients. If they are accepted, respected, and supported for their work, their ability to relate more therapeutically with patients is apt to be increased.

Comprehensive mental health programs, including the aspects of prevention, treatment, and rehabilitation, cannot be accomplished without the acceptance, support, and participation of the community as a whole. Mental illness may be reduced if the person in trouble is helped sooner by community resources—school, church, employment, public and private agency counselors. Psychiatric hospitalization and prolonged illness may not be necessary if the patient is treated early in his illness in available community facilities—general hospital, nursing home, outpatient clinic, doctor's office. Prolonged psychiatric hospitalization and illness can both be avoided if the patient can be returned to the community sooner for followup care.

An active program where community members come to the hospital and patients and staff go out into the community offers the best opportunity to break down old barriers and correct misunderstandings. Such programs may include educational, recreational, industrial, and social activities in which people from the hospital and the total community participate together. These programs offer a greater variety and depth to treatment approaches in psychiatric care than programs limited to the hospital itself. In such programs, there are closer personal ties, greater understanding, more mutual trust and support, and deeper involvement in community and hospital affairs alike. The psychiatric hospital in such a community is truly a part of it, and as such, is of greater service to it.

THE NURSING PROCESS: USE OF THE PROBLEM-SOLVING TECHNIQUE IN PLANNING NURSING ACTION

Some problems which nurses encounter in their work are never really resolved. As a result, they recur, perhaps in a slightly different form, and often become sources of discontent and low morale. To be successful in nursing, we must be able to identify problems, gather the pertinent facts concerning them, and work out constructive solutions to them. One way to do this is to apply the problem-solving steps in planning nursing action, instead of using the trial-and-error method over and over again. This is called the nursing process.

1. Assessment—Identification of the Problem. This first step consists of the collection of data and the nursing diagnosis. Nursing is faced with supplying the help that is required in order for the patient's needs to be met. That means that the nurses must

determine what the patient's needs are, what the patient can do for himself, and what the nurse must do in order to insure that his needs are met. This assessment requires alert and scientific observation on her part because his needs, as well as his abilities to meet them, fluctuate during the day and according to the circumstances. It requires, as well, healthy communication among the staff in which observations may be shared in order to get the whole picture, not just a piece of it. The nursing problem can be stated in terms of symptoms, syndrome, or diagnosis. For example, the problem may be described as "the patient cannot dress himself in the morning," or "the patient is confused and disoriented until he has been up and about for a couple of hours," or "the patient is suffering from acute brain syndrome and his sensorium is clouded until he re-establishes his contact with the environment." However it is stated, it should be in terms that are clear to all of the nursing staff involved so that they will know what is required of them.

2. NURSING CARE PLAN—DECISION AS TO THE COURSE OF ACTION. After all of the facts are gathered, the various circumstances which alter behavior investigated, all the observations, thoughts, and feelings of the staff discussed, then it is time to consider possible solutions to the nursing problem. From these discussions should come the decision as to the course of action so that all staff members can follow the same general plan. Only then does the patient's care become consistent, comprehensive, and complete.

3. INTERVENTION—IMPLEMENTATION OF THE SELECTED PLAN. The effectiveness of the implementation depends largely upon the understanding, involvement, and commitment of the nursing staff to the selected plan. If they do not understand what is to be done, obviously they will not be able to carry it out. If they have not participated in the planning and decision-making process, they are less likely to be concerned about the success of the implementation. If they do not agree with the course of action to be taken, they may consciously or unconsciously undermine the effectiveness of the selected plan, or even insure its failure with the attitude, "I told you so" or "I knew it wouldn't work."

4. EVALUATION OF THE EFFECTIVENESS OF THE SELECTED PLAN. This fourth step might be called the nursing audit or reassessment. Again, the nurse's purpose must be to supply the help that is required in order for the patient's needs to be met. As the patient's needs and abilities change, the nursing care plan must be altered accordingly. The nurse, through communication with the patient, other nursing staff, and other team members, must determine how well the nursing intervention helps the patient, where it fails, and what must be done to close the gap. Thus, the nursing process or problem-solving steps begin again: An assessment is

made, the nursing problems are identified, and the nursing care plan is outlined so that a course of action can be taken. Only if a nursing care plan is modified does it remain viable, useful, realistic, and effective.

QUESTIONS FOR DISCUSSION

Following are a number of actual situations which include nursing problems that are commonly encountered. See if you can identify the problem areas in each case and suggest possible courses of action to resolve the problems. There are no "right" answers, but there are a number of alternatives which might resolve each problem.

Situation 1. The evening nurse in charge of a readjustment ward fails to report or deal directly with any negative behavior on the part of patients; instead, she tries to ignore it. As a result, patients are not being dealt with therapeutically, there is a lack of consistency in carrying out the prescribed treatment program, and there is increasing conflict among the nursing staff.

Can you identify the problems involved and suggest ways in which they might be resolved? What do you think is behind the evening nurse's lack of effectiveness? How would you go about helping her?

Situation 2. The patient is a 24-year-old girl who has had severe emotional problems all of her life and has been hospitalized for 12 years. As a small child she would bang her head against anything solid. She started having serious problems in school in the fourth grade and became such a severe behavior problem that she was taken out of school the next year. Her mother could not handle her at home. She refused to obey, attacked her mother, and became sexually promiscuous. She was sent to a correctional school for girls and from there was referred to the psychiatric hospital for treatment.

In the hospital, she continued to have problems. She made several serious suicidal attempts resulting in self-mutilation, was extremely destructive, and was physically threatening to others. At one time, for example, she broke 22 windows on the ward, resulting in severe lacerations on her hands and wrists with subsequent scarring.

At first the nursing staff were very permissive in their approach to her and she did almost as she pleased. As a result, she became increasingly threatening and aggressive until this behavior culminated in her throwing a mop bucket through the nursing station window.

She was placed in seclusion and her activities were severely limited. A very restrictive treatment regime was planned by the day shift and the doctor, in which each step was carefully spelled out. Gradually, as her behavior became more appropriate, she was given increasing freedom of movement. However, it was agreed upon (and explained to her) that whenever she harmed herself or others, she would return to the first step which entailed her remaining by herself until her behavior warranted her moving on to the second step.

There was an increasing feeling on the part of the evening shift that the patient's regime was unnecessarily restrictive. At first, their dissatisfaction was not directly expressed but appeared in the form of sarcastic, critical remarks about members of the day staff. Over a period of a month, the feelings of friction among the nurses were heightened to the point where the evening shift accused the day shift of "punishing" the patient. The day shift retaliated by saying the evening shift was "spoiling" the patient. In the meantime, the patient had injured herself seriously enough on at least two occasions to require surgical treatment.

Can you identify the problems involved and suggest ways in which they might be resolved? Why might the evening shift have felt as they did? How does the conflict between shifts affect the patient and her behavior? What part does the patient's behavior play in promoting the disagreement between nursing staff?

Situation 3. The nursing supervisor brought a newly-employed nurse to a busy ward and asked the charge nurse to orient her. It was time for the nursing report customarily given between shifts and the charge nurse was upset at the interruption in her demanding schedule. She felt that she should carry out the supervisor's request to orient the new nurse, but she also felt that she should attend the report.

What would you do in such a situation if you were the charge nurse? How do you suppose the charge nurse really felt? What could the supervisor have done to alter the situation? How might the new employee feel?

Situation 4. On a particular hospital ward where patients were in bed most of the time and required full nursing care, linen was ordered once a day and the amount based on average daily needs. Since the need fluctuated from day to day, it was often necessary to borrow linen from other wards. Some days, as a result, there was an excess amount of certain items on hand. A routine check was made weekly by the supervisor to determine if the nursing staff were ordering properly or were overstocking the ward. On one particular day, there was an excess linen supply, and the supervisor took the charge nurse to task in front of her entire staff for not ordering properly.

If you were the charge nurse, how would you feel? What do you see as the real problems involved? What are some alternate ways of resolving these problems?

Situation 5. A young female patient was badly in need of clothing, and the family had been contacted many times by the social service department to send her either the needed clothes or the money necessary to purchase them herself. Finally, one afternoon the family arrived on the ward with two large boxes filled with clothes. One of the nurses took the boxes back to the patient's room and helped her open them while the family waited in the visiting room. The boxes were filled with soiled, old-fashioned, completely inappropriate clothing for the young girl, and she burst into tears.

How would you handle the situation with the patient? What would you do about the family? What prompted such behavior on the part of the family? How do you suppose the patient felt, and how might it affect her?

Situation 6. On a hospital ward where 60 elderly patients are housed, there is a total of 28 wheelchairs. Five of the 28 are privately owned by patients, and half of the remaining ones are in poor repair and unsafe for use. That leaves 12 wheelchairs that can be used by 55 patients. Most of the patients need some assistance in ambulation, and the nursing staff are encouraged to get them up and around the ward. Despite repeated requests, the wheelchairs go unrepaired, and there is not enough money in the budget to buy replacements. As a result, the nursing staff feel resentful and discouraged because they cannot fulfill one of the basic requirements in the care of the elderly—sustained ambulation.

What do you see as the problems involved? What alternative ways might the nursing staff ambulate patients? How would you react to the situation?

Situation 7. A college psychology class made a field trip to the psychiatric hospital in the community. A panel of staff members from different departments met with them to discuss the modern approach to mental illness and psychiatric treatment used at the hospital. The group was then taken to various wards where the patients had extended them an invitation to visit. Upon completion of the visits, the instructor of the class asked the escorting nurse, "Don't we get to see any of your violent wards?"

How would you react if you were the nurse? What prompts such a question? What might be done to avoid such a problem? How can the problem best be resolved?

REFERENCES

Atwood, Aileen H.: "The mentor in clinical practice," *Nursing Outlook, 79* (November, 1979) pp. 714–717.

Davis, Ellen Donnelly, and E. Mansell Pattison: "The psychiatric nurse's role identity," *American Journal of Nursing, 79* (February, 1979) pp. 298–299.

Diers, Donna: "A different kind of energy: nurse-power," *Nursing Outlook, 78* (January, 1978) pp. 51–55.

Gordy, Helen E.: "Gift giving: its effect on the nurse-patient relationship," *American Journal of Nursing, 78* (June, 1978) pp. 1026–1028.

Kalkman, Marion, and Anne Davis: *New Dimensions in Mental Health—Psychiatric Nursing,* McGraw-Hill, New York, 1974.

Kubler-Ross, Elizabeth: *Questions and Answers on Death and Dying,* Macmillan, New York, 1974.

McDonagh, Mary Jo, et al.: "Nurse-therapists in a state psychiatric hospital," *American Journal of Nursing, 80* (January, 1980) pp. 102–104.

McMorrow, Mary Ellen: "The manipulative patient," *American Journal of Nursing, 81* (June, 1981) pp. 1188–1190.

McShane, Nancy Gerberding, and Elizabeth McDowell Smith: "Starting a private practice in mental health nursing," *American Journal of Nursing, 78* (December, 1978) pp. 2068–2070.

Pisarcik, Gail, et al.: "Psychiatric nurses in the emergency room," *American Journal of Nursing, 79* (July, 1979) pp. 1264–1266.

Rawnsley, Marilyn M.: "Toward a conceptual base for affective nursing," *Nursing Outlook, 80* (April, 1980) pp. 244–247.

Smith, Christine Spahn: "Outrageous or outraged: a nurse advocate story," *Nursing Outlook, 80* (October, 1980) pp. 624–625.

Steel, Jean E.: "Precepts for practitioners," *Nursing Outlook, 78* (August, 1978) pp. 498–499.

Williamson, Janet A.: "Mutual interaction: a model of nursing practice," *Nursing Outlook, 81* (February, 1981) pp. 104–107.

Zangari, Mary Eve, and Patricia Duffy: "Contracting with patients in day-to-day practice," *American Journal of Nursing, 80* (March, 1980) pp. 451–455.

Chapter 9

Treatment and Care Planning

TREATMENT AND CARE PLANNING

Although we have talked about psychiatric treatment in general and the nurse-patient relationship in particular, it seems important at this point in time to go back and talk more specifically about the whole treatment planning process. It is no longer acceptable to assume that the patient who is hospitalized, attending a mental health clinic, or involved in some other kind of mental health program is being adequately treated. Funding agencies, public and private, and regulatory authorities now require a written treatment plan for each patient, documentation of the services performed, and the response of the sick person to the treatment given.

The Department of Health, Education, and Welfare* and the National Institute of Mental Health have published a detailed guide for treatment planning for psychiatric patients, called *Individualized Treatment Planning For Psychiatric Patients.* In this publication they list the following reasons for developing an individual, comprehensive treatment plan:

1. It forces the focus of attention on the patient as a unique individual.
2. It provides a systematic approach to care of patients and the documentation of what happens to them.
3. It assists the staff in their understanding of the patient and his or her needs.
4. It is necessary to meet the requirements for funding and accreditation.
5. It is in keeping with legislative and court concerns about appropriateness of treatment.

The Social Security Administration's Medicare program re-

*Renamed the Department of Human Services in 1979.

quires a recorded individual comprehensive treatment plan that is based on an inventory of the patient's strengths and disabilities; a diagnosis from the American Psychiatric Association's Diagnostic and Statistical Manual III (see Appendix B); short- and long-range goals; specific treatment modalities used; and the responsibilities of each member of the treatment team.

The Joint Commission on the Accreditation of Hospitals (the accrediting agency for all hospitals, including psychiatric) requires that "each patient shall have a written, individualized treatment plan that is based on assessments of his or her clinical needs, . . . [including] the patient's presenting problems, physical health, emotional status, and behavioral status."

In addition, the general public is much more aware and knowledgeable about health, illness, and treatment. There is an increasing concern in society about health care and health delivery systems. As a result, patients are more apt to inquire about their treatment plans, rather than passively accept whatever is done for them without knowing why it is done or where it is leading. Also, the individual treatment plan may serve to satisfy court and legislative concerns about the appropriateness of admission, diagnosis, treatment, and discharge of hospitalized psychiatric patients.

The treatment plan, then, needs to be individual, comprehensive, and goal directed. It should cover the patient's treatment from admission to discharge, with specific times designated for periodic review and modification. The planning process should involve all of the staff who have direct contact with the patient, the individual patient, and the family or significant others if possible.

Assessment. Initial and ongoing assessment of the patient's condition is based upon information gathered from the patient, family, staff, and any other significant person in the patient's life. Likewise, it is based upon information gathered from specific tests, which help to determine the physical, mental, social, and psychological status of the patient. Such assessment usually includes the reason for admission, medical history, including laboratory and diagnostic tests, psychiatric history, mental status, social history, nursing history or assessment, and any other pertinent information. There also may be additional information of importance from other agencies, treatment personnel, or previous hospital records.

Patient Participation. Involving the patient in his own treatment is an important aspect of successful treatment, not only in psychiatry but in any kind of health care. The advantages of patient participation are obvious, but are nevertheless often overlooked in our hurry to get the job done. We no longer are in the position of doing things to a patient or even for a patient. Instead we are working with the patient to provide a service which will help him move in the direction of optimum health or functioning. The very fact that we now often refer to the patient as a client reflects this concept.

Both the American Hospital Association and the Joint Commission on Accreditation of Hospitals have published documents detailing patients' rights (see Appendix D). Among these rights is the patient's right to know about his treatment, including what medications he is taking, why he is being given them, and what effects he may expect from them. Many hospitals have patient education programs that teach patients about their health and illness, including topics such as medications—what they are, how they are supposed to help the individual, what undesirable effects to look for, and the importance of staying on medications as prescribed; how to move toward optimum health; and how to adapt and cope with disabilities.

It is a well-demonstrated fact in any undertaking, including treatment, that the more the affected people have to say about what and how things are done, the more effort they put forth to see that success is insured. This is true of patients and staff alike. The response to treatment then is more positive if the patient and his family are included in the decision-making. Also, the patient's sense of worth and dignity are maintained and promoted if what he thinks and feels is taken into consideration. If a patient understands what is happening to him and why, there is less anxiety and resistance on his part. Some degree of control over one's life and state of health promotes healthier behavior on the part of the patient and insures greater treatment success. Finally, the patient is the only one who really knows what he thinks and how he feels, so his input makes the treatment plan more realistic, practical, and achievable.

Staff Participation. All of the staff who have direct contact or significant interaction with the patient should be included in the development of the treatment plan. Although the treatment team is often thought of in terms of professional staff only, more and more auxiliary or nonprofessional staff are directly involved with the treatment of psychiatric patients. For example, former addicts and former alcoholics are often primary therapists, particularly in community mental health programs. Sometimes volunteers, such as those connected with half-way houses, are involved in the treatment of psychiatric patients. It is just as important to involve these staff members in treatment planning as it is to involve the patient, and for some of the same reasons. The more involved the members of the treatment team are in decision-making, the more invested they are in seeing that the treatment plan is carried out and working. Also, their ideas and observations add an important dimension to the knowledge and information about the patient.

If for some reason all treatment staff cannot be included in the planning process (and this is often unrealistic, if not downright impossible), it is important that the plans and the reasons for them be communicated to others. Also, the ideas and observations of these absent staff members should be included in the planning process.

For example, in the hospital, conferences should be scheduled with afternoon and night shifts, or staff in other departments, who cannot attend the planning conference. In the community, other agencies dealing with the patient should be advised and consulted about the patient's treatment. Also, treatment plans should be written, so that they are clearly understood by all staff using them—the simpler the better.

Patient's Problems, Needs, and Strengths. The diagnosis alone can no longer be used to determine the patient's treatment. Treatment must be based upon the individual patient's problems, needs, and strengths. Just as all patients with heart surgery cannot be treated in exactly the same fashion, so all schizophrenic patients cannot be treated in exactly the same fashion. Successful psychiatric treatment is aimed toward the resolution of the individual patient's problems that brought him into treatment in the first place. The treatment plan then takes into consideration what the patient's problems are; what his needs are; what his strengths are (how much he can do for himself); and what is required from the staff in order for the patient's needs to be met (see p. 138). It is important for the patient to do as much for himself as possible, in order to add to his self-esteem and feelings of worth, accomplishment, and wholeness. Problems and needs are determined by making an assessment with the patient of what his current physical, emotional, and social status is. It may be necessary to list only those problems and needs that take priority in the present situation in the patient's life. Then, again with the patient, a determination is made of the patient's ability to meet those needs; in other words, of what strengths he has that can be used to resolve the problems and meet the needs. In the past we have focused on illness and symptoms; now it is being recommended in all kinds of health services that we focus instead on the patient's degree of health and wellness that can be used to help him move toward optimum functioning.

Problems that frequently bring patients into psychiatric treatment are revealed by the patient's history and behavior. The patient's history may show that he is unable to sleep, is up all night pacing around, sits and cries most of the time, fights with family members, fights with the neighbors, can't take care of house or family, thinks people are going to kill him, abuses drugs or alcohol, thinks a lot about taking his life, or is unable to care for his personal hygiene.

The patient's needs must be determined. Perhaps he needs to learn how to care for himself in areas such as personal hygiene or activities of daily living; needs to have a successful work experience; needs to share his feelings and thoughts with others; needs to feel more adequate, more important; needs to have vocational training or formal education; needs more family and community contact; needs to learn how to relax and how to relieve tension and anxiety in healthy ways; needs more physical exercise and outlets; needs to have one successful relationship with another person.

The staff can identify the patient's strengths by determining such things as who provides his support system (family, friends, church, job, etc.); what his intellectual skills, social skills, communication skills, and physical skills are; what his interests and preferences are; what he likes to do and not do; how he relieves his tensions and anxiety; what kind of formal education and learning experiences he has had in life; what kinds of things give him pleasure or discomfort; and what kinds of achievements (successes) he has had in life.

Examples of strengths can be even more specific. The staff may note that the patient can express feelings, can share with others, likes other people, is able to listen to others' ideas and problems, is friendly, makes others feel comfortable, has taught adults physical education, has a sister who visits and is willing to take him into her home after discharge, likes physical exercise, particularly walking, and is physically healthy.

Long- and Short-Term Goals. After the patient's problems, needs, and strengths have been identified, then long- and short-term goals can be determined. What, realistically, can the patient expect to accomplish in the way of resolving whatever problems have brought him into the treatment situation? It is important to select short-term goals that can be accomplished soon after admission, so as to give the patient that re-enforcing feeling of success. Nothing is so healing to the emotionally suffering person as some demonstrated accomplishment ("I can do that"), no matter how small it may seem to others. The process of saying to one's self "I can do that" is sometimes referred to as personal affirmation, and can be very helpful in building or repairing one's self-image.

As in learning objectives, goals should be stated in terms of expected behavior, so that success can be measured. Also, goals should be stated in a time frame—how soon, how often, how long is it expected to take before the patient can accomplish a particular goal. We have stated goals in the past which were not clear, measurable, or even achievable, such as "develop insight." It is better to say, "In one week, with a staff member, the patient will be able to identify what problems in his behavior interfere with his feeling good about himself."

Examples of long-term goals to consider for the treatment plan project that the patient will be able to leave the hospital within six weeks, will be able to live with his sister, will be able to go to a mental health clinic once a month, and will be able to return to work on medication.

Short-term goals help the patient more immediately with daily living; for example, treatment can be planned so that he will be able in one week to bathe, shave, shampoo, and do other personal grooming once a day without reminders from the staff; will talk about feelings and problems for fifteen minutes once a day with an assigned staff member; will participate in a patient activity group for thirty minutes once a week; will be able in one week to join a patient group studying for GED for one hour, once a week; and will be able, starting tomorrow, to participate in tension/anxiety–relieving exercises, fifteen minutes daily.

Goals need to be reviewed and modified as the patient's problems, needs, and abilities change, so that they are relevant, current, and achievable. In fact, the whole treatment process changes in relation to changes in the patient's condition. Frequent conferences with staff and patients help to keep the treatment process up to date. These conferences should be scheduled at regular intervals and documented so that patient and staff alike can keep abreast of the current treatment situation.

Additional information may be gathered which adds to or changes the patient's needs, strengths, or treatment plan. This information may come from additional input from the patient, his family, or significant others; changes in the patient's behavior, ability to function, or degree of health; observations of staff interaction with the patient; or previous health records.

Goals should be stated, if possible, in positive rather than negative terms or, put another way, in terms of healthy rather than sick behavior. The goal states what the patient is to do, or how he is to function, rather than what he is *not* to do. For example, "In one week, the patient will be able to talk to a staff member for five minutes at a time in terms of what he has been able to accomplish that day," rather than what he has failed to do. The establishment of goals may be a step-by-step process with increasingly difficult or more complex goals, but it is well to start off with the simpler, more easily achieved, most essential goals.

Implementation of Treatment Plans. Whatever treatment modalities are selected, they should relate specifically to the individual patient involved: (1) whatever problems led to admission; (2) what his individual needs and strengths are; and (3) what the long- and short-term goals to be achieved are.

Specific assignments of staff members should be made to specific parts of the treatment program. Identify who is responsible for what, including the patient's responsibility. Sometimes this is done in the form of a contract with the patient, in which each party agrees to act in certain ways either toward one another or toward the world at large. In this way, the patients' needs are not overlooked, and they are not left to sink or swim by themselves. Someone is assigned to help the individual patient in specific ways. Patients in this way become individuals: treatable, important people to be given whatever help is required in order for their needs to be met. When specific, individual assignments are made in this fashion, the patient knows to whom he can go (or upon whom he can depend) for certain things. He may go to the physician for medication change; or to the social worker for contact with his family; or to the activity therapist for an exercise schedule; or to the nurse for assistance in expressing his feelings about his hospital stay. Such assignments identify who is going to do what when, and how and why. When these things are fully understood among staff and patients, there develops an atmosphere of mutual trust, shared responsibility, and progress toward health.

Evaluation and Modification of Treatment Plans. From admission to discharge, the patient's treatment plan should be reviewed, evaluated, and modified at regular, specified times as the circumstances and the patient change, so that it is ongoing, relevant, realistic. It is important to consult with the patient, family, and staff to make sure the state of the patient's healthy functioning is clearly reflected and understood by all involved, so that they may interact effectively. Planning for discharge should begin with admission, so that family, friends, and community resources are all made available to the patient from the beginning of treatment. This also sets up the expectation for all who are involved in the patient's treatment that he will be moving toward health or optimum functioning and return to the community.

Documentation. This kind of individualized, comprehensive treatment planning lends itself to problem-oriented or goal-oriented records. (An example of a treatment plan is seen in Figure 7.) Whatever method is used, problem-oriented or goal-oriented or the traditional source-oriented recordings, it is important to document what is done, by whom it is done, why it is being done, what the effect upon the patient is, and what the future course of treatment should be. Without this kind of documentation, it is impossible to identify the treatment program and its results.

Summary. To be effective as well as accepted by funding and regulatory agencies, the planning process for the patient's treatment plan should do the following:

1. Involve the patient in the planning.
2. Identify the patient's problems, needs, and strengths.

Patient's Name and Vital Information	Reason for Admission	Diagnosis
Doe, Jane	Overdose of Thorazine Trouble at home Hallucinations and paranoid ideas	Schizophrenic disorder
Date of Admission		
3/16/81		

Problems	Needs	Strengths
Feels like a failure. Presents herself as helpless, childlike. Tends to get out of anxiety-provoking situations—sick behavior. Voices telling her to kill herself.	Needs to be successful at something. Needs to be independent. Needs to talk about feelings rather than act them out.	Young—21 years old. Has had some clerical training. Is aware of her behavior and wants to change it.

Goals	Therapeutic Action	Responsible Staff
Short-Term (1) Will be able to copy nursing procedures 15 min. daily M–F starting 3/17. (2) Will be able in 1 wks. time to talk with Nurse Smith about her feelings and successes 30 min./day. *Long-Term* (1) In 1 mo. will be able to talk about her problems rather than act out. (2) In 2 mos. will be able to do copy work without direction. (3) In 3 mos. will be able to leave hospital and attend MH Clinic 1×/wk. (4) On discharge will be able to participate in Voc. Rehab.	Find job in nursing office copying procedures. Regular conference 1×/wk. to talk about accomplishments and feelings. Medication to relieve anxiety, hallucinations—Thorazine, Stelazine. **Treatment Review** Once a month consult with staff and patient. Revise treatment plan as indicated.	Nurse Jones will make assignments and consult with her 1×/day for 15 min. Nurse Smith will set up regular meeting schedule with her to talk about success rather than failure 1×/wk. for 20 min. Social worker Murphy will arrange for consultation with Voc. Rehab. Dr. Brown will prescribe meds and supervise treatment regimen.

Figure 7. Treatment Plan (developed at Eastern State Hospital, Medical Lake, Washington).

3. Establish short-and long-term goals that are behavioral, measurable, and achievable within a certain time frame.
4. Involve all staff directly caring for patients.
5. Establish who is responsible for what.
6. Provide for regular, ongoing review and modification.
7. Relate treatment to needs and strengths, and direct toward the resolution of problems.
8. Document what is done, by whom it is done, why it is done, what the effect is upon the patient, and what is required or expected in the future.

NURSING CARE PLANNING

The most effective treatment planning includes all of the staff who are in direct contact with the patient, including nursing staff, or at least those who are directly involved with the treatment of the patient. Team planning provides for a more intergrated and comprehensive approach to treatment with less chance of fragmentation or working at cross purposes. In some situations this may not be possible because the structure or philosophy of the institutional setting prevents it, or because the nurse is the primary therapist in individual or group therapy in a noninstitutional setting. However, in any situation in which nursing staff are involved in patient's treatment, nursing care planning is an essential part of the nursing process.

ANA Standards of Psychiatric and Mental Health Nursing Practice. (See Appendix E.) The American Nurses' Association sets standards for nursing practice in all of the clinical areas. Of the standards they set for psychiatric and mental health nursing, the first three are particularly relevant to nursing care planning, so they are quoted here:

> Standard I. Data are collected through pertinent clinical observations based on knowledge of the arts and sciences with particular emphasis upon psychosocial and biophysical sciences.
>
> Standard II. Clients are involved in the assessment, planning, implementation and evaluation of their nursing care program to the fullest extent of their capabilities.
>
> Standard III. The problem-solving approach is utilized in developing nursing care plans.

Nursing Process. The nursing process is a problem-solving technique which consists of a number of steps—assessment (or collection of data and nursing diagnosis), planning, intervention, evaluation, and modification. Since assessment is the cornerstone of the nursing process, we will discuss it at some length. It is wise

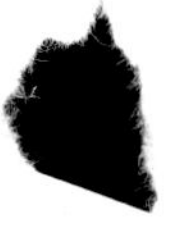

to keep in mind that the nursing care plan and subsequent nursing actions or interventions evolve from the assessment. Assessment consists of observation, interviewing, and measurement regarding the patient's state of health. It includes the identification of his problems, needs, and strengths in relation to his condition and life style. Not only does the nurse interview the patient and record what he tells her about himself, but she collects data as well from significant others (family, friends, other health care personnel). In addition, she uses her own observations and those of other staff members to make a series of judgments about the patient's health status and ability to function.

It is imperative that the nurse and patient enter into a problem-solving relationship from the very beginning, in order to progress as rapidly as possible toward the patient's highest achievable level of wellness. Plans for discharge begin at admission, so that the patient understands from the very beginning that this treatment situation is a temporary one, meant to restore him as soon as possible to independence and self-care. During the initial interview the nurse and patient begin a relationship based upon trust, respect, concern, and responsibility. The interview sets the tone for his stay in the hospital, represents his introduction to the staff and treatment situation, and sets the stage for his response to treatment. It is important, then, that the nurse do this interview as soon after admission of the patient as possible. The patient should feel from the way the nurse behaves toward him that she is truly interested in him as a person, that she is concerned about his welfare, that she recognizes and respects him as a partner in identifying and meeting his needs, and that she feels a sense of responsibility in helping him move toward a common goal of restoring his ability to function at his highest level of competence.

Assessment means identifying the needs of the individual patient, determining his ability to meet them, and making recommendations for the kind of help that is required from nursing staff in order for his needs to be met. The process begins with observation, which includes both subjective and objective data about a patient—what he says and does, as well as what the nurse thinks is the intent of the behavior. The nurse uses her knowledge and experience to interpret the patient's behavior and make a series of judgments or decisions about the nature of the patient's problems. Using validation the nurse checks with the patient to get corroboration from the patient about her assessment, so that there is an agreement between the patient and the nurse. In the assessment, the nurse determines what the patient's central problems are, what his critical needs are, and what his functional strengths are.

Interview Guide. The interview should be so conducted that upon completion the nurse will understand the patient's problems, needs, and capabilities. Through the interview the nurse will also gain insight into how the patient sees his illness and how it affects him and his life style.

It is important that the nurse establish rapport with the patient early on. If the patient can feel comfortable and accepted by the nurse, he will be better able to talk about those things that bother him. A friendly, courteous, nonthreatening approach that demonstrates sincere interest in the patient will do much to facilitate the assessment process. The nurse's behavior and attitude throughout the interview convey to the patient what she thinks of him. The way she conducts the interview should set up the atmosphere of attitudinal healing—"I'm here to help you." Her questions will fall short of the mark if she indicates in any way that she is hurried or disinterested or that the patient is in some way unacceptable to her. As the interview proceeds, the patient begins to develop trust in the nurse, and it becomes easier for him to discuss sensitive issues later in the interview. Thus, it is better to start out with physical facts, or questions that are not emotionally charged.

The patient should be afforded privacy in order that he understand that his communications are confidential as well as important. Provide a quiet area where you will not be interrupted; make the patient and yourself comfortable; pull up a chair and sit down in order to be on the same eye level; don't put a barrier between you, like a desk. Begin by introducing yourself and saying to the patient, "In order to give you the best possible nursing care, I need to ask you some questions. If it is all right with you, I will do that now."

Along with the manner and tone of voice of the nurse, the following guidelines provide the basis for the interview:

1. Let the patient tell his story in his own words.
2. Avoid leading questions that require a yes or no answer.
3. Ask one question at a time, and give the patient time to answer.
4. Keep questions brief and simple.
5. Use language understandable to the patient.
6. Clarify the patient's response.
7. Inquire about episodes or symptoms that deviate from the patient's normal pattern of behavior.

Decision-making and judgment on the part of the nurse are particularly important during the interview. The nurse decides what to ask, when to ask it, and how to ask it. The nurse decides when to listen, how to listen, and how long to listen. The nurse uses her judgment throughout the interview in focusing on some areas in depth and by passing more briefly over others. The nurse determines when there may be more to the meaning of the topic than that which the patient has given. The nurse summarizes all available data collected in the interview, makes an assessment of the patient's health status, and determines what is required of the nursing staff in order for his needs to be met.

When the interview is terminated, the patient should know who the nurse is; who will be responsible for his care; that someone knows what his views, fears, concerns, and expectations are; that someone knows the basic human needs that he fulfills for himself and those he needs help with. He knows how to summon the nurse, where to find the nurse, when and how he can communicate with the nurse, and when he will see the nurse again.

After the data are collected from the patient, the nurse may seek additional relevant data from family members or significant others, such as other members of the treatment team, appropriate members of the health services community, and from available records and reports.

Areas to Cover in Assessment. Figure 8 is an example of a nursing assessment form. It is divided into four areas, covering the patient's general appearance, general state of health, ability to function, and any problems that he has and his perception of his illness. This kind of nursing assessment assumes that other members of the treatment team are gathering more detailed information regarding his physical condition, mental status, and social history. It is meant for the primary use of the nursing staff; therefore, it focuses upon those areas of the patient's condition that are of importance to the nursing staff in providing the best possible nursing care.

The first area to cover is the patient's general appearance. This is one of the most important parts of the assessment because it not only tells you something about the physical status of the patient, but it also has to do with the way the patient feels about himself, thus how he presents himself to others. Sometimes his appearance says more about him and his condition than what he tells you verbally about himself. It is important to observe the patient's facial expression, such as sad, serious, happy, smiling, masked, grimacing, etc.; personal hygiene, such as clean, body odor, unshaven, bad breath; posture, such as erect, slumped, stooped, tense, relaxed; dress, such as appropriate, neat, clean, dirty, bizarre, disheveled; signs of anxiety, such as restless, pacing, wringing hands, gesturing, hyperactive, shaky, agitated.

The second area of importance to cover is his physical state of health and ability to function. Describe his general state of health, which cues the nursing staff as to what kind and how much help the patient requires to promote maximum independence for him in the activities of daily living. It also identifies the patient's preferences and habits that will help to individualize the nursing care. Take his vital signs: temperature, pulse, respiration, and blood

Patient's Name ______________________________ Date of Admission______

I. *General Appearance:* Circle or write in.

Facial Expression: sad, serious, happy, smiling, masked, grimacing, __________
Hygiene: clean, body odor, unshaven, bad breath, ______________________
Posture: erect, slumped, stooped, tense, relaxed, ______________________
Dress: appropriate, neat, clean, dirty, bizarre, disheveled, ______________
Signs of Anxiety: restless, pacing, wringing hands, gesturing, hyperactive, shaky, agitated, ______________________________________

II. *Physical Health and Function:* Write in any problems or preferences.

Vital Signs: T P R B/P ______________________________
Physical impairment: ______________________________
Skin: ______________________________
Personal Hygiene: ______________________________
Breathing: ______________________________
Eating: ______________________________
Sleeping: ______________________________
Activity: ______________________________
Elimination: ______________________________
Senses: ______________________________
Sexuality: ______________________________

III. *Perception of Illness and Treatment:* Write in patient's words.

What current problems does the patient express?

What is the patient's understanding of his illness and events leading up to illness?

What are the patient's expectations of the hospital, treatment, and staff?

What will help him feel more secure, comfortable, safe, cared for?

IV. *Ability to Function Emotionally, Mentally, Socially:* Circle or write in.

Mental Clarity: oriented, disoriented, stuporous, confused, clear, impaired intellectual function, ______________________________
Mood: euphoric, cheerful, apathetic, sad, hopeless, dejected, angry, __________
Speech: talkative, silent, rapid, slurred, clear, doesn't speak English, __________
____
Thought Content: delusional, fearful, morose, flight of ideas, ______________
Perception: hallucinations, expressed or suspected, illusions, ______________
Suicidal: thoughts, gestures, intent, ______________________________
Drug/Alcohol Problems: ______________________________

Figure 8. The Nursing Assessment (developed at Eastern State Hospital, Medical Lake, Washington).

pressure. Identify any physical impairment. Does he have any signs of skin problems: color? rash? bruises? sensitivity? What is the state of his personal hygiene? Does he have any difficulty breathing? Is he coughing? bringing up sputum? choking? Does he have any difficulty eating? any food preferences? any special eating habits? any allergies? any special diet? Does he have any difficulty sleeping? any trouble falling asleep? waking up? take any medications for the problem? What is his usual level of activity? any problems? any restrictions? Does he tire easily? Does he have any problems with elimination? any bowel or bladder problems? Is he using any medications for them? Does he have any hearing loss? sight loss? any other sensory problems? Does he have any sexual problems? Feelings about the opposite sex? same sex?

The third area of importance to cover is the patient's perception of his illness and what he expects from treatment. What current problems does the patient express? What is the patient's understanding of his illness and the events leading up to his illness? What is the patient's expectation of the hospital, treatment, and staff? What will help him feel more secure, comfortable, safe, cared for? The nurse gets some understanding of how the patient sees himself and his illness, what his expectations of staff are, and at the same time the nurse is given an opportunity to offer him immediate assistance and explanation. Ask questions like: What brought you to the hospital? Have there been any sudden changes in your behavior? Have you had anything like this before? When? Where? What happened to you? Have you ever been in psychiatric treatment before? When? Where? How long? What caused your difficulty? What do other people think is wrong? Do you have any problems at home? at work? with other people? with the law? What needs to be corrected in order for you to function better? What would you like to know about the hospital? treatment? staff? (Tell him who will be caring for him and what they will be doing for him.) What can I do for you right now that will make you feel more comfortable? safe? secure?

The fourth area of importance to cover is significant data about his ability to function emotionally, mentally, socially. Also, describe his present psychological state, which cues the nursing staff as to what kind of and how much help the patient requires in order for him to deal effectively with his environment. What is his mental clarity, such as oriented, disoriented, stuporous, clear, impaired intellectual functioning? What is his mood, such as euphoric, cheerful, apathetic, sad, hopeless, dejected, angry? What is his speech like, such as talkative, silent, rapid, slurred, clear? What is his thought content, such as delusional, fearful, morose, flight of ideas? What is his perception like, such as hallucinations, expressed or suspected, illusions? Does he have suicidal thoughts, gestures, intent? Does he have any problem with drugs or alcohol?

Remember the kind of assessment we have described here is based upon the assumption that other team members will do more detailed accounts of the physical, mental, and social history of the patient. This will eliminate duplication of effort, since these records will be available to the nursing staff and used in the total care of the patient. If there is not a treatment team supplying further

Patient's Name and Vital Information	Reason for Admission (Nursing Diagnosis)	Date of Admission
Smith, John	Wrecked his room. Not taking care of himself.	4/31/81

Problems	Needs	Strengths
Delusion that man inside directs him. Poor personal hygiene. Unable to develop friends. Has never held job.	Needs to learn how to direct energy constructively. Needs to develop personal health habits. Needs to be able to share ideas and feelings with others.	Young—22 years old. H.S. graduate. States he wants to improve himself.

Goals	Nursing Interventions	Responsible Nursing Staff
Short-Term (1) In 1 wk. will be able to spend 20 min. daily on his personal hygiene. (2) Starting tomorrow will be included in physical activity program 30 min./day. (3) In 1 wk. will be able to share ideas and feelings with 1 person 15 min. 2×/wk.	Assist him in improving his personal hygiene 15 min. daily. Include him in activity-oriented group 30 min. daily. Establish 1–1 relationship with him to improve trust and communication skill 15 min. daily. Provide job assignment doing janitorial job 20 min. daily. Include him in group discussion meeting 2×/wk. for 30 min. **Nursing Care Review** Review with all nursing staff and patient once a week. Each assigned nurse will review progress with patient in their sessions each day as they work with him.	Nurse Smith will spend 15 min. each morning teaching him how to do personal hygiene. Nurse Jones will spend 20 min. 1×/wk. to plan and review physical activity program. Nurse Brown will spend 15 min. daily with him encouraging him to talk about himself. Nurse Murphy will teach him how to do janitorial job and supervise him in this work 20 min. daily. Nurse White will make out referral to Voc. Rehab. and see that he follows through.

Figure 9. Nursing Care Plan (developed at Eastern State Hospital, Medical Lake, Washington).

information, it may be necessary for the nurse to obtain more detailed and specific information about the patient's physical, mental, and social status than we have indicated here.

Nursing Care Plan. The nursing care plan flows from the assessment done by the nurse. With the patient, identify his current problems, needs, strengths. What are the short-and long-term goals in treatment? What nursing actions, assistance, or intervention needs to be taken to help the patient reach these goals? The nursing staff should be directed as to how to help the patient meet his needs at this time. Assign responsibility to specific nursing staff for specific nursing interventions. Additions and modifications can be made later as the patient's needs and abilities change, and as the nurse gets more input from the patient and other treatment staff. Specific times should be designated for review of the nursing care plan, and the patient should be included in the review. What has been said before about treatment planning in general holds true as well for nursing care planning, so it will not be repeated here. There are many different ways to document the nursing care plan; one example is given if Figure 9.

REFERENCES

American Nurses' Association: *Nursing—A Social Policy Statement,* American Nurses' Association, Kansas City, Missouri, 1980.

American Nurses' Association: *Standards of Psychiatric and Mental Health Nursing Practice,* American Nurses' Association, Kansas City, Missouri, 1973.

Blount, Mary, et al.: "Documenting with the problem-oriented record system," *American Journal of Nursing, 78* (September, 1978) pp. 1539–1542.

Brands, Alvira, ed.: *Individualized Treatment Planning for Psychiatric Patients—* A Joint Publication of the Health Standards and Quality Bureau and National Institute of Mental Health, U.S. Department of Health, Education and Welfare—National Institute of Mental Health, Rockville, Maryland, 1977.

Dodd, Marilyn J.: "Assessing mental status," *American Journal of Nursing, 78* (September, 1978) pp. 1500–1503.

Forman, Mary: "Building a better nursing care plan," *American Journal of Nursing, 79* (June, 1979) pp. 1086–1089.

Harris, Ruth B.: "A strong vote for the nursing process," *American Journal of Nursing, 79* (November, 1979) pp. 1999–2000.

Inzer, Frances, and Mary Jo Aspinwall: "Evaluating patient outcome," *Nursing Outlook, 81* (March, 1981) pp. 178–181.

Jacobs, Kathy D.: "Does the nurse practitioner involve the patient in his care?" *Nursing Outlook, 80* (August, 1980) pp. 501–555.

Jacoby, Muriel K., and Doris J. Adams: "Teaching assessment of client functioning," *Nursing Outlook, 81* (April, 1981) pp. 248–250.

Joint Commission on Accreditation of Hospitals: *Consolidated Standards Manual for Child, Adolescent, and Adult Psychiatric, Alcoholism, and Drug Abuse Facilities,* 1981 Edition.

Krozy, Ronna: "Becoming comfortable with sexual assessment," *American Journal of Nursing, 78* (June, 1978) pp. 1036–1038.

Minor, Harriett E., and Cecelia A. Macauley: "The nurse as admission evaluator," *American Journal of Nursing, 81* (January, 1981) p. 118.

Nursing Service Policies and Guidelines, Eastern State Hospital, Medical Lake, Washington, 1980.

Chapter 10

Reactions to the Stress of Adolescence

We have briefly discussed the stage of adolescence in Chapter 4. However, it is such a critical period of development that we will discuss it further in this chapter in order to better understand both healthy and unhealthy reactions to the stress and anxiety of this and other periods that follow. From this stage of growth the individual emerges as the kind of person he will be as an adult. The stress of the period tests all the strength the individual has acquired in the few short years of his life. This is a period of transition from the expectations and competencies of childhood to a whole new set of expectations and competencies for adulthood. Erikson (1968, p. 244) describes the overwhelming stress in adjustment at this time: "In no other stage of the life cycle, are the promise of finding oneself and the threat of losing oneself so closely allied."

Adolescence may be defined as the transitional stage of growth and development between the end of childhood and the beginning of adulthood, roughly 12 to 18 years of age. Puberty in its strictest sense refers to that time in the adolescent's life when his sexual organs are sufficiently developed physiologically to accomplish reproduction. Pubescence refers to the period of time when the major developmental changes occur. Adolescence may be divided roughly into three periods—early, middle, and late—sometimes referred to as prepuberty, puberty, and postpuberty. During adolescence major physical, emotional, and social changes occur in the individual. Changes are occurring in all three of these areas simultaneously or in a series. They are interrelated and affect one another. However, in order to identify and understand the major changes, we will discuss them separately, keeping in mind that they do not occur this way in real life.

PHYSICAL GROWTH AND DEVELOPMENT

Throughout childhood the reproductive organs have not changed much, but in adolescence pubescent growth toward sexual maturing follows an orderly sequence. Pubescent growth is initiated by the hypothalamus, which stimulates the pituitary gland. The pituitary gland controls all growth, stimulating hormone production of the ovaries, testes, and adrenal glands. The specific agents of pubescent growth are the sex hormones—estrogen from the ovaries and androgen from the testes. Girls are generally two years ahead of boys in reaching sexual maturity. Their average age of puberty is between 11 and 14 years, with boys following between 13 and 16 years. Each individual has his or her own growth timetable, so there may be wide variations in time, but the normal maturational sequence follows the same order.

The dramatic development of the reproductive system leads to sexual arousal and desires, but there are very rigid restrictions governing the sexual behavior of adolescents. Although they are mature in physiological function, they are still regarded as children emotionally and socially. Adolescents are frightened and confused by these new sexual feelings, which they (and parents) frequently think of as "bad." They need the opportunity to discuss such feelings and learn how to control and channel their sexual desires.

At the same time that sexual growth is taking place, there is a general spurt in physical growth. The adolescent seems to grow overnight. The average growth during puberty for a boy is about 8 inches, and a girl 3¼ inches, with the growth peak for girls being from 12 to 13 years of age and for boys 14 to 15 years of age. There is not just an increase in height and weight, but in other dimensions as well—head, chest, hips, hands, and feet. All parts of the body do not grow at the same rate, so the adolescent looks awkward and somewhat disproportionate. Often his pants legs or shirt sleeves are too short, which gives him a gangling appearance.

Both boys and girls worry about their appearance and spend hours in front of the mirror, studying the changes that are taking place. Girls often want to be shorter and boys want to be taller than they are. Often there is a spurt in the growth of their feet, and the earlier it happens, the bigger their feet seem. This sometimes poses problems for parents as well as adolescents because of the frequent need for new shoes. Any period of rapid growth is a time of vulnerability, and the adolescent needs extra food and rest. He needs all the strength and energy possible to master the problems of this stage of growth. His calorie needs alone are tremendous. The average boy between 16 and 19 years of age needs more than 3600 calories daily, more than he has ever needed before or ever will need again. The average girl between 13 and 15 years of age needs 2600 calories daily, a need exceeded only by that of the nursing mother. The adolescent may literally never get filled up if his stomach is too small to hold all he needs. As a result, it seems to his parents as if he eats all the time. There is rapid growth in all bones, muscles, joints, and tendons, which makes them particularly susceptible to strain. In the growth of the cardiovascular system, the heart may be too small to withstand the stress and strain, so the adolescent needs to be protected from overexertion. He needs all of the nutritional elements for growth—vitamins, minerals, and proteins—not just carbohydrates and fats for energy. Deficiencies in diet can have an adverse effect upon energy level, resistance to disease, behavior, emotions, and appearance. One of the greatest difficulties is in helping the adolescent to meet his nutritional needs and not eat large amounts of junk food because he is hungry. Also, he needs to be independent and make his own decisions, so he cannot be constantly supervised or "preached at," which creates problems for both adolescents and parents.

His motor development continues, and he gains in strength, coordination, and endurance. His awkwardness is related more to his appearance, increased self-consciousness, and frequent uncertainty than it is to neuromuscular inability. Athletic success is a social asset to boys and a major source of satisfaction from which he learns a sense of adequacy as well as physical mastery. This is becoming increasingly true of girls as well as boys. The newest trend in physical education for both boys and girls is to give them experiences in adolescence that they can use throughout life for recreational, social, and health purposes—activities like tennis, swimming, dancing, and bicycling.

The adolescent is introduced to a whole new way of thinking. For the first time he is able to achieve abstract thinking or formal thought, which is really a culmination of what he has been building toward throughout childhood. All of his thought processes are reorganized on a higher, adult level. As a child, he thought in terms of concrete things and events and what existed at the present time in reality. As an adolescent, he is able to think in abstract and symbolic terms, entertaining concepts and ideas with which he has had no experience—like infinity. He begins to build systems and theories regarding the explanation of events, rather than just accepting and describing them. Probably the main distinction between adolescent and childhood intelligence has to do with the adolescent's ability to think in terms of hypotheses—"what if" propositions, which open up a wide expanse for thought. The ability to carefully consider one aspect at a time and each part's relationship to the whole, the ability to relate real experiences to what might be possible, and the ability to entertain new ideas and replace or modify the old ones are all extremely fascinating new intellectual experiences for the adolescent. They change his whole perception of himself and the world in which he lives. He spends hour after hour caught up in this new world of thought, often much to the annoyance of his parents. He is not just "daydreaming," as he is often accused of doing, but experiencing, exercising, and growing in his thought processes—a vital development.

Related to his new intellectual experiences is a disturbance in the experience of time, a disturbance that Erikson (1968, p. 169) calls the "diffusion of time perspective." The adolescent experiences a feeling of urgency but acts as if time is not important. In fact, it appears sometimes from his actions that he has lost all track of time. It is hard for him to stop activities that he is engaged in, and equally hard for him to get started. For example, it is as difficult for him to go to bed at night as it is to get up in the morning. Another dimension of time new to adolescence is the need to be future-oriented. The adolescent must develop the ability to delay immediate gratification in order to gain more pleasure in the future, an ability that is one measure of adult adjustment.

The adolescent's ability to consider his own thinking and the thinking of others enables him to construct an imaginary audience. It is easier to understand some of the adolescent's behavior when we realize that he is both actor and audience. One way for him to learn new behavior is to act it out and see how it fits. Sometimes he has difficulty differentiating between his own thoughts, feelings, and desires and those of others. As he becomes more adept at this, he begins to see himself in relationship to others more realistically. Self-discovery does not come easily because he tends to think of himself either as someone very special or unique (the prince or princess) or as someone no good or unwanted (the stepchild). However, self-discovery is essential to the establishment of independence.

At this time also there is a general increase in the adolescent's vocabulary for communication and thinking purposes. He develops as well a particular kind of vocabulary and manner of speaking peculiar to adolescents, which comes directly from his peer group. The language does more than just convey an idea or information, it also distinguishes an individual as a member (or nonmember) of the group. It sometimes serves as a kind of mask for the real thoughts, feelings, and actions of the adolescent, so that others, particularly parents, will not discover what is really happening to him.

During adolescence also there is a resurgence in fantasy or imagination. It is a time for idealistic, impractical dreams of glory about himself and the universe. He has lots of ideas about how the world ought to be and how it could be made better, some of which he may try to put into action. Adolescents need experiences that promote independent thinking and creative behavior. Creativity in the adolescent is fostered when he is respected, trusted, and encouraged to explore and enjoy himself and the world around him.

EMOTIONAL GROWTH AND DEVELOPMENT

Adolescence is one of the most difficult times of adjustment in our lives. The child has learned to live comfortably in a world of adults and is doing pretty well until all of a sudden, as an adolescent, he is expected to change drastically in every part of his being. He must develop his own sense of identity—who he is, what he can do, and where he fits in relationship to others. Erikson defines identity as "the sense of persistent sameness within oneself and a persistent sharing of some kind of essential character with others." In order to find himself, the adolescent must reject his own childhood self and the people most closely associated with that part of himself, his parents. He must establish himself as an independent person, directed and guided by himself rather than someone else. He must carve out his own future—what he is going to do and what he is going to be. All this poses a very real conflict within the adolescent and between him and others, particularly parents. It is a period filled with anguish and suffering for both adolescents and parents, as well as a period of extreme highs and lows in terms of fulfillment and pleasure.

Adolescence puts to the test all he has learned so far about satisfying his needs in acceptable ways and handling the anxiety that results from lack of success. At each stage in his life he has been expected to master certain developmental tasks. How well he has managed this will influence how well he manages the task of adolescence: developing the sense of identity.

Let us review what we have already said in Chapter 4 about stages in the life cycle. At each developmental stage the individual faces a crisis, a turning point, which when mastered adds to his strength and competency as a person. With the development of each sense or perspective about life, we have the components of the growing personality. The most fundamental of these is the sense of basic trust, which precedes all others and begins in infancy. Without a sense of basic trust in oneself and others, there can be no successful relationships with others; there can be no sense of identity. In early childhood, the child must develop the sense of autonomy he learns that he is a separate person with certain abilities of his own. He begins to experience the rudiments of independence, his first experience with freedom. Now that he knows he is a person in his own right, he moves on to find out what kind of person he is to become. In the play age he must develop the sense of initiative that gives direction and purpose to his life. He tries to do what he sees others doing and begins to investigate the reasons why things are as they are. During the school age, he develops the sense of industry, the ability to produce things. This development is the forerunner of his ability to be a worker, provider, and parent.

If in the first stage he has developed the basic sense of trust, then in adolescence he looks for people in whom and causes in which he can invest his trust and also attempts to prove himself trustworthy. At the same time he is afraid of being betrayed and expresses his distrust of parents and society in a loud voice. If in the second stage he has developed the sense of autonomy, then in adolescence he looks for opportunities to make his own decisions. He is mortally afraid of being forced into doing things that would expose him to self-doubt or ridicule from his peers. He would rather make his own mistakes and take his own chances. If he has developed the sense of initiative, then in adolescence he will put his trust in those who support his ambitions. At the same time that he fiercely defends his right to potential glory, he is terribly afraid of punishment or destruction and can be easily defeated. Finally, if he has developed the sense of industry, then in adolescence his choice of an occupation and his preparation for it is of extreme importance to him. It is so crucial that sometimes young people postpone making the choice as long as possible and go through a period of searching for answers or "finding themselves."

All that has gone before, then, is a part of his emerging identity in adolescence, just as the development of a sense of identity is essential to the development of a sense of intimacy in young adulthood. It is not possible for the adolescent to give himself to another in love and fulfillment until he has become his own self. So until he is an adult, his love relationships are apt to be temporary.

In our society, the children are expected to grow up, leave home, and start their own family—the nuclear family. To do that, the adolescent must free himself from the protection and direction of his parents, learn to make his own decisions, think for himself, and be responsible for his actions. The stage of adolescence is bound to be full of confusion, frustration, and conflict, and out of this turmoil must come the independent, giving, and cooperative adult. At the same time that he is rejecting childhood and striving toward independence and identity, the adolescent needs the love, comfort, and guidance of his parents. In interaction with them he gets his sense of identity; in interaction with them he determines what kind of a person he is; in interaction with them he learns to relate with others on an adult level.

For an adolescent to grow toward maturity in a healthy fashion, he needs first of all parents who care about him, not just because he is their son or daughter, but because he is a person. Adolescents who get in trouble often say that their parents didn't pay any attention to them, weren't interested, or didn't seem to care about them. How can you find out who you are, where you're going, and how you stand in relationship to others, if the important people around you demonstrate no interest in you? Adolescents need reasonable limits placed upon them, so they can learn to control and direct their behavior in constructive ways. Again, adolescents who get into trouble often say they wish their parents had set some limits for them or stuck to the limits they set for them, instead of giving in to them all the time. Often youngsters behave in more and more inappropriate ways just to get their parents to exhibit enough interest to restrict their activities. When they get no positive response from parents, they feel unloved, unimportant, and insecure.

To learn to make wise decisions that affect one's life and sometimes the lives of others, the adolescent needs some practice. The best kind of opportunity is in his relationship with his parents. Things need to be discussed with him, his ideas must be listened to, and a shared decision should be made. He needs to have sufficient trust and freedom from his parents to make decisions on his own, especially when his parents are not available. These decisions need to be respected, even if he makes a mistake. The important thing is that he can learn from the whole process, not that he has made a mistake, and parents can help him see that. Conflict and misunderstanding stem most often from not seeing the other person's point of view. Communication and relationships are enhanced when parents and adolescents respect and sincerely care about each other.

Adolescents are influenced by the feelings and relationships of their parents toward them, toward each other, and toward other people. Parents are the adolescent's models for men and women, husbands and wives, and mothers and fathers, and adolescents tend to be more like parents than unlike them. Adolescents learn to treat others as they are treated, relate to others as they are related to, and behave generally in accord with the behavior they see demonstrated in their daily lives by their parents. Youngsters are particularly sensitive to and critical of dishonesty, so they tend to believe what they see rather than what they are told.

Parents often have ambivalent feelings toward the child's growing up. Often it represents a loss to the parents, particularly the mother, of a major source of satisfaction, as well as of responsibility. The critical thing for parents to know is when to let him go on his own and when to guide or protect or restrict him. Parents have to have particularly keen insight into what constitutes opportunity for growth and what may result in certain devastation. Many parents are uncertain about themselves and their own beliefs, which makes it difficult for them to guide the searching, questioning adolescent.

Adolescents are particularly sensitive to their parents' feelings about them and about each other. Because of the intense emotional pitch of the adolescent, sometimes even a hint of criticism is devastating, so it is important that he be guided lovingly and carefully. Often parents are unwittingly cruel in making fun of the behavior or appearance of their youngsters. Sometimes parents complain about the financial burden of the adolescent in terms of the cost of food, clothes, school, and recreation, making the youngster feel guilty and unwanted. Parents' feelings about each other influence the adolescent's feelings about himself and others. If the parents love and care for one another, then the youngster learns to feel and behave this way, too. If there is constant strife and bickering between the parents, the youngster learns this behavior.

The development of the sense of identity includes the development of sexual identity as well. Although there has been recent modification of the typical male and female roles, masculine identity is still most often defined in terms of activity and achievement, whereas feminine identity is defined in terms of sensitivity and interpersonal competence. As a result, boys are often given more opportunities for achieving independence and the realization of their potential than girls. Girls have some difficulty developing their potential because of the attitudes of society. So much emphasis is placed upon preparation for marriage in the development of the feminine role that the adolescent girl's popularity with boys becomes more important than achievement. Sometimes girls do not have an opportunity for self-realization until after they have established a lasting love relationship. The search for new values and a redefinition of male and female roles have moved us toward greater equality for women and will no doubt affect the development of adolescent girls in the future.

Girls want to be whatever is beautiful, and they spend hours searching for it in movie stars, television personalities, models, parents, teachers, and peers. The right blouse or dress is an absolute essential that must be taken care of before the girl can go to school, or anywhere else for that matter. Physical appearance is a matter of real concern to both girls and boys. However, boys generally want to be whatever represents assertiveness and independence, as well as to be handsome. Sexual expression of the adolescent may range from masturbation to homosexual or heterosexual activities in an attempt to find his place in relationship to others.

Changing from a child to an adult, the adolescent must also learn to adjust to a whole new body image. He needs to come to terms with his new body—see what it is, what it can do, how to control it, and how it looks to the rest of the world. He needs to see himself as he is—not bad or ugly, but good and beautiful. He needs to see where he ends and the rest of the world begins. He needs to see himself as the child he was and the adult he is to be, in order to achieve the sense of identity necessary for healthy adjustment.

SOCIAL GROWTH AND DEVELOPMENT

Parents, teachers, other adults, and peers all exert influence on the adolescent. Next to parents, teachers have the most opportunity to exert considerable influence on adolescents. Many youngsters model themselves after teachers or other adults, such as scout or religious leaders. It is the period of hero worship and "crushes," which may provide conflict with parental values and authority. Part of the "letting-go" process for parents is to allow their youngsters to have other meaningful adult relationships.

For most adolescents the peer group becomes very influential. The amount of influence depends upon whether the adolescent sees himself as more like his parents or his peers. He makes an identification with his own age group in terms of dress, speech, manners, appearance, and behavior. He may spend less and less time at home, and more and more time with his friends. "The crowd" is usually made up of school friends, since school is where most of the social interaction for adolescents occurs, and it may consist of members of the same sex or of mixed sex. Within the crowd is the "clique," a small group of close friends. Within the clique is the "best-friend" relationship. From all these social relationships, the adolescent gains in his knowledge of himself and others. The crowd provides him with a group identity, gives him opportunities for self-assertion, and provides him with an audience and an essential source of support in trying out new roles. In the crowd he is understood and accepted because the others are like him, not like adults or parents. Best-friend relationships are important in developing a sense of identity. They are same-sex relationships, and often the two adolescents build a common identity for strength and security. It is possible in a best-friend relationship to project oneself into any number of roles and test out various possibilities in safety and comfort. Often such a relationship is the forerunner of more permanent relationships required in the development of a sense of intimacy. Boys get help from a few close friends in handling conflict and aggression, and girls get help from their close friends in handling their emotions and relationships with others. Early dating or going steady may prevent the formation of deep same-sex friendships and thus interfere with the development of a sense of identity.

Just before adolescence, boys and girls generally thoroughly dislike each other and avoid anything having to do with the opposite sex. With pubescence come covert interest, taking a quick look when others aren't noticing, and provocative, teasing behavior. Then come group activities, group dating, double dating, and pair dating. Dating at this time is more of a social relationship than one of courtship. It promotes the development of the adolescent's sense of identity. He may have considerable experience with the opposite sex before choosing a marriage partner. One danger is having sexual relations before he is ready for intimacy, which may cause him to regress in anxiety and guilt. Adolescents are ripe for romantic love because of their idealistic view of a fantasy world where everything is beautiful and harmonious and they live happily ever after. Even though there is an increase in premarital sex, the majority of girls do not engage in it. Often the boy is faced with a double standard in which he is expected to try to have intercourse with his date, but if he succeeds he may break off the relationship in disappointment over her lack of virtue.

There are a number of problems that can result from marrying too early. The young people may not have sufficiently developed their own senses of identity and thus are not able to care enough for the other's thoughts and feelings to sustain a permanent relationship. There is often a curtailment of education and aspiration, which interferes with the development of the adolescent's full potential. Children of such a marriage often do not have the benefit of stable parent models, so they may grow up with severe inadequacies in handling the stress of life.

An important part of social growth in adolescence is the development of self-direction and a sense of responsibility. The adolescent needs to experience the feelings of adequacy and accomplishment in the work he does at home and at school, so the jobs he is assigned by his parents and teachers must be seen through his eyes as important, valuable, and productive. He will develop standards of performance in accord with expectations, if he is treated with respect and dignity. If he is expected to do well, parents and teachers must have faith in him and give him the opportunity to work out his problems in his own way. A major concern for adolescents is choosing their life's work and becoming prepared for it.

Increasing self-direction includes the development of moral judgment and action. The adolescent develops his moral sense of justice from the experiences he has. He may have significant religious interactions with people or ideas that guide his search for the meaning of life. An important part of his adjustment is his concept of himself as a moral person, behaving responsibly and acceptably in his own eyes and the eyes of others and being able to control himself and the environment.

COMMON DEVELOPMENTAL PROBLEMS IN ADOLESCENCE

There are some common problems that occur during adolescence related to the many physical, emotional, and social changes that are taking place in the individual. Because of the adolescent's hypersensitivity and his great need for approval and a feeling of adequacy, these problems, if not resolved, may become major sources of stress that can overwhelm the youngster. One of these problems is the skin condition of acne, present in 75 to 80 per cent of adolescents. The primary lesion is the plugged sebaceous gland, which becomes secondarily infected. The condition, all too familiar to youngsters, is characterized by open and closed whiteheads and blackheads, mostly on the face and neck, consisting of an accumulation of fatty material and bacteria that dilates the follicular duct. The cause of the condition is the increase in hormonal and glandular secretions in pubescence, particularly those of the male hormone, androgen. Many kinds of treatment have been employed with little success. The best care is (1) not squeezing the pimples, because this can cause the lesions to spread and scar the surrounding tissue; (2) thorough cleansing of the skin surface involved, including careful expression of the contents of the lesions by instrument, not fingers; (3) ultraviolet light or sunlight in small amounts; and (4) a balanced diet, excluding large amounts of fatty foods, chocolate, nuts, and cheeses.

Another problem of adolescence is obesity, particularly in girls, who are rather desperate in their desire to be attractive. Obesity is the accumulation of an excess of fatty tissue in the body, resulting in overweight. It is caused by taking in more calories than are needed for energy requirements. Any number of factors, physical and emotional, may be involved, but what usually happens is that the adolescent is unsuccessful in his endeavors and begins to withdraw and regress. He becomes less and less involved in activities and turns more and more to food as a compensation and source of comfort. Sometimes the youngster is unconsciously assisted in the development of this problem by the overprotective parent who wishes to hold onto the child. Treatment consists not of just putting him on a reducing diet, but of assisting the adolescent in resolving his interpersonal difficulties, resuming his activities, and reestablishing his control over himself and his environment.

There are a number of problems that can occur during adolescence in the sexual sphere, but probably the most common ones are those surrounding masturbation. Masturbation refers to sexual gratification through self-stimulation. It is not a new experience for the adolescent, since it is a part of the investigative process of the child's growth and development. However, it takes on a new significance in adolescence. The adolescent has achieved sexual maturity biologically, but he is not yet ready for adult sexual relations. He has the physical desires and drives without a sanctioned way of expressing his feelings outwardly, so he turns them inward and derives sexual pleasure and relief from tension through masturbation. Also new in this stage of adolescence are the accompanying erotic fantasies, which have a preparatory effect for adult sexual relations. If he learns that masturbation is a bad and forbidden pleasure, he may suffer tremendous feelings of guilt and unworthiness, which he cannot share with anyone, especially his parents. It is important, therefore, for parents to understand and accept masturbatory activity as part of the growing-up process. The only reason to be concerned about it is if it begins to interfere with other sources of satisfaction and his progress toward adult sexual relations.

Another problem for adolescent girls is that of difficult menstruation, or dysmenorrhea. Usually the incapacitating "cramps" are related to other difficulties in the girl's adjustment to the adult female role, rather than to some physical abnormality. It is particularly important that the adolescent girl be properly prepared for the onset of menstruation. Otherwise, it can be a frightening and guilt-producing experience. She needs to be told in a matter-of-fact way how her sexual organs function and how menstruation fits into the reproductive cycle. The attitude of her mother toward menstruation will make a lasting impression on the adolescent.

A great problem for adolescents, parents, and society alike is the inconsistent, unpredictable behavior of the adolescent. One moment he wants to be held and cuddled by his mother, and the next he is embarrassed by any show of affection from her, particularly in public. One moment he is obedient and compliant, and the next he is fiercely defiant and rebellious, refusing to follow suggestions or directions from his parents. At times he is loving and respectful toward his parents, and the next minute he is critical and rejecting of them because they are ignorant and hopelessly old-fashioned. He is often generous, kind, and considerate of others, but suddenly becomes selfish, cruel, and cunning. One moment he is a likeable, affable youngster, and the next he is a threatening, riotous teenager. His behavior stems from his need to act out his conflicts and experiment with different roles, and like the pendulum, it swings from one extreme to the other before winding up somewhere in the middle. The adolescent is serious, intense, and sensitive in his actions as well, which makes it even more difficult to react to his extreme behavior in a constructive way. It takes great strength, patience, and faith for parents not to react in punitive or rejecting or ridiculing ways. It is the lot of parents, and in some cases society as well, to determine when the behavior will be allowed and when it will not be. A very important part in the resolution of this problem is how restrictions are placed on the youngster. If the restrictions are fair, honest, reasonable, and understood, then he will profit from the experience; if they are not, he will likely suffer.

Accidents are the greatest single cause of death of adolescents, the most vulnerable period being between 15 and 24 years of age, and most accidents involve cars. The automobile has become a necessity to most families in the United States—to get to work, school, stores, and essential services. The automobile has also become a status symbol in our society. Without a car, a person becomes dependent on or alienated from others and is often seen as a second-class citizen. To have a powerful car, or a sporty car, or a foreign car gives a person prestige and status and makes him popular with others. It becomes essential, then, to adolescents, especially boys, to have a car, as much for approval and esteem as for transportation. It is particularly important that the adolescent be taught safety and responsibility before he begins to drive. Most schools now have driver education classes that help youngsters learn the principles and mechanics of safe driving. Parents are in a position to teach them how to behave responsibly while driving, which means obeying rules and regulations, being courteous on the road, and knowing how to deal with emergencies. Firm restrictions must be imposed until the adolescent can handle himself in a responsible way while driving.

Unhealthy Reactions to the Stress of Adolescence

The surprising fact is that most adolescents (as well as most parents) cope successfully with the stress and problems of this stage of growth and development and go on to healthy adjustment. Some do not, however, and it is about those youngsters and the most common kinds of unhealthy adolescent reactions that we want to talk now. According to the Joint Commission on Mental Health in Children (1970, p. 372), "There is no symptom of the disturbed adolescent that does not in one way or another fit into the category of normal adolescence." The identification of unhealthy behavior follows the same process here as it does in all stages of the life cycle. If the behavior fails to accomplish its twofold goal, the satisfaction of needs in socially acceptable ways, then we say it is unhealthy. In other words, if the adolescent behaves in ways that fail to get him the satisfaction that he needs, or if his behavior is outside the boundaries of society's rules and regulations, we say he is sick and in need of psychiatric care and treatment. In 1966, there were 93 million young people under the age of 25 years in the United States. The survey of the Joint Commission showed that at least 1,400,000 of these youngsters under the age of 18 years were in need of psychiatric care.

We will discuss three major kinds of psychiatric disorders that occur in adolescence: (1) antisocial behavior, including delinquency, use of alcohol and other drugs, and sexual deviations; (2) depression and suicide; and (3) autistic behavior and schizophrenia.

Delinquency. Juvenile delinquency has become a very serious problem in our society. According to the Joint Commission, it is estimated that 11 per cent of all children in the United States will reach juvenile court by the time they are 19 years old—one in every nine youths (or one in six males). These figures are from 1966, so they without a doubt would be much higher now because of the alarming increase of crime among youngsters, especially those under the age of 15.

Delinquent behavior is defined in different ways by different authorities. For our purposes, we will define it as antisocial behavior that gets the adolescent in trouble with the law, is contrary to society's rules and regulations, and is symptomatic of underlying emotional conflict. The kind of behavior we see varies from minor crimes, such as petty theft, truancy, vandalism, and running away, to major crimes, such as auto theft, arson, burglary, and murder.

There are a number of factors that contribute to the development of antisocial behavior (see Chapter 14), but we want to talk here about those particularly related to adolescence. There are three things, among the many the adolescent has to learn, that are critical in preventing the development of this kind of unhealthy reaction. First, he has to learn to incorporate into his own personality the rules and regulations of society that act as a governor on his behavior. Second, he has to learn to postpone the satisfaction of his own needs in deference to other people or circumstances in his life. Third, he has to learn how to handle his natural reactions to frustration—hostility and aggression—in socially acceptable ways. If he fails to accomplish these all important tasks, he may continue to behave in ways characteristic of the child rather than of the adult, or he may act out his conflict in attacks upon society and wind up in difficulty with the law.

Most frequently what has happened to him results from a lack of parental love, respect, and guidance. Either the parents (particularly the father) give him very little attention or they are punitive or authoritarian in the way they relate to him. He feels unloved, inferior, and inadequate, and he covers these inner feelings with acts of bravado that are sometimes a cry for help. Very often his attempts to succeed in scholastic efforts, athletics, and interpersonal relationships fail, and he tries to compensate for this in antisocial ways. In so doing, he sets up a vicious circle of repeated failure in which he behaves in ways that get him the opposite of what he wants. Further rejection and punishment create increased frustration and anger, which in turn increase his unacceptable behavior, and so the wheel turns. Unless somebody intervenes, he is on his way to a life of crime.

Unfortunately, there are few sources of help for the delinquent youngster. The lack of success of reform schools is largely due to the continued failure of the adolescent to learn those three lessons mentioned earlier that are essential to healthy adjustment. Most correctional institutions serve only to incarcerate the young offender and more often than not only add to his problems. The answer, of course, is to find better ways of satisfying his needs and correcting his behavior. We will discuss this further in the section on care and treatment (p. 159).

Drug Use and Abuse. Another major area of social concern is the increased use of drugs by the youth of our country. It used to be that drug users were young adults from emotionally and socially deprived backgrounds. Now 15- and 16-year-olds, even 10- and 12-year-olds, are experimenting with and generally knowledgeable about drugs, including marihuana, LSD, and narcotics. Also, these young people come from all socioeconomic levels of our society—upper, lower, and middle. It is difficult to estimate the number of young drug users, but it is probably conservative to say that approximately half of our teen-agers have tried some kind of drug, including alcohol.

Many factors contribute to the development of this kind of behavior, but let us concentrate on a few major ones. First of all, we have become a drug-oriented, pill-taking society. The medicine cabinet in the average home contains over 30 drugs. We take pills to keep us awake and put us to sleep, pep us up and calm us down, increase and decrease our appetite, speed up and slow down our elimination, and stimulate and inhibit our hormonal production. We even have "The Pill," which can control the very creation of life itself. Young people are products of our society; they see what adults do and imitate them.

Youngsters take drugs for different reasons. A great many just experiment with drugs, taking them once or a few times to satisfy their curiosity, display rebellion or courage, or identify with the group. Most youngsters feel at some time that their parents do not really understand, accept, or care about them, and they may turn to drugs and one another for solace and comfort. But some young people take drugs regularly for comfort, to feel good, or to experience some of the joy and pleasure they do not have in real life. Those most likely to become addicted already have serious emotional problems, which include unsuccessful relationships with others, a fear of adult responsibility, and lack of parental love and support. These youngsters turn to drugs for a solution to life's problems, for relief from the desperate struggle to achieve, and for the solace and ease they do not find in their relationships with people. But it doesn't work; they do not succeed. Instead of making things better, the use of drugs makes things worse. The chronic drug user finds himself increasingly unsuccessful, unwanted, and alienated from others. He is outside the boundaries of social acceptance and healthy adjustment.

The youth of today have been called the "turned-on" generation. This is partly due to their inclination to take anything they can get their hands on—not only marihuana, LSD, and heroin, but antihistamines, glue, barbiturates, amphetamines, tranquilizers, cold remedies, heart stimulants, nasal inhalants, and aerosol ingredients. Recently, there has been increasing concern about the number of youngsters who have turned to alcohol. One of the factors in the increased use of alcohol is the fact that it is easier and cheaper to obtain than other drugs. Most parents drink, at least socially, and have alcohol in their homes. In addition, it is often possible for an older adolescent to buy alcoholic beverages across the counter and share them with his friends. Because of its social acceptance, the consumption of alcohol by the adolescent is much less frightening to parents, and they raise less "fuss" about it. Alcoholism has become a major health problem in the United States, with an estimated four to eight million people addicted to alcohol. Again, adolescents follow the example that parents and other adults set for them, and they begin to experiment with alcohol, sometimes at a very early age. Some of them become alcoholics, and without outside help they are doomed to a life of misery and suffering.

Sexually Deviant Behavior. Promiscuity is often a way for adolescents, particularly girls, to act out their conflicts with parents and society. Sometimes it is an attempt to achieve in sexual relations what the adolescent has been unable to achieve in social relationships—some degree of love and closeness. Sometimes it is an expression of rebellion and hostility toward the too rigid, inhibiting influence of parents or society. Sometimes it is an attempt to find themselves in relationship to others. Sometimes it is a symptom of more serious underlying emotional disturbances, such as depression or schizophrenia. One of the serious complications of sexual promiscuity is that of pregnancy in the unmarried teen-ager. Often the teen-ager is ill-prepared physically, emotionally, and socially for parenthood. Rather than receiving the love and acceptance she is seeking, she is often rejected, ridiculed, and even punished by others—both her peers and her parents.

Homosexuality is an unhealthy reaction to the stress of adolescence and is often a symptom of underlying emotional problems. Youngsters enter adolescence with a diffuse sexual orientation, and they have to move through the stage of homosexual feelings to heterosexual gratification. Teen-agers often feel anxious and guilty about their homosexual feelings, and they should be helped to accept and understand such feelings as part of the growing-up process. Many factors contribute to the development of homosexuality, including the fear of adult heterosexual relations. The youngster may retreat to relationships with his own sex if he has unsuccessful or traumatic heterosexual experiences. He may feel safe and secure with his own sex and not want to leave that source of satisfaction. He may have inappropriate or pathological role models in his parents and make an identification with the opposite sex, such as the effeminate boy or the tomboyish girl does. The adolescent needs help and guidance in developing a healthy attitude toward himself and sex in order to move in the direction of adult sexual identity.

Depression and Suicide. Probably most adolescents, like most adults, have had feelings of depression. It is difficult to distinguish between the wide swings in mood, the feelings of utter despair, that are characteristic of the adolescent's painful struggle toward adulthood and symptoms that indicate serious disturbance. However, if the degree to which the behavior interferes with his successful functioning and the satisfaction of his needs is great, then this is an indication of more serious problems than normal. It is a mistake for parents to think he will "just grow out of" the symptoms—he needs psychiatric help.

Adolescents must have socially acceptable ways of expressing their reactions to frustration, such as hostility and aggression. If they do not, they will find unhealthy ways, by turning it outward in attacks on society, such as in antisocial behavior, or by turning it inward in attacks upon themselves, such as in depression and suicide. Often in the development of depression, the adolescent suffers repeated failure because too high expectations are placed upon him, either by parents, by teachers or by himself. Achievement is a major source of satisfaction to the adolescent, from which he derives status, self-esteem, and approval. When he fails, and fails repeatedly, he falls from favor in his own eyes, the eyes of his peers, and the eyes of his parents. He develops feelings of worthlessness and hopelessness that often immobilize him. At the same time, he has diffuse feelings of anger over his inability to gain what he needs. Depression may also be a reaction to loss, real or fantasied, of a parent, of love, or of esteem.

The symptoms that we see vary from physical problems, such as eating, sleeping, and motor disturbances, to behavioral problems, such as disobedience, running away, and truancy. Often the depressed adolescent is described as moody, angry, uncommunicative, sullen, bored, or fatigued. He is frequently on the fringe of activities rather than actively involved. Usually the fact that he is in trouble becomes apparent because of a significant drop in his school performance.

Suicide is the most severe form of acting out one's aggressive and angry feelings on oneself and punishing others at the same time. The death rate from suicide rises during adolescence, so that it becomes the fourth leading cause of death late in this period. There is also a great deal of evidence that many accidents are essentially suicides, either conscious or unconscious, and accidents are the number one cause of death in adolescents. The suicidal act may be a long, thought-out decision to end a lifetime of unhappiness, or it may be a sudden, impulsive reaction to overwhelming stress. It may be a cry for help that comes too late. Whatever the forces are that cause an adolescent to take his own life, the action has a devastating effect upon all concerned. Parents of such youngsters often carry a very heavy burden of guilt and anger that may even interfere with their own successful functioning.

Schizophrenia and Autistic Behavior. There is some controversy about the development of schizophrenia in adolescence. Some authorities believe that if the psychotic episode is confined to adolescence, it is some other form of mental illness, sometimes called borderline psychosis. Other authorities believe that the roots of the illness come from faulty interactions in childhood and break through in the stress of adolescence. Still others believe that schizophrenia is a major psychiatric disorder of adolescence.

We will discuss it here as an unhealthy reaction to the stress of adolescence with roots in the past experiences of the individual.

All youngsters do not move into adolescence with the same kind of experience in the world, and they may come ill-equipped for the major struggle toward adulthood. If the individual has not successfully developed the senses of trust, autonomy, initiative, and industry, then he will not be able to develop the sense of identity required in adolescence. If he has not successfully negotiated the previous stages of growth and development, mastered the major tasks, and met the expectations, then he has not grown into a healthy, well-adjusted individual and will not be able to cope with the changes, demands, and turmoil of adolescence. If he has not learned that all in all the world is a pretty satisfying place and that he is a worthwhile, competent person, then dealing with the confusion and frustration of adolescence will be impossible for him to manage.

In the development of schizophrenia, the individual may not have learned the basic sense of trust. In his interactions with significant other people, he may have learned instead to fear and mistrust his feelings and the feelings of others. Frequently, he has experienced repeated failures in his attempts to obtain the love and approval he needs, because of the loss or rejection of his parents. As a result, he withdraws from the real world and retreats to one of his own making. This may not interfere with his development too much in the dependent world of childhood, but the demands and expectations of him in adolescence are different. He is expected to become his own person and move into the responsible world of adulthood. He is expected to accomplish the major task of adolescence, developing the sense of identity. These things he cannot do without the basic sense of trust—trust in himself and other people. In fear and frustration, he retreats further and further into his own world.

Distinguishing between autistic behavior and healthy behavior in adolescence is sometimes difficult and most often a matter of degree. In normal adolescence we see the individual interacting with his fantasy world and excluding the world around him. We also see the extremely self-centered, narcissistic behavior of the healthy adolescent, fascinated with himself and what's going on with him rather than paying attention to the needs and demands of others. However, when the behavior begins to seriously interfere with his relationships with the world and other people, then he is no longer able to satisfy his needs in socially acceptable ways and we say he is sick.

In addition to not being properly equipped for coping with stress, other things may happen to the adolescent that can make him falter and retreat from the world. Just as at any other stage of life, the individual may have traumatic experiences that simply overwhelm him, and he may not be able to react with healthy behavior. One of these traumas is the loss of a parent or significant others. Parents serve as a major source of support and satisfaction to the adolescent even while he is trying desperately to free himself from parental domination. Without that support and satisfaction he is handicapped in the adolescent struggle to establish himself as an independent person. Other traumatic experiences have to do with the lack of healthy opportunities for physical, emotional, and social development. Poverty, racial discrimination, and lack of recreational, educational, and vocational resources deprive the individual of essential experiences that help him learn to behave so that his needs are satisfied in socially acceptable ways. Physical illness or injury may further handicap him in his attempt to cope with the stress of adolescence and emerge as a whole and healthy adult.

Probably the most common psychotic reaction is that of acute catatonic schizophrenia (see Chapter 11). The symptoms vary from highly excited, hyperactive, destructive behavior to almost complete immobility, autism, and regression. Frequently, the schizophrenic adolescent suffers from severe feelings of fear, distrust, and loneliness. His distorted thinking, delusions, and hallucinations often center on sexual conflicts, good and evil, and a desire to make the world a better place to live. Fortunately, his behavior is generally not so threatening that people further isolate him, as in paranoid schizophrenia. As a result, the individual is often more successfully treated in adolescence than adulthood.

Care and Treatment

The psychiatric care and treatment for adolescents follow the general principles of care and treatment for the particular kind of reaction to stress—antisocial behavior (see Chapter 14), depression (see Chapter 12), or schizophrenia (see Chapter 11). However, there are some special areas in the treatment of adolescents that we want to discuss here. Any effective psychiatric treatment must take into consideration a number of factors, including (1) the overt symptoms in the adolescent's behavior; (2) the individual adolescent's development; (3) the peer group influencing the adolescent; and (4) the interaction of the adolescent's family. The treatment approach should be multidimensional and adapted to what the individual and the circumstances require. It should include individual, group, and family therapy in an outpatient setting, circumstances and where a structured environment is necessary. Crisis intervention should be used in acute or repetitive episodes of illness, when the youngster can be maintained at home. Chronic illness may require a change of environment in a foster or group home until some of the problems can be resolved with the adolescent and his family.

Individual Psychotherapy. Individual therapy poses some problems in the treatment of a disturbed adolescent, because it is often difficult for him to form a trusting relationship with an adult. In the first place, the therapist cannot relate positively if he is seen by the adolescent as authoritarian, "square," or in collusion with the patient's parents. Secondly, the therapist has to be able himself to withstand the challenging, rebellious, testing behavior of the adolescent. Thirdly, the therapist has to respect the adolescent as a person in his own right and treat him as such.

The first aspect in individual therapy is the establishment of rapport. What kind of person the therapist is becomes particularly important. Sometimes it is easier for the adolescent to relate to the family doctor who treats the football team than to the psychiatrist whom the adolescent sees as coming from a different world. The therapist has to be stable, consistent, and firm in his interaction with the adolescent, and at the same time caring, considerate, and flexible. It is important to treat the adolescent as the person he is. For example, it may be a good idea to see him separately and independently from the family, make appointments with him, not his parents, and keep confidential information that he does not want divulged.

Another important aspect of individual therapy is helping the adolescent understand things about himself and what is happening to him. In order to dispel fears and fantasies, he needs to have the facts about himself in relationship to the world around him. He needs to know about his body and how it functions, about his sexual desires and how to express them. He needs to know what is expected of him and how to achieve it. He needs to know how to relate to others in order to get his needs satisfied. He needs to know that he is a person of essential worth and that the world is not too bad a place to live.

The adolescent must experience therapy as something worthwhile to him; otherwise he is apt to drop out. If he sees that therapy helps him achieve certain things he wants—freedom, privileges, acceptance—then he will probably continue. Many therapists are reluctant to treat adolescents individually because of the common problem of their dropping out of therapy.

Group Therapy. Group therapy is probably the treatment of choice for adolescents because of their natural identification with the peer group. The group can provide a protected environment in which the individual can learn about his shortcomings and practice new ways of behaving in safety. Also there is a great feeling of support for the adolescent in hearing others talking about problems and feelings that he thought were his alone because he was different from the others. The experience facilitates personal involvement and the sharing of feelings. It is easier for the adolescent to open up to a group of his peers than to adults in general, or to one adult in particular, as in individual therapy. Often the therapist becomes a facilitator who encourages free exchange to get the problems out and then helps the group and the individual deal with them in a constructive way. In some cases there may be a need for structuring and limit-setting to help the individuals assume responsibility for their own behavior. With older adolescents, "rap sessions" are particularly helpful in expressing concerns, correcting misconceptions, and opening up new ways of thinking, feeling, and doing. In groups of the same sex, particularly appropriate for younger adolescents, a group leader of the same sex may serve as a role model. Also, in groups with younger adolescents, activities to relieve tensions and promote healthy social interaction may be the focus, rather than discussions. Whatever kind of group it is, it is important that the adolescent know the ground rules and preferable that he participate in the decisions about what those ground rules will be and what will happen if they are violated.

Family Therapy. Although the symptoms may be manifested by one person, the illness may stem from faulty family interaction. Not infrequently the combination of a domineering, overprotective mother and a passive-aggressive father forces the adolescent son to act out in dramatic fashion his need for acceptance, guidance, and support. In such cases, the family may be the most suitable focus for intervention and should be helped to define the problem in interpersonal terms and try to change the interaction. If the family becomes a problem-solving group, the crisis may be resolved quickly as they arrive at a rational solution. It may be necessary to combine individual and family therapy, often carried out by the same therapist, to provide continuity. It may also be effective to have parents placed in a group with other parents to help them see that others have similar problems, to share in the solution of these problems, and to develop new skills in handling their own problems.

Hospitalization or Residential Treatment. There are times when full-time, inpatient service is the desired treatment because of the severe disturbance of the youngster and the inability of the family to give him the needed support and protection. It is preferable to have a specialized treatment unit just for the adolescent, where he will receive accurate assessment, sensitive understanding, and adequate psychiatric treatment. Corrective experiences that will help him change his unhealthy ways of behaving and move in the direction of healthy adult behavior are essential. That means planning occupational, recreational, social, educational, and interpersonal activities with him that are appropriate to his level of functioning.

The residential milieu provides a variety of necessary services to the seriously disturbed adolescent. In the first place, it removes him from his overwhelming stress situation and provides him with support and protection. It presents him with appropriate, consistent, and predictable external controls that allow for regressive, dependent behavior in the acute phase of illness and help him restore his own controls as he gets better. It provides him with a variety of healthy people from among the psychiatric staff with whom he can identify and work through his problems. Residential therapy makes available the appropriate intensive psychotherapy, including individual, group, and family therapy. It also offers the adjunctive therapies mentioned earlier. Generally, the supportive nature of the staff and hospital help the adolescent resolve his problems in a short time so that he can return to his life with his family.

Psychiatric Nursing. The psychiatric nurse may be the primary advocate for the disturbed adolescent through individual, group, and family therapy in the hospital, home, or community. She may be a consultant in mental health to other service agencies, such as the schools, public assistance, or juvenile court. She may teach or supervise others in providing direct care to adolescent patients and their families. The nurse may be the most appropriate person to provide psychiatric care for the disturbed adolescent and his family, because she is generally more acceptable to them than other members of the treatment team. She is generally less threatening, less of an authority figure, and less formal. She may also seem more practical, more like the adolescent and his family, and more concerned with both physical and mental health (see p. 344).

Trends in the Treatment of Adolescents. A variety of nonresidential, community-based services for young people in trouble have been established, such as hotlines, drop-in centers, runaway houses, and free clinics, probably partly in response to the increased use of drugs by young people. These services are generally provided by youthful, nonprofessional, volunteer staff who are somehow more acceptable to troubled youngsters. They generally focus on the here and now, what the individual needs right now—a place to sleep, a hot meal, or someone to listen to his troubles.

Community mental health centers have made it possible for many youngsters to be treated at home, or close to home, rather than having to be hospitalized (see Chapter 17). It is possible to provide intensive psychiatric treatment for individuals and family members using the full facilities of the mental health center—chemotherapy, psychotherapy, and activity therapy.

Now let us look at some case examples of adolescents in serious difficulty.

Case Example No. 1

At the age of 16, John was arrested for stealing a car and sent to reform school. He had a long history of repeated difficulty with the law—at school, at home, and with the neighbors. He began stealing money from his parents when he was about six, and efforts on the part of his parents to stop this kind of behavior ended in frustration. In school, he took things from other children, especially younger ones, but always seemed to have some kind of explanation when he was confronted. Neither his father nor his mother seemed able to curb his antisocial behavior or direct him into constructive behavior.

John had one older brother, age 26, who had little contact with John because he joined the service when he was 18. Father was a mild-mannered man who left the discipline up to mother. Mother was a perfectionist, expecting great things of John, which he was never able to accomplish. She was at a loss to know how to set limits for him and usually ended up by ignoring the behavior.

At the age of 12, John and two other boys entered a neighbor's house while they were away on vacation and wrecked the place. They emptied all the drawers in the middle of the rooms, turned over furniture, and poured flour, sugar, and water on the floors and tracked it all over the house. They also stole a coin collection and some antique guns. They were arrested and sent to juvenile court. John was held in a facility for the treatment of juvenile offenders for a period of 16 months because of his previous history of difficulty. He seemed to respond to the treatment and was returned home.

He wasn't home six months when he began running around with a gang of boys who had the reputation of being tough. His parents were unable to control his behavior; in fact they were afraid of him because he had threatened to kill them if they interfered or sought help. When he was 14, he was picked up by the police for illegally entering a business place after hours and returned to juvenile court. After another 16 months he was sent home again. In less than six months he was again in trouble—this time for stealing the car—and because of his long history of repeated difficulty, he was sent to the reformatory for a two-year period.

Case Example No. 2

Sheila was 14 years old when it was discovered that she was consuming large amounts of alcohol. She had her first drink at age 12 when she and some other girls found her parents' liquor supply and had a small party. She hadn't paid much attention to her parents' drinking until then, but she began watching them as they had several drinks before dinner and at their frequent parties. At first she just watched, but before long she was draining the unattended drinks. Frequently, she passed out on or behind the sofa, and her parents would put her to bed thinking she had just fallen asleep there.

Sheila was an only child. Her parents were well-to-do, entertained frequently, and were often gone in the evenings to social affairs. Father owned his own business and worked long hours; in his free time he enjoyed being with other people. Mother was ambitious for her husband and socially inclined. Neither of them spent much time with Sheila, leaving her to the care of a baby sitter, or to her own devices as she grew older.

Sheila's schoolwork began to suffer; she could no longer concentrate in class and frequently she was physically ill and could not go to school. She lost interest in glee club and debating and seemed no longer to have any friends. She spent more and more time in her room, and sometimes her parents had difficulty waking her or getting her to eat.

One day she showed up at school obviously intoxicated. She was taken home by the counselor, who talked first to her mother and then to both parents. They decided they all needed help, so Sheila and her parents sought family counseling. It was difficult at first for Sheila and her parents to admit that drinking was a problem and face it squarely. Once they did, it became easier for them to talk together and they began to resolve other problems that had led to their turning to alcohol in the first place. After a few sessions with the psychiatrist, the family decided together to abstain from alcohol and offered support to one another in this effort. Once Sheila had the love and support of her parents, it was no longer necessary for her to drink. Her school work improved; she began to participate in activities again; and her popularity with other youngsters increased.

Case Example No. 3

Jim was 15 years old when he killed himself. He shot himself in the head with a hunting rifle his father had given him for his birthday just two days before. For the past year he had been having considerable difficulty at school and at home. He had always been a better than average student, but for some reason this year he found it hard to concentrate, and as a result his grades were going down.

Jim was the oldest of three children. His father and mother were both teachers and they put great emphasis upon academic achievement. They set particularly high standards for Jim and were extremely critical of his poor performance. His father had talked to him several times and expressed his disappointment in Jim's poor schoolwork. Lately, Jim's father had become increasingly strict with him, limiting his after-school activities and visits with other youngsters. Rather than help Jim, this had made him feel less and less successful, until he had begun to question the whole purpose of living.

On his birthday, his father had given him the rifle with the understanding that he would raise his school average one letter grade. This seemed to Jim more than he could manage, and when he flunked an English test he went home, put the gun to his head, pulled the trigger, and ended it all.

Case Example No. 4

Paul was 19 when he was admitted to the psychiatric hospital. He had joined the Air Force after his eighteenth birthday and had spent most of his time in the service at different Air Force bases in the United States. He had gotten along fairly well in the service, but his constant complaint was the lack of work to do. He seemed to have a lot of free time on his hands, and since he didn't participate much in the recreational activities available, he spent considerable time in idleness and boredom.

When he was admitted to the hospital, he was extremely suspicious and thought the food was poisoned. He had to be forcibly fed, in order to keep up his nutritional intake. At times he was extremely agitated and aggressive. He also became destructive of property at times, tearing up mattresses, throwing furniture around, and once knocking a door off its hinges. However, he never attacked other people.

Paul had been a quiet, well-behaved boy, showing a particular interest in work. It seemed as if he always had some kind of paying job. He was an average student, very conscientious, and always on time. Although he was a big, husky boy, he didn't care for sports, preferring to spend his after-school hours engaged in some form of work. He did not have many friends, except for his brother, two years younger, and they were constant companions. He did not participate in the usual boy and girl parties, but did lots of fun things with his brother.

When he was 12 years old, his mother and father began having difficulty, and there were some unpleasant arguments between them before they finally separated. Shortly after this, his father was killed in an airplane crash that looked suspiciously suicidal. The brothers talked together about their feelings, but there was little discussion with their mother.

Paul was treated at the hospital with Thorazine 100 mg. q.i.d., Stelazine 5 mg. b.i.d., and Cogentin 2 mg. daily. His mother and brother visited daily and he began to improve soon after his admission. He was discharged at the end of six weeks on Prolixin Decanoate 25 mg. I.M. q. 2 wks. and was to be seen regularly in the community mental health clinic.

According to the Joint Commission, most disturbed youngsters still do not receive adequate psychiatric care and treatment. "A whole network of diagnostic, treatment and care facilities must be available, including: a service information and referral center, physical and mental health clinics with special services for children and youth, mental health and special educational services in the schools, day-care and homemaker services with mental health consultation and supervision available, halfway houses for disturbed adolescents, residential treatment and other forms of group care centers, special child and adolescent units in psychiatric hospitals, vocational rehabilitation and protected work situations, and family counseling services."

Most of all, the Joint Commission recommends an advocacy system be set up by the Federal government that will guarantee that educational, vocational, economic, medical, and social services are provided to needy youngsters and their families. This system would assure them these basic rights: to be wanted, to be born healthy, to live in a healthy environment, to have satisfaction of basic needs, to have continuous loving care, to acquire the intellectual and emotional skills necessary to achieve individual aspirations and cope effectively in our society, and to receive care and treatment through facilities that are appropriate to their needs and that keep them as closely as possible in their normal social setting.

REFERENCES

Aichhorn, August: *Delinquency and Child Guidance,* International Universities Press, New York, 1967.
Armour, Richard: *Through Darkest Adolescence,* McGraw-Hill, New York, 1963.
Bettelheim, Bruno: *The Empty Fortress,* Free Press, New York, 1967.
Bettelheim, Bruno: *A Home for the Heart,* Alfred A. Knopf, New York, 1974.
Erikson, Erik: *Identity: Youth and Crisis,* W. W. Norton & Co., New York, 1968.
Glasser, Paul: *Families in Crisis,* Harper & Row, New York, 1970.
Greenfeld, Josh: *A Child Called Noah,* Holt, Rinehart & Winston, New York, 1972.
Greenfeld, Josh: *A Place for Noah,* Holt, Rinehart & Winston, New York, 1978.
Hart, Nancy A., and Gladys C. Deidel: "The suicidal adolescent," *American Journal of Nursing, 79* (January, 1979) pp. 80–84.
Joint Commission on Mental Health in Children: *Crisis in Child Mental Health: Challenge for the 1970's,* Harper & Row, New York, 1970.
Kandell, Netta: "The unwed adolescent pregnancy: an accident?" *American Journal of Nursing, 79* (December, 1979) pp. 2112–2114.
Kaufman, Barry Neil: *Son Rise,* Warner Books, New York, 1976.
Koehler, Mary Frances: "Child psychiatric nursing option," *Nursing Outlook, 81* (March, 1981) pp. 174–177.
Sheehy, Gail: *Passages,* Bantam Books, New York, 1977.
Vonnegut, Mark: *The Eden Express,* Praeger Pubs., New York, 1975.

Chapter 11

Schizophrenic Reactions to Stress

According to Dr. William Menninger, more people are in hospitals with mental illness at any one time than with all other diseases combined, including cancer, heart disease, tuberculosis and every other killing and crippling disease. Of all mental illnesses, schizophrenia is the most prevalent, most complex, most serious, and takes the greatest toll in human lives and productivity. It is the number one health problem in the United States. Over half of all the hospital beds in the country are occupied by patients suffering from this mental disorder. Among its victims are people of all ages—from very young children to the elderly; people of all cultures—from the highly sophisticated to the more primitive; people from all levels of achievement—from the intellectually superior to the mentally retarded; people from all races and both sexes and from all walks of life.

When this illness was first described by Kraepelin it was called dementia praecox. This name was based upon the knowledge and understanding of behavior and mental illness over one hundred years ago. It was thought to be an inherited, or genetic, organic disorder of the brain, leading to a progressive deterioration of intellectual or mental functioning, that is, dementia. In contrast to senile dementia, it was observed to begin early in life, hence it was called praecox, meaning early.

In modern psychiatry, there are still many questions about this illness, but we have found some answers along the way that have drastically changed the picture in regard to the nature of the illness and what constitutes effective treatment.

There are changes in the physiological functioning of the

schizophrenic patient, but they offer inconclusive evidence as causative agents. Rather, they may be interpreted as resulting from psychological factors. No established specific brain pathology has been found in the exhaustive post mortem studies done on the brains of schizophrenic patients.

Although the illness may begin very early in life, so early that it seems the person is born with it, there is no direct evidence that it is inherited. It is generally believed to result from early faulty relationships between the child and his parents. Further, the concept of regression has replaced that of deterioration. The schizophrenic patient either remains at an infantile level of development or returns to infantile, even primitive behavior when he is faced with severe stress later in life.

In response to recent developments in psychiatric treatment, many patients who have been ill with schizophrenia for years have returned to health and productive functioning both inside and outside of the mental hospital. Using combined physical, emotional, and social kinds of treatment, patients who were thought to be hopeless in terms of recovery have been discharged from the hospital.

The following example is characteristic of hundreds of patients who have left state mental hospitals after prolonged illness:

> A 45-year-old woman who had been a patient in the state mental hospital for twenty-five years was discharged a year ago. She was admitted to the hospital when she was a young woman of twenty, and spent the prime years of her early adult life as a patient. Her diagnosis was that of paranoid schizophrenia, and she received the care and treatment available at the time—Metrazol, apomorphine, and epsom salts.
>
> A great deal of her twenty-five years was spent in restraint and seclusion because of her violent behavior. Most of the time she was not able to have visitors, and her family and friends gradually drifted away from her. Until recently she had not been out of the hospital or even off the hospital grounds for years.
>
> She received a course of therapy with psychoactive drugs, began to benefit from more therapeutic relationships with doctors and nurses, moved to a self-care ward and participated in the various social activities offered to patients there.
>
> She visited her first supermarket a couple of years ago, and made her first visit to a major city shortly thereafter. She had never even seen, let alone ridden on, an escalator; she had never been in a large department store; she had never tasted a pizza pie; she had never smelled or smarted from the city smog; she had never heard a jet airliner taking off.
>
> One of the staff members was looking for someone to live with his elderly mother who was recovering from a broken hip. This woman fit the requirements, took the job, and has been there ever since. She visits her friends at the hospital on her day off, is happy with her work, reportedly is doing a good job, and looks and acts like a new person.

There has been increasingly successful use of psychological and social methods in the treatment of schizophrenic patients in conjunction with the primary somatic method of drug therapy. Harry Stack Sullivan and others associated with The Washington School of Interpersonal Psychiatry have made great contributions toward the use of psychotherapy in schizophrenia. Thus it is that nowadays schizophrenia is no longer considered an inherited, organic, and progressively hopeless illness.

However, there is a resurgence of an effort to find biological causes for mental disorders, and a great deal of research has been done in this area. Part of the problem is that because of the complexity of man, his behavior, and his physiology, it is difficult to distinguish between cause and consequence. There is, however, general agreement that in certain cases, there seems to be a genetic predisposition to schizophrenia, manic-depressive disorders, and alcoholism. It is likely that the cumulative effect of genetic predisposition, parent-child relationship, and social pressure produces the symptoms.

Also, there is a definite interrelationship between the psychological and biological functioning of any individual. Disturbances in blood chemistry, metabolism, and hormonal secretions can produce secondary disorders of mental and neurological function. Now we are learning about brain peptides, such as endorphins, that may be linked not only with pain but with depression, for example. There is a linkage between an upset in the body's own timing mechanism and the behavior of the individual. For example, in "jet lag," in which the body's own biological clock has not yet adjusted to the environmental clock, we often find symptoms of disorientation, and confusion. Biofeedback is one of the techniques used to help the distressed individual re-establish homeostasis by achieving a degree of voluntary control over certain body processes, such as blood pressure and heart rate.

The current emphasis on holistic healing, that is, treating the whole person rather than his physical, psychological, and social parts, has added impetus to genetic, biological, and neurological research.

DEFINITION

Schizophrenia can be defined as a psychotic disorder of psychogenic origin, characterized by (1) a lack of correlation between the thinking, feeling, and doing of the individual; (2) a severe disturbance in his ability to distinguish between reality and his own subjective experiences; (3) a serious disruption in his relationships with other people and his environment.

Schizophrenia is popularly referred to as split personality; this term often results in misconceptions about the nature of the illness. When Bleuler named and described the illness as schizophrenia, he referred to the "splitting of psychic functions," meaning the lack of correlation between the thinking, feeling, and doing of the individual. For example, it is not uncommon for the schizophrenic patient to laugh, we say inappropriately, when the situation calls for a sad or serious response. A schizophrenic patient who has positive feelings toward you may express them in negative ways. He may hit, or spit, or scowl at you as a sick or schizophrenic way of saying he likes you or that you are important to him.

We need to make a distinction between schizophrenia and multiple personality, which is a neurotic illness classed as a dissociative reaction (see Appendix B). In multiple personality, we see the existence or the emergence of distinct personalities or patterns of behavior within one person, for example, the literary classic of Dr. Jekyll and Mr. Hyde. Here, one part of the dual personality was kind, good, generous; the other was selfish, aggressive, amoral. In healthy behavior, we sometimes see a different side or facet or personality of an individual under the influence of alcohol. For example, the quiet, considerate, model husband may suddenly become a loud, self-centered Don Juan after a few drinks. We will discuss the details of the multiple personality at greater length in Chapter 15.

Every schizophrenic patient, like every individual, is both similar to and different from other people, healthy and unhealthy. He is a person with a specific kind of illness that takes on his individual characteristics, and to which he reacts somewhat differently from any other person with the same illness. Each schizophrenic patient must be considered and treated in accord with his individuality as well as his illness. However, we will discuss the similarities in the way in which the illness develops and progresses; the form that it takes in types and symptoms; and the methods of treatment that seem to be most successful. At the same time, let us keep in mind that each of these generalities must be applied to the specific person who is ill, and altered or modified accordingly.

TYPES

The common types of schizophrenia are disorganized, catatonic, paranoid, undifferentiated, and residual (see Appendix B). The process of development and symptoms are similar in all types, but there are some distinguishing features of each.

In the disorganized type, the prominent symptoms are marked incoherence and flat or silly affect. There is an absence of systematized delusions, although fragmentary, disorganized delusions and hallucinations are common. There may also be grimacing, mannerisms, and odd behavior. Characteristically, there is extreme social impairment, an early and insidious onset, and a chronic course of illness.

In the catatonic type, the symptoms may vary from extremely withdrawn, stuporous behavior to wild, destructive excitement. A patient may exhibit the most resistive, regressed, negativistic, and ambivalent behavior of all schizophrenia. However, his response to treatment is often better than with paranoid schizophrenia, perhaps because he is usually younger and more acutely ill. In addition, his behavior is generally not so threatening, and people often continue to interact with him, even take care of him, instead of avoiding or rejecting him.

In the paranoid type, the predominant symptoms are those of a suspicious, aggressive, hostile patient who suffers from grandiose and persecutory delusions, and hallucinations. Frequently, this person gets into difficulty with the law because he interacts with others in a threatening way. For example, a patient who believes his next door neighbor is poisoning his shrubs may take matters into his own hands and retaliate in some fashion. A patient who believes the Mafia are after him may repeatedly call the police for protection. A patient who believes her husband intends to kill her may take to sleeping out-of-doors in all kinds of weather.

The most common type is that of undifferentiated schizophrenia, either acute or chronic, because of the mixture of symptoms. We most frequently see a combination of withdrawn, regressed, and suspicious behavior. Common symptoms are prominent delusions, hallucinations, incoherence, or grossly disorganized behavior. However, it does not meet the criteria of any of the previously listed types.

In the residual type at least one episode of illness has occurred, but without prominent psychotic symptoms; yet the signs of illness persist. The common symptoms are emotional blunting, social withdrawal, eccentric behavior, illogical thinking, and looseness of association. It is a chronic or subchronic illness.

Occasionally, we see another combination of symptoms—those associated with paranoid schizophrenia, and those associated with depression, which we will discuss in the next chapter. This type is sometimes called schizo-affective and is most commonly seen in older patients reacting to the stress of the middle years or the process of aging. Often the presenting picture is that of depression; as a patient is treated, the depression lifts and we see the suspicious, aggressive, hostile behavior of paranoid schizophrenia.

Schizophrenia can occur at any age—childhood, adolescence, adulthood, middle age, or later life—and as a reaction to the physical or psychological stress one experiences in life. When the symptoms are evident very early in life, before puberty, it may be called childhood schizophrenia. It includes the withdrawn and autistic behavior of children who are so grossly outside the limits of normal growth and development that they are not able to participate in healthy interaction with the objects and persons in their environment.

PROCESS OF DEVELOPMENT

Every child must have his physical, emotional, and social needs met in order to maintain survival and attain security. From the way in which his needs for food, love, and belonging are satisfied, he gets the feeling that he is worthy, that he belongs, that he is an individual in his own right, or the opposite. He needs approval because his self-esteem, self-image, and sense of identity are built upon it. He develops his perception of himself and the world he lives in from the way he is treated by significant other people in his environment. If his parents are accepting, loving, and sympathetic toward him, he will develop the same attitude toward himself and others. If he is cared for gently and with respect, he develops the initial sense of trust basic to healthy adjustment and mature responsibility.

Most serious illnesses, like schizophrenia, occur in patients who have been neglected, abused, or otherwise deprived of consistent and appropriate love in infancy. Every child experiences disapproval, frustration, and disappointment to some degree in the process of growth and development, in interaction with his parents. However, if he experiences love and acceptance from his parents, he can survive these blows and even further strengthen his sturdiness. If he receives constant nagging, scolding, or criticism from his parents, he may develop the feeling that he is bad or worthless. The child who experiences ridicule, lack of encouragement, unfulfilled promises, outright rejection, and instability from his parents may develop extreme anxiety, insecurity, and sensitivity. If he experiences unconscious hostility from his parents masked with love, a contradiction in their response to his needs or distorted communication, that may make it impossible for him to determine a safe course of action. In any case being unloved or rejected or betrayed is not conducive to developing a sense of trust in adults or one's own self.

Typically in the history of schizophrenic patients, one finds that both parents have failed the child, often for different reasons. Frequently, mother is domineering and hostile while father is dependent and weak or the opposite. The child is often overwhelmed with ambivalent feelings that are extremely anxiety-provoking and destructive. For example, if the child is sensitive and overreacts, the already anxious mother may become more anxious and express her anxiety in the form of hostility toward the child. The child begins to cry and she tries to quiet him, he begins to wail or shriek and she slaps him, and they (and often even those around them) wind up in terrible turmoil. The child responds to mother's inadequacy, anxiety, and hostility with even more disturbing behavior which makes mother feel guilty, more inadequate, and even more anxious. And so the vicious circle is formed.

The child has great difficulty developing his own identity—the "me" of him, the self of his personality, the individual person he is to become. He fails to develop the sense of trust, autonomy, initiative, industry, and identity essential to successful living. He tries to remain anonymous and win approval by behaving like a baby, but this doesn't work either. He feels that his parents are bad to treat him as they do, but this makes him feel guilty, so often he believes that although his parents are bad, he is worse. His behavior fails to get him the approval he needs so badly, and as a result, he becomes very sensitive to the slightest sign of oncoming disapproval. He doesn't know who he is or what he should be or how he is supposed to behave, and he hurts all over from the repeated bruising for his efforts. He tries to find some way of relieving the frustration and hopelessness he experiences in his repeated failure to obtain parental love and approval. Finally he gives up and turns to an aloof, detached, withdrawn posture meant to protect him by maintaining a safe emotional distance. It seems to him to be the only solution, the only possibility of survival. Unfortunately, it doesn't work, as we shall see in the course of our discussion of schizophrenia.

In developing schizophrenia, the individual takes a series of steps which we call the schizophrenic process. The first step is the development of fear and distrust, the inner, subjective basis of schizophrenia. The child finds that his needs are not adequately met, and he experiences strong feelings of ambivalence as a result. He feels bad about his hostile feelings because they further jeopardize the parental love and approval which he so badly needs. He learns that it is not safe to have such feelings; they are not to be trusted; they are too painful.

The second step is to separate from himself and his environment those unsafe feelings, using the mechanism of dissociation. He withdraws his emotional investment from the environment, and as a result he feels even more misunderstood, lonely and unhappy.

In an attempt to gain some satisfaction, he takes the third step in the process and transfers his emotional interests to himself, using the mechanism of displacement. His own self-love, or narcissism, is meant to take the place of the desired thing, parental love.

Because he can no longer cope with the real world and its trauma, he takes the fourth step in the process and creates a world of his own, using the mechanism of fantasy. He gives up his place in the outside world and retreats to the inner world of his own subjective experiences.

He goes further, takes the fifth step, and replaces the real world with his own, using the mechanism of projection. Then he proceeds to interact with his own world as if it were the real one, and we see the symptoms typically attached to schizophrenia.

SYMPTOMS

Characteristic of schizophrenic behavior is the failure to externalize emotional attachment, relate successfully with others, and test one's behavior and emotions in reality; this is the core problem. There are severe disturbances in the patient's thinking, feeling, and doing. He is unable to satisfy his basic needs, and the way he goes about it is not only unacceptable but bizarre and inappropriate. Common distortions in the schizophrenic patient's thinking are reflected in the symptoms of delusions, hallucinations, and blocking. Delusions are ideas contrary to reality, based upon underlying emotions, and are not commonly held by a group of people, not previously held by the sick person, and not changed by logic. We say a patient has delusions of grandeur if he believes he is some great and important figure in history when he is not. We say he has delusions of persecution if he believes people intend to harm him when they do not. Hallucinations are sensory perceptions without external stimuli based upon underlying emotions, and are not commonly experienced by a group of people, not previously experienced by the sick person, and not changed by logic. Such perceptions may affect one or all of the senses: auditory—hearing; olfactory—smell; visual—sight; gustatory—taste; tactile—touch; kinesthetic—space and motion. Delusions and hallucinations often occur together and serve to reenforce each other. For example, a person may have experiences in life that lead him to the conclusion that other people will hurt him if given a chance. A schizophrenic patient goes several steps further. He has delusions of persecution that the Mafia are out to kill him. In addition, he can smell the gas they are shooting into his room, or taste the poison they are putting into his food, or hear them plotting against him at night.

Blocking is a sudden disruption of the thought process. It is reflected in the abrupt cessation of the individual's speech or action. To produce an idea or a thought, a person goes through a series of steps called the cognitive process—sensation, perception, attention, memory, association, and thought. In schizophrenia, there is a characteristic failure in the person's ability to put the present together with the past and come out with a logical or realistic thought or idea. It is referred to as blocking, or loosening, or disturbance of association. We see this sometimes in healthy behavior, for instance, when in reaction to stress, we suddenly stop talking because we have forgotten what we were about to say, and even sometimes what we have already said.

Common disturbances in the schizophrenic patient's feelings are reflected in the symptoms of extreme ambivalence, sensitivity, fearfulness, distrust, loneliness, and flattened, blunted, shallow, dulled affect, or apathy. Often the patient is so ambivalent that he cannot carry through with simple actions, such as eating, dressing, going to the bathroom. He isn't sure whether or not he should do or say or think or feel various things. He may not be able to make up his mind about anything. In addition, he is particularly sensitive to the unexpressed or nonverbal expressions of the other person's feelings even though he may behave with indifference. For example, disagreements among staff are keenly felt by the schizophrenic patient even though the staff may be unaware that their feelings are showing. Patients usually react to such covert feelings by increasingly disturbed behavior.

We have said the schizophrenic patient is fearful of feelings, his own and those of others. His experiences have led him to the conclusion that no matter how he feels, it will turn out not to be right. He will be hurt or disappointed, rejected or betrayed. Therefore, he does not trust himself or others. It is very difficult for him to believe the unsuccessful relationships he has had with others will not be repeated. He has no reason to think that things are different from what he believes, that the world and the people in it are not all bad. As a result of his fearfulness, sensitivity, and distrust, he suffers from extreme loneliness; he is not loved, and loves no one. He is in the world though not a part of it. He is unable to attain peace within himself or harmony with others and he is afraid to try.

Affect means sustained feeling or mood and is reflected in the emotional response of a person. The schizophrenic patient feels deeply because of his extreme sensitivity, but he cannot express those feelings because that might lead to further suffering and he cannot tolerate any more. So he keeps them locked up inside himself, and remains aloof, detached, apparently disinterested in what goes on around him. He may show little or no emotional response when such response is ordinarily expected, a condition described as flattened, blunted, shallow, dulled affect or apathy. He may laugh when the occasion calls for tears, or cry when laughter is expected, and this is called inappropriate affect.

Common disturbances in the schizophrenic patient's actions are reflected in the symptoms of autism, regression, and negativism, which result in inappropriate, impulsive, unpredictable, ritualistic behavior. Autism means thinking unduly directed toward one's self to the exclusion of reality. Autistic behavior is a kind of primitive, infantile way of behaving. Often, if a child has angry, hostile feelings about mother, he feels guilty if she cuts or hurts herself, as if he had inflicted the injury. If he has sexual thoughts or impulses which he thinks are bad, he may feel they are the cause of his misfortune or that of others. The schizophrenic patient thinks, feels, and acts in similar fashion. As a result, we often see ritualistic behavior on the part of the patient in an attempt to undo or protect against the wrongdoing. For example, a patient stands with his hands up over his head, trying to keep the world from crashing down around him. Another patient dances in great, swirling circles to get the evil spirits off his back. Still another patient carefully collects and eats bits of dirt to rid the environment of threatening forces.

Sometimes very sick schizophrenic patients or those who have been ill for a long time regress to very early levels of development and function. They may curl up in positions resembling those of the fetus. They may be incontinent, and have to be changed and toilet trained like a young child. They may have to be fed and exhibit sucking movements like those of an infant. They may have to be dressed, and display negativistic behavior like a youngster who does the opposite of what is requested of him. They may be so lacking in initiative, preoccupied, ambivalent, or apathetic, that even the simplest actions must be directed by someone else. Very often schizophrenic patients not only act, but also look much younger than they actually are. It is always somewhat startling to see a patient who has been very regressed begin to look older as he begins to get better.

Often, because schizophrenic patients do not respond in expected ways or sometimes do not respond at all, other people act in their presence as if they did not know what was going on in their immediate environment. It isn't that patients are unaware of their surroundings or others around them, because they can often recount events that occurred during their illness in great detail. However, if a person has left this world, rejected it as undesirable or unsafe as the schizophrenic patient has, then the social standards and expected behaviors do not apply and have no influence or real meaning. For the schizophrenic patient, his own world becomes reality, and his thoughts, feelings, and actions are guided by, and are responses to, what is going on there. His behavior as we see it from the outside appears to be inappropriate, impulsive, and unpredictable because we do not understand or experience life as he does in terms of his inner world. We say he lacks insight because he does not seem to realize, or at least admit, that he is sick.

The behavior patterns of life styles commonly seen in schizophrenic patients are exaggerations of the withdrawn, regressive, and suspicious patterns already discussed in Chapter 6. Because of his fear and distrust of others, a sick person becomes increasingly unsuccessful in his relationships. The more unsuccessful he becomes, the less he relates to others. As a result, it becomes more and more difficult for him to test the reality of his feelings and actions. Without this corrective feedback, his behavior becomes unrealistic. In addition, he becomes reluctant to take the chance of failing in his attempts to relate, and he draws further and further away from others, more and more into himself. He becomes more unsuccessful in his attempts to satisfy his needs, and the final result is gross interference in the organization and function of his personality. He begins to rely more heavily upon the use of the coping methods of fantasy, regression, dissociation, and projection. The resulting behavior, rather than satisfying his needs, interferes further, causes even greater distress and even more bizarre behavior. Although a person may have been sick for many years and usually has been, this spiraling disruption generally reaches a climax when there is an event of some personal significance in a sick person's life. At this point there is usually some kind of intervention by family or members of a community, which results in his receiving treatment, usually in a psychiatric hospital.

Now let us look at some actual case histories of schizophrenic patients that will demonstrate the types, symptoms, process of development, and progression of the illness as we have discussed it.

Case Example No. 1

The patient is a 25-year-old, single young man, living at home with his parents. According to them, for the past several weeks he has become increasingly uncooperative around the house, refused to go to work, wandered aimlessly over the countryside, and is preoccupied with bizarre fantasy. On the weekend before admission, the patient ran off to another state, demonstrated poor judgment by selling his car, was jailed for inappropriate behavior, and his parents had to go get him and bring him home. Upon return, his parents convinced him he should go to the psychiatric hospital and ask for admission. The admitting physician felt he should be committed so as to insure his stay in the hospital, and his father did this.

Upon admission to the hospital, he was described as haggard-looking, wide-eyed, superficially calm. He exerted considerable self-control to prevent the emergence of underlying anger and anxiety, manifested by marked tremor, pronounced facial redness and grimacing directed toward his father when discussing touchy subjects. When interviewed alone, he was calm, organized, and for the most part, appropriate at a superficial level. Bizarre ideation and loose association were evident under pressure. He felt he could predict things, was a football hero, composed songs and was a writer. He heard voices saying "there goes that Harvard boy." He considered the present difficulty to be a misunderstanding between himself and his father, not related to mental illness and not requiring hospitalization. His description of circumstances surrounding his admission was tangential. He was oriented as to time, place, person. His intellectual functions appeared intact. Physical examination and results of laboratory tests were within normal limits.

The patient was born and raised in a small town, the second child, with an older married sister. His father has a small business and makes a comfortable living. His father is a modest, meek person who communicates very little with his son, and then mainly through his wife. His mother is a domineering housewife who runs the home. According to her, the patient's sister developed normally, but the patient was always a shy, quiet, withdrawn, sensitive person. The patient feels his sister has always dominated him, and says this is the reason for his shy, sensitive behavior toward girls.

He received average grades in high school and was considered an honor student in college. In college he did very well socially, became outgoing, had many friends, and participated in sports. He feels he was happy there. He has worked for his father during the summers since he was 16. He attended church when he was a child but now says he is agnostic and that he was an atheist before. He believes in a supernatural power but he does not believe in various religions.

The patient has a poor self-image; he feels inferior, lacking in confidence, inadequate and weak. His assets are good physical health and normal intelligence. His lack of motivation and insight are his liabilities. Emotionally, he is a cold, distant person with shallow affect, and rather marked withdrawal. His relationship with his parents consisted in getting them to take care of him and make the major decisions concerning him. They were supplying his every demand, particularly his mother.

He became manifestly ill two years ago. He had functioned reasonably well as a student until then. After his rejection by a girl to whom he had proposed marriage, he became increasingly disturbed. About two months ago he became frankly delusional, withdrawn, and eventually completely disorganized. He spent a great deal of time at the beach alone, refused to work, and was very uncooperative at home, sleeping in the daytime and walking and listening to records all night. He wandered aimlessly around the countryside, being gone for several days at a time, sleeping in his car, and coming home dirty, hostile, delusional, and most uncooperative. There was marked regressive behavior; he could not take care of himself adequately, and sometimes he behaved in a silly, inappropriate fashion.

Diagnosis: Schizophrenia, undifferentiated type.

Case Example No. 2

The patient is a 48-year-old, divorced mother of two children, who has lived an isolated existence for several years. Her home recently burned down, and she was placed in a nursing home by the Department of Public Assistance because she was unable to care for herself. There she became quite suspicious, thought she was being deprived of her property and belongings, and walked away from the nursing home. She caused enough significant disturbance in the community that she was considered for a more supervised setting for treatment and evaluation. Since she refused voluntary admission to the psychiatric hospital, commitment proceedings were instituted, and she was brought to the hospital by the sheriff.

Upon admission to the psychiatric hospital, she was described as slightly disheveled. She was quite cooperative during the admission interview and examination and answered all questions rapidly in a vague, circumstantial manner. She had no awareness or insight concerning what led to her hospitalization and tended to give as a reason for commitment that her home had burned down. Her intelligence appeared to be average or normal, but she displayed an inordinate lack of sophistication about usual personal hygiene and habits. She was fully oriented as to time, place, person. She had no motivation whatsoever to be admitted to the hospital, but she did not resist. She seemed to understand that this was done to aid her, but she could in no way speculate as to what kind of help she needed. She did feel that people were depriving her of her property, but she cast this in the context of being a welfare recipient who could not own property while on welfare. She had no distinct hallucinatory or delusional behavior. Physical and laboratory examinations were within normal limits.

Not too much is known about her past history, since she is not sufficiently trusting to reveal much about herself. Apparently she completed the eighth grade but never held a job. She was married when she was 19 and had one daughter, who is now married. The child was reared by the patient's mother until her death and then was taken by a maternal aunt. The patient's husband left her after four years of marriage and got a divorce. She was married again two years later and had a son by this marriage; her second husband also left her after three years of marriage and got a divorce. Both husbands obtained their divorces on the grounds of mental cruelty. The patient's son was taken from her by court order and placed in a foster home. She maintains an interest in her son and realizes that she cannot rear him, but she is distrustful of the foster parents.

She came to the attention of the Department of Public Assistance about two years ago, and the rest of the information comes from them. She was living in an old wooden trailer, unfit for habitation, on a small acreage in the country. She had no furnishings except a kerosene stove. She slept on a bundle of rags on the floor, with one blanket for cover. She was known in the neighborhood as a recluse who distrusted people, liked to live in the woods, and roamed about in them day and night. She did not accept advice or counsel from others, had a violent temper, and would use force when angry.

She was moved into a furnished cabin in town, where she did not heat the house or use a fire to cook on. She ate out or bought prepared food. She did not bathe or wash her clothing or bedding. She wore her clothes until they were in rags and then bought new things. She had a long white raincoat which she wore constantly for several years. Her bedding consisted of one blanket. Her landlady cleaned her house when she could gain entry, every three or four months. Because of her strong body odor, she was denied use of a post office box and entrance to several stores. Recently, the house in which she was living burned down, and the landlady gave her shelter in another cabin, but said she could not stay there.

A home visit was made by a community case worker. When the worker called at the house, she was beckoned inside by the patient. The cabin in which she was staying was colder than out of doors. The patient's appearance was frightening to the worker, but at the same time, the patient herself appeared frightened and, of course, cold. She wore clean clothes but her hair was long, snarled, matted, and filled with lice. The patient stood throughout the visit, but offered the worker a chair.

Arrangements were made for commitment because the patient could not stay where she was any longer. Awaiting legal action, it was thought that a nursing home was the best solution for temporary shelter. After two hours in the home, she ran away. She was apprehended by the sheriff and taken to the general hospital under physical restraint. At the hospital, she was given sedation, a bath and haircut, and held until she could be taken to the psychiatric hospital.

Diagnosis: Schizophrenia, undifferentiated type.

Case Example No. 3

The patient is a 35-year-old railroad worker, married, father of a young child, whose wife is in the process of getting a divorce. Although he has shown signs of mental illness for a number of years, this is his first hospitalization. He became progressively disturbed, emotionally, and socially maladjusted over a number of years. He developed strange notions which appeared delusional and had a definite grandiose flavor. Socially he has become more and more withdrawn. He acted erratically and strangely, displayed much suspiciousness and secretiveness. His judgment in general matters has become progressively poor. He made threatening remarks and his behavior and attitude toward others caused them to be afraid of him. He failed to accept his wife's divorce intentions, refused to cooperate with physicians, psychiatrists, lawyers, employers, and relatives, so it was necessary to commit him.

Upon admission to the psychiatric hospital, he was described as emotionally blunted, rather distant and aloof, as well as haughty and quite suspicious. He was most evasive, vague, and circumstantial and talked about his work as a fireman on the railroad. He expressed a variety of markedly grandiose notions about his abilities and skills, and seemed convinced about his strange ideas. For example, he has been convinced for years that he was able to understand others and to predict the future by means of assorted letters which he cut out of newspapers. He has pestered relatives, family members and others with absurd schemes. He readily explained that he felt persecuted and singled out. He was oriented, his memory was intact and his intelligence average. He showed no insight whatsoever and seemed unaware of his situation and difficulties. Physical and laboratory examinations showed no evidence of pathology.

He was born to a schoolteacher mother and a father who was a conductor on the railroad and a part-time fisherman. He described his mother as affectionate but a person with whom it was difficult to communicate. While he was very respectful and admiring of his father, whom he described as an active and dynamic man, he was quite fearful of him.

The patient completed high school and began working for the railroad on a part-time basis shortly after his graduation. Due to the decrease in business, he has never held a full-time job with the railroad, even though he has worked up to the position of assistant engineer and fireman. No full-time, permanent position will be open to him for approximately eight to ten years due to lack of train runs and seniority. He also worked on a part-time basis fishing with his father. He and his father got along poorly, and on one occasion they had a violent altercation in which the patient severely beat his father.

He was married for the first time at age 22, had one child by that marriage, but was divorced by his first wife because of his violent, hostile behavior. He married his present wife approximately six or seven years ago and has one daughter, now aged six, by that marriage. This marriage is currently undergoing dissolution because the wife states that she can no longer live with her husband's threatening attitude and unpredictability.

He has had a gradual onset of delusional thinking over a number of years. He was well-known in his community as an aggressive, hostile, threatening individual. Over the last several months he has become increasingly unpredictable and disorganized, concomitant with a reduction in the number of work hours available to him and the impending divorce from his wife. His railroad foreman revealed that he was doing such things as standing behind the engineer during a train run on which the patient was fireman, sharpening his knife in such a threatening manner that the engineer was fearful of working with him. When confronted with this incident, the patient stated, "Everyone carries a knife and sharpens it; and I certainly did not mean to frighten anyone."

Just prior to admission, he became obsessed with the color orange and destroyed items of that color in his home. He also believed that there was a system of communication using a certain series of numbers through which people were trying to get in touch with him, if he could only understand it. He also felt that his wife's work was somehow tied in with his work for the railroad, and he thought this was the reason that the number of working hours available to him had been decreased. He had also questioned the parenthood of his daughter and accused his wife of infidelity. Because he had become so threatening in demeanor that he could no longer work for the railroad, and his actions were so bizarre in his family situation, a commitment was sought and obtained by his family.

Diagnosis: Schizophrenia, paranoid type.

Case Example No. 4

The patient is a 27-year-old, single young man, unemployed, living with his mother and family. He has been ill for many years and has been previously admitted to mental hospitals, once two years ago and again a year ago. He was brought to the hospital by his mother because he was unduly tense, apprehensive and tremulous. According to his mother, he became this way a few weeks prior to admission. She emphasized that he is not different mentally than he has been for a long time; in fact, he seemed more calm and reasonable than he had been prior to his previous admissions to mental hospitals.

Upon admission, he was described as physically neglected, dirty, unkept, unshaven. He is of small body build and markedly feminine in appearance. He showed marked coarse, rapid tremors of hands, arms, knees, and marked rigidity of the lower back. He complained of restless legs and during the interview, he continuously moved his feet and legs. He has been taking Stelazine 10 mg. t.i.d. (or 20 mg. t.i.d., patient was not altogether sure of the dosage), and it appeared that he was suffering from a resulting parkinsonian reaction. Otherwise, the physical and laboratory examinations were negative.

Emotionally, he had severe blunting, withdrawal, seclusiveness, lack of spontaneity and very impoverished thought processes. Patient was agreeable and cooperative; however, he seemed mildly suspicious and distrustful. He answered all questions in monosyllables, showed no signs of perspective thinking, and did not seem to have any plans about the future. He said he was totally content just sitting and watching TV all day long, and accepted hospitalization without question. He was correctly oriented and his memory was intact. His verbal skills were fair, and he seemed to be of average intelligence, if not above. He revealed no evidence of delusional thinking, explained that he had heard voices in the past but not at the present time. His lack of ambition, drive, and initiative are marked, and he seemed totally disinterested in what was going on in the world. He was without insight and markedly regressed.

Patient is the youngest of three children, seventeen years younger than his next older brother. His early childhood was described as normal by his mother. In his teens he began to show a tendency to be high-strung, nervous, and unduly shy. At age 16 he had some teeth pulled and according to mother, he has been disturbed ever since. Previously he had been reluctant to go to school, and unable to learn well because of "nervousness." He refused to go back to school after he had his teeth pulled and never went back. The patient's family has been described by various observers as "good but strange." His older siblings are unmarried. One brother is overtly mentally ill, has been described as a paranoid schizophrenic, and is considered by observers to be more sick and disturbed than the patient. The older sister is shy and withdrawn, suffers from severe asthma, but has been a clerical worker for periods of time in the past.

The patient's father, who was 55 years old when the patient was born, died eight years ago. He is described as a very shy, quiet, passive man who had little influence in family matters. The mother is a practicing Christian Scientist who impressed observers as somewhat strange. She is the organizing, dynamic force in the family, holding them together to the best of her ability. An uncle and aunt live with the family, sharing a large, old, partially-unfurnished home, and pooling their social security benefits with the mother. According to her, the family has moved throughout the United States a great deal, mainly to live in climates more suitable for the daughter's asthmatic condition. During the past eight years, the family has lived in four different states.

Four years ago the patient came to the attention of the Department of Public Assistance. At that time he was considered mentally defective and for reasons not quite understood, also epileptic. He was taken for two weeks to a hospital where he was thoroughly studied from a psychiatric as well as a neurological point of view. There was no evidence of epilepsy, no gross evidence of physical abnormalities, and a diagnosis was made at that time of chronic undifferentiated schizophrenia.

Two years later the patient became acutely psychotic. He was delusional, heard voices and felt that the dog was "saying terrible things" to him. He was admitted to a psychiatric hospital where he stayed several months and was released as improved. Approximately one year later he again became disturbed and was admitted to a psychiatric hospital in another state. At this hospital he was described as withdrawn, apathetic, lethargic, unmotivated and disinterested. He was released as slightly improved, with the recommendation to continue on Stelazine 10 mg. q.i.d., and Artane 2 mg. q.i.d. According to the patient and his family, he has taken these medications regularly since then.

He continued to show much the same behavior and attitude that he had displayed for some years. He remained withdrawn, seclusive, inactive, spent the day watching TV, doing no work whatsoever, conversed with no one, and neglected his appearance. When he began to develop marked tremors and became restless and shaky, his hospitalization was brought about by the community mental health coordinator.

Diagnosis: Schizophrenia, catatonic type.

CARE AND TREATMENT

Physical. There are two basic factors upon which care and treatment are based—the first pertains to the nature of the patient's needs and his level of competence, and the second pertains to the nature of the therapy best suited to the individual and his illness. In schizophrenia, the first kind of physical care and treatment is related to the individual patient's degree of detachment from reality. He may be so withdrawn, or regressed, or suspicious that all his physical needs have to be met for him. In other words, he may have to be cared for like an infant or a child. He may have to be fed, clothed, sheltered, and activated. For another patient whose contact with reality is intact, the physical care and treatment may consist only of providing opportunities so that the patient may take care of himself and meet his own needs. The nature of the physical care and treatment to be given is determined by ascertaining the patient's needs, assessing his ability to meet them, and providing only the amount of help that is required.

The patient may be treated on an outpatient basis, in the doctor's office or mental health clinic, or he may be treated on an inpatient basis in the general hospital, nursing home, or psychiatric hospital. If the illness seriously disrupts the patient's ability to care for himself, as schizophrenia usually does, he is most apt to be cared for in the psychiatric hospital.

The modern approach treats the acute psychiatric illness like the medical emergency that it is. The patient is usually admitted to the hospital, and treatment begins immediately so that his emotional turmoil and disorganization are relieved in a matter of hours. The somatic therapy of choice in the treatment of schizophrenia is a combination of psychoactive drugs, antipsychotic and antianxiety, which proves most effective for the individual patient. ECT may be added to the drug therapy if there are disturbances of mood or activity level in the patient's illness. Very often the treatment plan consists of two phases, intensive care and readjustment or convalescence, sometimes with a third phase of extended care or continued treatment.

Intensive care is sometimes called crisis intervention or intensive tranquilization. The patient may be given psychoactive medications either I.M. or orally depending upon the severity of his disturbance. He might be given a combination of drugs, for example, Thorazine q.i.d., Stelazine b.i.d., and a sedative such as chloral hydrate at bedtime. If the patient responds well to treatment, that is, becomes more calm and better organized, he moves into the readjustment phase.

In the readjustment phase of the treatment plan, he will be actively involved in re-establishing an effective pattern of living, learning to use medications as an outpatient would, and preparing to return home. He is expected to act in socially acceptable ways, helping to keep the ward tidy and clean, going to meals on time, taking care of his own personal needs and environment, making his own appointments, arranging for his own work and recreation, and participating in the ward government and group meetings. He is assigned a counselor with whom he makes plans regarding his discharge and who works out with him whatever problems stand in his way. He usually carries his own medications and contacts his physician for another prescription whenever he needs a refill. The length of time he stays in the Readjustment Area is an individual matter. It depends not only upon the response of the patient to treatment, but upon the living situation which confronts him as well. However, it is usually from two to three weeks. During that time he is encouraged to go home for visits, and usually goes home on weekends.

When he is discharged, in approximately one month's time, he usually continues the drug and counseling therapy, either returning to the psychiatric hospital as an outpatient, or using the outpatient facilities in his community that offer the best services to him. He may be referred to or seek help himself from the private psychiatrist, general practitioner, mental health clinic, vocational, rehabilitation or recreational centers, special education or training programs, public health or public assistance departments, or other counseling and consultation services offered by various individuals and organizations in the community.

Emotional. Emotional care and treatment of the schizophrenic patient is crucial to his recovery and centers around helping him relate more successfully with other people. Various kinds of psychological approaches are employed, ranging from psychoanalytic techniques to the "buddy system," in which one patient who is fairly capable assumes some responsibility for another patient who is less capable, like taking him for walks. The effectiveness of the treatment can be determined by how successful it is in helping the patient resolve the core problem of his illness, and how well suited it is to the individual patient's needs and his ability to meet them. In general, the treatment must help him build trust in himself and others before he will be able to invest something of himself in his environment. It must help him turn toward reality rather than fantasy for his basic satisfactions if he is to relate successfully with others. It must help him correct his distortions about himself and the world by providing him with opportunities to safely test his old behavior patterns and helping him acquire the necessary new ones to be more successful.

One form of psychotherapy in current and common use is counseling. The counselor may be any one of the traditional members of the helping professions or some of the newer members of the treatment team as discussed in Chapter 7. The counseling techniques vary according to the individual needs of the patient and the training and experience of the counselor. For example, as we shall see later, for one patient the counselor may use directive techniques, advising him what he should and should not do. With another patient the counselor may use permissive techniques, allowing the patient to decide what he will and will not do. For still another patient, the counselor may use confrontation techniques, reflecting or interpreting reality to the patient and showing him how his behavior affects other people. The way the counselor interacts with the patient constitutes corrective feedback in the patient's distorted communication system, aimed toward helping him alter his behavior or way of communicating so that he is more successful in satisfying his needs and more socially acceptable. This is sometimes called reality orientation, or reality therapy.

With a schizophrenic patient, family therapy is of particular importance and usefulness because schizophrenia is often a family illness. The faulty patterns of thinking, feeling, and doing are directly related to, and reenforced by, the faulty interactions with significant people in a schizophrenic patient's life situation. Unfortunately, it is often difficult for members of a sick person's family to admit or realize, let alone understand or seek help for, their individual contributions to the illness. It is much safer and more comfortable to isolate the illness and quarantine an individual who exhibits the symptoms of the whole family. A patient then becomes the scapegoat which protects the self-esteem or self-respect of the other members of the family. Thus, while an individual patient may be treated successfully, if he returns to the same family situation, he is most apt to have repeated schizophrenic episodes for which he requires hospitalization and intensive care.

In the treatment of schizophrenic or autistic children, family therapy is often a requirement. A sick child will often not be accepted for treatment unless the whole family, particularly parents, agree to individual, group or family therapy as well. There is not space to deal adequately here with the treatment of children and their families, so the student is referred to the following sources: Dorothy Baruch's *One Little Boy* and Bruno Bettelheim's *The Empty Fortress: Infantile Autism & the Birth of the Self.* Each contains graphic accounts of the illness and treatment of youngsters, including family and play therapy.

Social. Social care and treatment of the schizophrenic patient is aimed toward providing him with opportunities to test his behavior and acquire (in a protected environment) the necessary social skills for successful living. It usually, therefore, includes some sort of program in remotivation, rehabilitation, or resocialization.

In such programs, an effort is made to include the patient in group activities which will help him express himself in more socially acceptable ways. Patients may participate in the problem-solving of the total patient group such as occurs in ward government meetings, or they may participate in various social activities in small groups. In many psychiatric hospitals, even schizophrenic patients who have been ill for a long time have learned to function fairly effectively in such small groups. These groups usually meet regularly with a particular member of the staff, often the nursing staff, and they direct their meetings toward some shared experience. Their focus may be upon verbal expression, and they might discuss current events, or their own problems, or great books. The group may be action-oriented, and go for walks, or rides, or shopping tours. Again, it might be educational in purpose and may have classes in good grooming or cooking or sewing.

A frequent method of promoting socialization and rehabilitation is through the use of O.T. and R.T. activities which are planned for individual patients, small groups, or the patient group as a whole. For schizophrenic patients, particularly, various arts and crafts may be useful in helping them express their feelings in acceptable ways other than verbal, such as painting, sculpting, and drawing, among others. Games also offer an avenue of expression that may be safer for the fearful, regressed, or suspicious patient than talking or person-to-person interactions.

One of the common problems with schizophrenic patients is the lack of successful work experience. Assignment to a job or to a training program leading to a job is often an extremely important part of the patient's rehabilitation and return to society as a contributing member of the group. Many psychiatric hospitals offer job assignments within the hospital community—in the laundry, in one of the offices, on the farm, on one of the maintenance crews such as painting, plumbing, electrical work, gardening, or in the cafeteria or kitchen. Also, there are many programs where patients live at the hospital and do work for the community, either in sheltered workshops, or going out into the community to work, or staying at the hospital and doing various kinds of piecework that are brought in.

All of these forms of treatment must be directed toward restoring optimum functioning in the individual patient, and this may be a very high level indeed for some and a very low level for others. Great effort is being made to prevent, and in many cases correct, an unhealthy or unrealistic dependency of an individual, particularly the chronically ill schizophrenic patient, upon the hospital. Such dependency may be a protective device for the patient by assuring him temporary safety and anonymity, but it is sure to lead to a helplessness and hopelessness that make life insecure and unbearable.

Let us look at the care and treatment plans and progress reports for each of the previous case histories.

Case Example No. 1 (See p. 177)

The patient was admitted to the psychiatric hospital and put on the following medications: Navane 10 mg. t.i.d., Navane 20 mg. h.s., Artane 2 mg. t.i.d. He was assigned to a counselor and an activity group. For the next four days he showed increasing activity, restlessness, and inappropriate pacing, packed and unpacked his clothes, and repeatedly washed his hands. Although his behavior was somewhat inappropriate, he responded well to verbal confrontation and seemed to be able to relate in a satisfactory manner.

Two days later he left the hospital without permission. He was returned to the hospital, and his medication was changed to Prolixin Decanoate* 50 mg. I.M. q. 2 wks. He had some difficulty adjusting, refused to take his medication on a couple of occasions, and became acutely psychotic. This seemed to convince him that he could not get along without medication, and he offered no resistance after that. About two weeks later, he asked to go home so he could go to work.

He has resolved some of his difficulties, offers no resistance to medication, and in fact seems convinced that he needs it. He has decided that there are more advantages to staying at home than living alone, although he is still angry at his parents for having committed him. He is well-organized, his associations are tight, and he does not seem preoccupied with any delusional ideas. He appears to have settled down in a fairly well-organized state, in which life is difficult but tolerable, and he will exist at a moderate level of social adjustment.

It is recommended that he have weekly conferences at the mental health clinic, and that he continue on medication for the time being. Family therapy is also recommended for his parents to help them stop the pathological dependency.

Case Example No. 2 (See p. 178)

The patient was admitted to the psychiatric hospital and put on the following medications: Thorazine 100 mg. h.s., Stelazine 10 mg. q.i.d., and Cogentin 2 mg. q.d.

Because of her extreme suspiciousness, she was not assigned a specific counselor, but rather treated by all staff with a passive friendliness. This allowed her to initiate the interaction with others; however, staff were always available to her. It was necessary for the nursing staff to be directive and insistent about her personal hygiene.

---

*This medication has the advantage of being an injectable drug which is given every two weeks, so that the patient can be maintained on drug therapy even though he is out of the hospital or somewhat unreliable in taking his own medication.

Although she showed improvement, it was felt that she needed further hospitalization and social training before she could return to the community on her own. She was transferred after two weeks of hospitalization to a self-care ward on medications: Stelazine 10 mg. b.i.d., Cogentin 2 mg. q.d. She was assigned to a vocational education group and given ground privileges. She walked away from the hospital grounds several times without permission, and it became obvious that she could not care for herself or assume the responsibility required of residents on a self-care ward. Therefore, she was transferred to a ward with more direct supervision, where she is beginning to make some progress toward caring for herself in socially acceptable ways.

Case Example No. 3 (See p. 180)

The patient was admitted to the psychiatric hospital and started on Loxitane 25 mg. b.i.d., Cogentin 2 mg. q.d. After eight days, it was felt that he remained basically unchanged except that he seemed more relaxed and at ease. He was put on Loxitane 25 mg. t.i.d., Taractan 100 mg. h.s., Cogentin 2 mg. q.d.

After a few days, he was cooperative and agreeable and had ceased the verbal expression of delusional material. He adjusted fairly well; however, throughout his hospitalization he remained distant, suspicious, and at times unpredictable and threatening to other patients. He was assigned a counselor, and it was felt that he might respond best to an authoritarian, directive approach. Therefore, decisions were made for him, and he was told what to do and what not to do and what results he could anticipate from certain of his actions.

It was initially made clear to the patient that he must take his medications, and that if he was not able to take his own, he would have to remain in the hospital until he could. He was further told that if he did well, the amount of medication would be gradually reduced, but that he would probably remain on some medication for a long time. He was then placed on self-medication. He was verbally resistant to taking his medications, but when he was checked out on several occasions, it was found that he was taking them rather faithfully. At times when he would miss one dose, he would even report this to his counselor. When he complained bitterly about having to take his medications, he was told he only had to take them, he didn't have to like them, and his complaints stopped.

Next he was desirous of a home visit, which was allowed under the condition that he was not to frighten people and not go near the offices or shops of the railroad. He did well on his first home visit according to reports. After two more successful home visits, he was discharged and referred to the mental health clinic. It was recommended that he remain on medication and find a job.

Case Example No. 4 (See p. 181)

The patient was taken off all medications, started on antiparkinsonism medication, and within a day recovered from his marked shakiness. He displayed the same attitude and behavior that he had for some time. He was assigned a counselor and a vocational group, but he showed no interest or initiative in what went on around him. He would sit in front of the TV all day long if allowed to do so, and was observed to be hallucinating when it was not on. He was cooperative and would do whatever he was asked or told to do. He was started on Moban 25 mg. b.i.d.

At the end of two weeks, it was felt that he needed direction and stimulation, so he was encouraged to participate in various O.T. and R.T. activities. He would do this but in a passive way, and then only if he were encouraged.

It was suggested that he be exposed to socialization and motivation efforts, with the hope that it would help him to mature socially to a point at which he might leave the hospital and lead a halfway meaningful existence. It was not considered suitable to release him to his home, as he would just return to the same withdrawn, seclusive, inactive, and asocial behavior pattern and life style that he had been practicing for so many years. So he was transferred to a halfway house.

He participated for approximately one year in a coeducational remotivation program, and was seen for counseling on a weekly basis. At the end of that time he appeared less withdrawn, more spontaneous, and was willingly taking part in recreational activities. He was friendly and had developed a friendship with another resident. His personal appearance was usually good, although he had to be reminded to bathe. He obtained a job in the community working in a restaurant, where he received his board and room plus $50.00 per month.

NURSING CARE AND TREATMENT

The nursing care and treatment of schizophrenic patients follows the same pattern as that outlined in the preceding section; however, since there are some functions and responsibilities peculiar to nursing, let us consider some of the general and specific applications.

Effective nursing is directed toward the accomplishment of a threefold goal in the care and treatment of all patients: (1) to help the patient maintain survival by relieving his suffering; (2) to help the patient attain security by seeing that his needs are met; (3) to help the patient regain his health by combating the disease. There really is no such thing as the "care of the schizophrenic patient" because each patient and each nurse is different. How a particular nurse interacts with a particular patient must be guided by the kind of person the patient is, the kind of person the nurse is, their particular relationship, and the particular life circumstances in which they find themselves together. There are many ways in which to help a patient, not just one right way and all the others wrong ways. It is not humanly possible for us to discuss all the ways that might be helpful, even if we knew what they were. However, we can talk in general about some of the facts that might be used as guidelines in the care of schizophrenic patients, keeping in mind that these generalities must be adapted to the individual patient's care and treatment plan.

The schizophrenic patient has the same needs as any other person—physical, emotional, and social—and his problem centers about his inability to satisfy those needs in healthy ways. The kind and amount of nursing care required is the difference between what his needs are and how capable he is of meeting them. If he did not need some help in this endeavor, he would not be considered sick, he would not be a patient, and nurses would not be taking care of him. The real art and science and skill in nursing involve determining the nature of the help required and possessing the ability to provide it.

Physical Care. In meeting the physical needs of a schizophrenic patient, there are some common problems that deserve comment. The important point to remember is that the nursing care should do more than just meet his needs for food, clothing, shelter, and activity. Effective care is given in such a way as to promote a patient's self-esteem and respect for others. If his physical needs are met gently and with respect, he develops, like a child, the essential sense of trust, and it is from the lack of trust that his illness has stemmed. If a patient's needs are met consistently by a warm, accepting, affectionate parent substitute (the nurse), then he may begin the perilous journey back to reality and health.

It is particularly important for the nurse to see that his intake and output are sufficient to maintain good health. If he is suspicious, he may not eat or drink for fear of being killed. It may be necessary for the nurse to provide food and fluids in ways that lessen his fear of attack. Food packaged in individual containers may help him accept the fact that it has not been tampered with—cartons of milk, cereal, soup; cans of vegetables, meats, prepared foods; packages or cans of desserts. Foods that come in their own containers may also be used—oranges, bananas, eggs, nuts. On the other hand, eating the same food that everyone else is eating may be the best and most realistic solution of all. For the very regressed or withdrawn patient, it may not be possible for him to tolerate solid food, let alone feed himself. He may have to be fed, by tube or by mouth, with a special formula, usually consisting of milk, reenforced with a protein supplement.

Elimination is often a problem, particularly with a regressed or withdrawn patient. He may be so preoccupied that he is not aware of having to void or defecate. He may have to be taken to the bathroom at regular intervals in order to avoid incontinence. His inactivity, or liquid diet, or tranquilizing drugs may lead to constipation, or impaction, or obstipation, unless he is toileted regularly, checked frequently, has some roughage in his diet, or receives cathartics or enemas as his condition requires.

His needs regarding clothing and shelter center chiefly around warmth and protection from environmental hazards. Again, if he is very preoccupied with his own thoughts, his physical health may be of little or no concern to him. In such cases, the nurse may have to see that he is appropriately dressed for warmth, appearance, good taste, personal hygiene, and so on.

For a very regressed or withdrawn patient, it may be necessary for the nurse to activate him. He may stand all day in one spot, or remain in bed, or sit in his favorite chair in the dayhall, unless someone actually engages him in some kind of physical activity. It may be a walk, or a game, or some kind of work, or exercises that provide the necessary activity to maintain healthy body function.

It is of particular importance that the nurse be observant of a patient's physical condition. Often, either because of his preoccupation or his inability to communicate verbally, his fear of attack or lack of trust, he will not be able to tell the nurse when he feels physically ill or when he injures himself. Very withdrawn patients may suffer serious injury such as fracture without reporting it or complaining of pain. Again, as with small children, with whom it is up to the observant mother or father to discover that they are sick or hurt, the alert nurse will discover what is wrong with the patient by observing some malfunction, such as limping, or cradling his arm, or holding his head stiffly. If a patient is warm, flushed, perspiring, the alert nurse may check his TPR to see if there is some other evidence of infection. Sometimes a patient just doesn't look as if he feels well, and the nurse needs to find out what the trouble is rather than wait for the patient to complain or show other symptoms.

The nurse plays a crucial role in the drug therapy of all patients. First she must know and carry out the rules and regulations that govern preparing, administering, observing, reporting, and recording the medications that patients receive in their care and treatment. With schizophrenic patients, she must be concerned as well with the way in which she is relating with the patient while she is carrying out her functions and responsibilities in regard to medications. She must know further how to modify and adapt procedures to meet an individual patient's needs, and still practice nursing safely and efficiently.

Let us take the five common rights to remember in giving medications—the right patient, medication, dosage, time, and route—and see how they may apply to a schizophrenic patient. First, there may be some difficulty in identifying the right patient. A very sick schizophrenic patient may not be able to give the nurse his name, or he may say he is someone else, or a patient next to him may say he is someone else. He may not have any identification bracelet or I.D. card or name tag on his bed, because he is often not in bed. What should be done? The best thing is to have a nurse who knows the patients give medications. If the medication nurse does not know the patients, the safest thing may be to have someone accompany her who can identify them.

Because of different individual reactions to the psychoactive drugs, it is very important that the nurse observe and report the effect of the medication on the patient so that the doctor may change it if it is indicated (see Appendix C). The dosage may be too much or too little for the individual patient, and the report of the nurse's observations will help the physician adjust it to make it most effective. If the nurse adheres too strictly to the correct time for medication, it may hinder rather than help her to be more efficient. Sometimes, with a suspicious or apprehensive patient, it is better to try to give the medication later, rather than to insist and have to force the medication upon a patient before he is ready to take it willingly. With psychoactive drugs, the physician may order the medication both by mouth and intramuscularly, so that the nurse is often in the position of determining by which route the medication should be given. For a suspicious, negativistic, uncooperative patient, the I.M. route may be best until such time as he is more amenable to suggestion. For an agitated, excited patient, I.M. may be the best route because it gets faster results.

When schizophrenic patients are receiving psychoactive drugs, there are some aspects of care to which the nurse must give particular attention. In the intensive care phase, for example, she must carefully check intake and output to see that the patient does not become dehydrated. She must also be sure that the patient is not developing retention of urine or feces. She must check the patient's vital signs frequently to see that there is no rapid drop in blood pressure that might lead to hypotension, shock, or other cardiovascular complications. She must make certain that other complications do not develop during the intensive care phase such as pneumonia or infection. She must be alert to both the desirable and undesirable effects of the drugs being administered. The desired effects of tranquilizers in the care of schizophrenic patients are the relief of anxiety and its effects, and the restoration of the patient to more calm, reasonable, organized behavior. The most common side effects are seen in the extrapyramidal symptoms of parkinsonism (muscular rigidity, masked facies, drooling, tongue rolling, lip smacking, peculiar gait) and CNS dysfunction (motor restlessness, involuntary muscle movements, muscle weakness and fatigue). The nurse needs to watch for jaundice, which would indicate blood dyscrasia or liver damage; paling or cyanosis, which would indicate anemia or shock; rash or photophobia, which would indicate a sensitivity to the drug; behavioral changes such as somnolence or agitation; or idiosyncratic reactions.

Emotional Care. The way in which a schizophrenic patient is cared for physically conveys to him whether or not the nurse cares about him. Again, as with children, he learns that he is loved, that he belongs, that he is important as a person from the way in which significant people in his environment treat him. If he is to turn toward reality, he must be convinced that reality is safer and more desirable than the refuge he has chosen, and that takes some effort. Everything and everyone around him has to work toward that goal if he is to turn outward instead of inward.

The usual procedure is for one member of the nursing staff to try to make personal contact and establish an emotional bond with the patient. Sometimes there is a certain intangible, non-verbal feeling or attraction that occurs between two people, and that is usually the beginning of a relationship. The point is, once a fearful, distrusting patient can learn to trust another person, he can learn to trust still others. It is the foot in the door, the chink in the armor, the beginning of the long road to healthy adjustment.

The nurse uses her own healthy personality, her own self, as a major method of treatment. That means she may need some help herself, through counseling and guidance, so that she does not hold expectations and make demands upon a patient which are unrealistic. It takes great strength and determination and faith for the nurse to meet with rebuff after rebuff from a patient. She is tempted to give up and seek out someone else more rewarding. She has to keep in mind that this is not like relating with healthy people in the usual give-and-take manner, where she can walk away from unsuccessful interactions. A patient has suffered his own rebuffs, and he has to test to see if the nurse can be trusted. Does she really care? Can she really help? These are questions which a schizophrenic patient must have answered if he is to reach out again toward other people in his environment.

When a withdrawn, regressed patient begins to improve, he has bad days in which he returns to the old, sick ways of behaving. Again, if the nurse is not careful, she will feel (and therefore communicate) disappointment, anger, or hurt by such recessions, and turn away from (and therefore reject) the patient. This kind of interaction only helps to prove to the patient that he was right all along—people are not to be trusted—and it serves to reenforce and justify his flight into a world of fantasy.

A suspicious, paranoid patient is often keenly sensitive to the other person's shortcomings (perhaps because he is so aware of his own) and sore spots. It is not unusual for him to pick at the nurse in his own sick way until she responds to him. If her response is filled with anger and the bitterness which sometimes comes from deep pain, it will serve to again reenforce the patient's own pain and distrust. Sometimes a patient satisfies his own need for importance by putting the other fellow down—he raises his own low self-esteem by attempting to lower the nurse's. To let him win the argument is to let him be the important person that he needs to be, and that is what the nurse would do for someone she loved, like her husband, daughter, or best friend, as well as her patient.

With a schizophrenic patient the nonverbal methods of communication are often most important. Often a sensitive patient can sense phoniness or dishonesty in the nurse even if she is unaware of it herself. Schizophrenic patients are especially sensitive to contradictory messages or faulty communication. They tend to put more stock in the intent of the message than in its content. (Many healthy people do just the opposite—they rely more upon what is said than what is done). It is extremely important that the nurse be consistent with a patient. Consistency means that the nurse in her interactions with the patient means what she says, and says what she means, rather than saying one thing and doing the opposite.

Sometimes people use the expression "tender, loving care" (often abbreviated to the meaningless letters TLC) as if it were an antidote for all the ills of the world. It is true that all patients, and particularly schizophrenic patients, need all the tenderness, love, and care they can tolerate if they are to return to health, or for that matter if they are to survive at all. But whether or not that care is helpful depends to some extent upon who gives it and a great deal upon how it is given. A schizophrenic patient is fearful, distrusting of the very love that he yearns for, and he must learn how to accept it and depend upon it if he is going to tolerate it at all. It is like feeding a person who has been gradually starving to death for months. It is not likely that he will be able to swallow or retain or digest a sumptuous feast, no matter how well prepared the food or how well intentioned the server. The food has to be offered in small, concentrated, easily-digested form until he adjusts to a healthier existence. Furthermore, he cannot be expected to be grateful or appreciative or return the compliment until he is sufficiently well-nourished to be able to function in that kind of reciprocal fashion. Likewise, if the love or compassion comes from someone who is not important to the patient, he is not likely to be very responsive. In fact, he may resist strongly any attempts to care for him by people who are either unimportant or threatening to him for whatever reason. It is best, then, that the love and affection that a patient so sorely needs comes from the most appropriate person in his environment, and comes in a form which he can accept.

Social Care. If a patient is to relate successfully, he needs an opportunity to test his behavior in a variety of social situations. Obviously, he cannot do that until he is ready, until he is sure it is safe to do so, and until he has gained enough strength and security in his ability to deal with others. What he has developed in a relationship with one person can then be transferred to other people individually and in groups.

Social interaction can occur on many different levels and it does not always require highly sophisticated people or equipment. For example, group sings are often a successful and spontaneous way of communicating socially. Sometimes all that a very sick patient can tolerate is just the presence of other people. Just to let the nurse sit beside him may require great effort and represent a degree of improvement for him. Just to attend a ward meeting, even though he doesn't say anything, may be a significant social interaction for him. Various activity therapies may be available to all patients through organized programs, but often, and especially for very sick patients, the nurse may provide these activities for a patient. Occupational therapy such as arts and handicrafts may be used to help a patient express himself and may also contribute to the welfare of the patient group through the making of things for the ward. Recreational therapy, such as pingpong and pool are often available for the use of patients who are not able to attend functions off the ward. Classes in homemaking and good grooming are often held on the wards by nursing personnel.

Ward meetings where patients participate in making decisions about problems in group living offer a protected setting for social interaction. They foster the participation of patients in assuming responsibility for themselves and others. They offer patients an opportunity to practice coming to grips with the small problems before they are faced with the big ones. They encourage patients to test their old patterns of behavior and acquire new ones that may be more successful in helping them interact in a socially acceptable way. Often the nurse can encourage a patient to attend the meetings or bring up particular problems or even accept an office in the group.

Frequently, a common job or project can serve as a vehicle for establishing a relationship with a very withdrawn, regressed, or suspicious schizophrenic patient. It might be popping corn together, or cleaning house, or sanding a table, or anything that allows the nurse and patient to be together, joined by some common purpose and sharing a cooperative effort.

Very often the nurse is engaged in teaching a schizophrenic

patient social skills that he has lost or never had. It may be encouraging a mute patient to talk again. It may be taking a chronically ill patient in to town to shop. It may be showing a patient how to do the latest dance steps. It may be teaching an illiterate patient to read and write.

Schizophrenia is the most severe, complex, and common disease of our times. It is a functional psychosis which results in severe disturbances in the individual's ability to think, feel, and act in an organized and appropriate way. The roots of the illness lie in early life experiences when in interaction with significant other people his basic needs are for some reason unmet. He reacts with ambivalence, fear, and distrust to the repeated failure of his relationships, and this causes him to withdraw his emotional investment from his environment and transfer it to himself. In a desperate attempt to compensate for the resultant loneliness and to meet his needs somehow, he creates his own world and interacts with it instead of the real one.

The most common symptoms of the schizophrenic illness are extreme ambivalence, autistic behavior, interference in association, and disturbed affect. His bizarre behavior is a gross exaggeration of the withdrawn, regressed, suspicious behavior patterns discussed in Chapter 6. Although he may have been ill for years, often some significant event in his life requires intervention by outside forces, family or community, and he is propelled into treatment, usually in a psychiatric hospital.

Each care and treatment plan is based upon the needs and abilities of the individual patient and is directed toward the resolution of the core problem of the schizophrenic illness: failure to (1) externalize emotional attachment, (2) relate successfully with others, and (3) test behavior and emotions in reality. Somatic therapy consists primarily of the use of antipsychotic tranquilizers, which relieve a patient's anxiety and symptoms. Psychotherapy usually takes the form of counseling and therapeutic relationships, which help him correct his distorted perception of himself and others and the resulting faulty interactions. Social therapy involves some kind of resocialization, remotivation, rehabilitation, or readjustment program where a patient learns the social skills necessary for him to live productively.

REFERENCES

Adelson, Pearl Yaruss: "The back ward dilemma," *American Journal of Nursing, 80* (March, 1980) pp. 422–425.

Arieti, Silvano: *Interpretation of Schizophrenia,* Basic Books, New York, 1974.

Arieti, Silvano: *Understanding and Helping the Schizophrenic,* Basic Books, New York, 1979.

Baruch, Dorothy: *One Little Boy,* Dell Publishing Co., New York, 1964.
Bell, Norak: "Whose autonomy is at stake?" *American Journal of Nursing, 81* (June, 1981) pp. 1170–1172.
Bettelheim, Bruno: *The Empty Fortress: Infantile Autism & the Birth of the Self,* Free Press, New York, 1967.
Boyajean, Anne: "Fighting despair," *American Journal of Nursing, 78* (January, 1978) pp. 76–77.
Chiland, Colette: *Long-term Treatment of Psychotic States,* Human Sciences Press, New York, 1977.
DiFabio, Susan: "Nurses' reactions to restraining patients," *American Journal of Nursing, 81* (May, 1981) pp. 973–975.
Fitzgerald, F. Scott: *Tender Is the Night,* Charles Scribner's Sons, New York, 1960.
Green, Hannah: *I Never Promised You a Rose Garden,* Holt, Rinehart & Winston, New York, 1964.
Hyde, Alexander: *Living With Schizophrenia,* Contemporary Books, Chicago, 1980.
Kesey, Ken: *One Flew Over the Cuckoo's Nest,* Penguin Books, New York, 1976.
Krauss, Judith Belliveau: "The chronic psychiatric patient in the community—a model of care," *Nursing Outlook, 80* (May, 1980) pp. 308–314.
Wisser, Susan Hiscoe: "When the walls listened," *American Journal of Nursing, 78* (June, 1978) pp. 1016–1017.

Chapter 12

Manic-Depressive Reactions to Stress

The major affective disorders compose the second group of nonorganic psychotic disorders and include bipolar disorder and major depression. Bipolar disorder is subclassified as mixed, manic, and depressed, and major depression is subclassified as single episode or recurrent. (See Appendix B.) In the bipolar disorder, mixed, the patient displays symptoms of both manic and depressed behavior or alternating periods of manic and depressed behavior. In the bipolar disorder, manic, the patient currently displays manic behavior. In the bipolar disorder, depressed, the patient is currently in a major depressive episode but has had at least one or more manic episodes previously. Major depression means the patient has had one or more depressive episodes but has never had a manic episode. Schizophrenia is a primary disturbance of thinking, with accompanying characteristic disturbances in feeling and doing, whereas the affective psychoses are primarily disturbances in feeling, with accompanying characteristic disturbances in thinking and doing.

We have said that affect means sustained feeling, emotion, mood, or emotional response. A person's feelings are reflected in his thoughts and actions. For example, if a person feels unhappy, "down in the dumps," his thoughts are likely to be gloomy and pessimistic and the whole thought process is slowed down. If he is feeling happy, his thoughts are apt to be gay and carefree, and the production process is speeded up. His actions are correspondingly slow, preoccupied, and dull, or quick, alert, and bright.

Sometimes when a person feels unhappy, he tries to shrug off the blues with increased productivity or forced gaiety, or increased social activity such as cleaning house, laughing it up, or going out on the town. We see something similar in the affective disorders, except that they are so exaggerated as to be abnormal and unrealistic. It was first thought that they were caused by an evil spirit or demon taking possession of the sick person, and later they were attributed to some physiological disturbance in the body. As a result, treatment often took the form of punishment or purgatives to get rid of the demon or toxin in the body. As with schizophrenia, as knowledge of behavior and mental illness increased, understanding of the nature of these illnesses and what constitutes effective treatment has changed with it.

In modern psychiatry, it is generally agreed that these affective illnesses are related to a person's psychological reaction to his experiences in life; hence they are called functional psychoses. They result from faulty perceptions that a person has of himself and the world he lives in, the ineffective use of coping methods, or the overwhelming stress of a particular life situation. The physiological changes in the functioning of the sick person may be either a result of the feeling disturbance, such as in manic-depressive psychosis, or a reaction to the physical changes in the body, such as in involutional psychosis.

If the illness occurs in the middle years when the person is going through the menopause or change of life, it is sometimes called involutional psychosis. At this time there are changes in the physiological functioning of the body, particularly involving the endocrine system. However, it is generally agreed that it is not the person's physical condition alone which causes the psychotic symptoms, but his reaction to the physical and psychological stress of this period in his life. For example, if a woman interprets the loss of reproductive function which accompanies menopause to mean that she is less likely to be loved or respected or accepted, this period represents a serious threat to her survival and security, and adds stress to her life. If the stress is too much for her to master, or if her methods are not effective, she may develop the symptoms of involutional psychosis. Although the presenting symptoms are usually those of depression, we may also see the symptoms of the suspicious, hostile, paranoid patient.

Let us take another life situation, pregnancy, which may represent a serious threat to the survival and security of a particular person. If the physical and psychological stresses of having a baby are more than the woman can master, then we may see the development of psychotic symptoms. Again, the reaction may take the form of psychotic depression or paranoid schizophrenia. This reaction is sometimes called postpartum psychosis, or psychosis associated with childbirth.

One more example may help to clarify the complicated mixture of physical illness and psychological forces at work in mental illness. An individual who has a serious physical disease such as cancer faces a threat to his survival and security. Again, if the resulting stress is more than he can master, we may see the development of psychotic symptoms, which may be diagnosed as psychotic depressive reaction or psychosis associated with physical condition, and may take the form of psychotic depression or paranoid schizophrenia.

Since the process, symptoms, and treatment for these psychotic reactions to stress, such as involutional psychosis, psychotic depressive reaction, and psychoses associated with physical conditions, can be understood in terms of psychotic depression and paranoid schizophrenia, we will not discuss each of them separately. We will discuss bipolar disorder and major depression because they are representative of the major affective disorders and are the second most common illnesses among the functional psychoses found in actual practice.

DEFINITION

Bipolar disorder may be defined as a psychotic disorder of psychogenic origin, characterized by (1) marked disturbances in mood, which result in the inappropriate emotional responses of elation or despair; (2) severe interference in ability to think and act in accord with reality, resulting in over- or underactivity; (3) serious disruption in relationships with others and the environment.

Since most people have experienced feelings of joy and sadness in their lives, it is often easier to understand and accept this kind of illness than schizophrenia. However, although it may be similar, it is not to be confused with healthy behavior. We are talking here about ways of behaving that are contrary to realistic or appropriate thinking, feeling, and doing. For example, if a person feels sad when someone he loves or depends upon dies or leaves him for some other reason, it does not mean that he is mentally ill or psychotically depressed. However, if his feelings seriously interfere with his daily functioning, if they continue over a prolonged period of time, or if his grief reaction is otherwise out of proportion to the life situation, then he may, indeed, be suffering from a psychotic depression. On the other hand, patients with the illness of manic-depressive psychosis may not have had any particular life situation which accounts for the illness. Instead it usually represents the person's faulty reaction to the ordinary stresses of life, which he handles in unsuccessful ways.

We need to make a distinction between major depression and the neurotic disorder which is called dysthymic disorder or, sometimes, neurotic depression. In disthymic disorder, there is not the same degree of disturbance in the person's mood or inappropriateness in his emotional responses. He does not lose his ability to function in accord with reality, and he is usually able to maintain relationships with others and his environment. In the development of dysthymic disorder, we usually see the evidence of previous neurotic symptoms in the individual, such as excessive anxiety, hypochondriasis, or neurasthenia, which we will discuss in some detail in Chapter 15. Also, in dysthymic disorder there is generally an identifiable precipitating life situation in which the individual experiences the loss of an important source of satisfaction in the form of a person, job, money, status, body organ, or physical function.

TYPES

Bipolar disorder is divided into three major subtypes—manic type, depressed type, and mixed type. The process of development of all three types as well as major depression is similar, although the symptoms may be different. We will mention the prominent features of each type briefly, and then discuss psychotic depression at some length, since it is the most common form seen in both bipolar disorders and major depression.

In the mixed type, we see alternating, severe swings of mood from elation to despair, combining the features of the manic and depressive types in the same person or illness. If we let line AB in Figure 10 represent an individual's normal or healthy mood, affect, or emotional response, then in the mixed type of bipolar disorder we see peaks above and valleys below the line, following each other, sometimes with few or no healthy or normal periods in between.

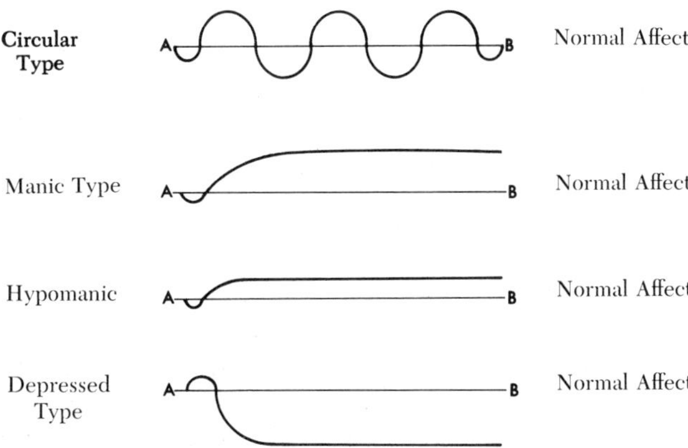

Figure 10. Disturbance of affect in manic-depressive psychosis.

In the manic type, there is an abnormal increase in the individual's feeling, thinking, and doing. He stays above the line in mood, or has a brief episode of depression, which often goes unnoticed, and then swings up into a prolonged mood characterized by elation and euphoria. In thinking, we see the characteristic symptoms of rapid association and flight of ideas. In doing, we see the characteristic symptom of overactivity.

The term hypomanic is used sometimes to describe hyperactive people, although more popular terms are "hyper" or "high." The term hypomanic means above normal in mood, thought, action, but below the level characteristic of mania or the manic type of bipolar disorder—hence the use of the prefix hypo- (less than).

It is important to remember that each person has a different level of functioning which is characteristic of him. That is to say, every individual has moods, thoughts, and actions which are a part of his particular life style. As long as they help the individual satisfy his basic needs in socially acceptable ways, we call them healthy or normal, and this allows for a great variety of individual levels of healthy functioning. To judge the degree of health, then, one must know not only what is normal for most people but what is normal for a particular person. For example, if a person who is characteristically a good listener suddenly becomes talkative, it may indicate that he is having some emotional problems. For another person who is characteristically a great talker, silence may be an indication of difficulty. In addition, what is overly talkative for the first person may be under-talkative for the second person. Normal and abnormal, healthy and unhealthy, behavior and functioning must be measured on a general as well as an individual continuum rather than on the level of functioning per se.

In the depressive type, both in bipolar disorder and in major depression, there is an abnormal decrease in the individual's feeling, thinking, and doing. He stays below the line in mood, or has a brief episode of elation which often goes unnoticed, and then dives down into a prolonged mood characterized by sad, morose, despondent feelings. His thoughts are slowed down and center on his unworthiness, sinfulness, and guilt. His actions are slowed down so that it may be difficult for him to complete even simple activities of daily living. This is the classical picture of retarded depression.

Sometimes we see a slightly different picture that is sometimes called agitated depression. This person stays below the line in mood, which is characterized by sad, morose, despondent feelings. His thinking is usually distorted by illusions and delusions that center upon his unworthiness, sinfulness, guilt, and body functions. His activity level remains the same or is increased so that we see restlessness, pacing, wringing of the hands, and so on. It is this kind of depression that holds the greatest threat of a successful suicide because the individual is capable of acting out his despair and following through with his impulse to end it all.

PROCESS OF DEVELOPMENT

The person who develops bipolar disorder experiences early in life repeated failure to measure up to the expectations, first, that his parents have of him, and then, that he has of himself. All people experience hostility or anger in response to such repeated frustration, but this individual finds these feelings frightening, intolerable, and wrong. He feels that he is bad or sinful to feel as he does. He turns these hostile, angry aggressive feelings inward and punishes himself for feeling as he does. Not only does he manage to punish himself, however, but he punishes as well the incorporated world and the people in it.

He develops an early sensitivity to any situation which challenges his competence or creates a feeling of doubt. When his parent's expectations are higher than he can reach, and his own internalized standards and expectations are more than he can manage, he establishes a pattern of failure. As a result, he repeatedly expects more of himself and others than it is humanly possible to accomplish. He fails, and others he depends upon fail him; his needs are not met, he feels angry, he feels bad for feeling angry, he punishes himself for it, and he feels even worse. He develops a sense of inadequacy and rejection accompanied by strong feelings of resentment and expected punishment. Any situation, then, in which he experiences high expectations engenders self-doubt, which in turn touches off the sequence of failure, rejection, hostility, guilt, self-punishment, and the resulting depression.

The core problem of bipolar disorder or major depression is the way in which the person handles his hostility and the aggressive feelings that result from threats to his security. He doesn't necessarily have any more hostility than any other person, but he tends to accumulate more because of his inability to accept such feelings in himself and cope with them directly. To him, it is not a natural response to threat; it is instead an unacceptable part of himself that he must deny, disguise, and atone for. His method of atonement is self-punishment in the form of feelings of despair, unworthiness, guilt, and sinfulness.

The depressed person develops a picture of himself that is unhealthy and distorted. He feels that he is inferior, inadequate, unworthy. If a person has been told all his life by significant other people that he is no good and his experiences confirm this, he tends to believe it. Because he has so little self-acceptance and self-approval, he tends to be overly dependent upon others for acceptance and approval. At the same time he resents having to be so dependent on others, and this adds to the accumulation of his hostility, which he dares not admit, let alone express. It obviously isn't safe to bite the hand that feeds you. In addition, the worst kind of security is that which rests too heavily upon the actions of other people. They seldom respond consistently with the kind of acceptance and approval that the other person needs so desperately. Successful human relations require an ability to give and take that this person usually does not possess. He may form relationships that are successful as long as the other person allows him to be dependent.

Very often in the history of patients who develop this illness, we find a background in which the child is brought up rather strictly. In such an environment he is apt to develop an oversized conscience which keeps him under such tight control that he is allowed very little freedom in expressing or satisfying his negative feelings or basic impulses. With such a rigid, domineering, punishing conscience he may have far fewer outlets or sources of satisfaction than the average person. This, of course, adds to the possibility of failure, frustration, and self-doubt and sets off the sequence which produces depression.

He usually carries a high degree of anxiety because of the conflict between his desires or needs and his expectations or conscience. He wants to be taken care of, loved, accepted, and approved of, but he wants also to be important, successful, and above all adequate, too. He strives for recognition and success, and when he fails, as everyone does on occasion, he punishes himself by feeling hurt, sad, disappointed. Those feelings interfere even further with his success and add to his failure and need for self-punishment and thus, the vicious circle is formed.

Arthur Miller's play, *Death of a Salesman,* is a classic picture of this illness. A father who had great ambitions for himself and his sons was repeatedly denied success. He could not admit his failures to himself and his family, punished himself and his family for not being more successful, and finally wound up by committing suicide.

The primary method of adjustment in depression, self-punishment, is healthier and more acceptable than the methods of withdrawal and projection used by the schizophrenic patient. The depressed person continues to interact with his environment; in fact, he tends to control it and the people in it with his behavior. There is nothing more controlling or punishing or threatening than the behavior of a moody person who is periodically depressed. All those in the family and even the environment try to alter their behavior accordingly. They try to please him, or cheer him up, and think up activities to help him prove his adequacy, or demonstrate their love for him. The ultimate in control, punishment, and the expression of hostility and aggression is the threat of suicide. It is a terrifying and powerful weapon that leaves family, friends, and community feeling bereft and somehow guilty if it results in death.

An interesting thing about the development of this illness is that the individual usually incorporates sufficiently healthy aspects into his personality that he may manage, with the right life situations, to live a fairly successful life. The illness tends to occur, later in life, in reaction to the stress of a particular adult stage or as an internal combustion of accumulated failure and hostility. Then we see the characteristic symptoms of psychotic depression.

SYMPTOMS

The core problem of the illness is that feelings of aggression and hostility experienced in response to threat are turned inward upon the self in a destructive manner. Life situations in which the patient experiences self-doubt touch off the chain reaction of failure, rejection, hostility, guilt, self-punishment, and depression.

The behavior patterns or life styles commonly seen in manic-depressive patients are exaggerations of the aggressive patterns already discussed in Chapter 6. Whether the patient turns the behavior inward upon himself or outward upon his environment, it is still aggressive, only the target is different. Directing the aggression outward in the form of manic behavior and inward in the form of depressed behavior can and sometimes does occur in the same person in the circular type of manic-depressive psychosis. Many people feel that this illness is closer to health than other psychotic reactions because the patient and his symptoms are closer to social acceptability. They are not so bizarre, distorted, covert, or foreign as those in other kinds of mental illness.

Manic type. We seldom see the manic type of the illness in clinical practice, but we need to know the symptoms of the manic type because it is the other side of the coin of the depressed type, which we see most often. Manic behavior is sometimes explained as an attempt on the part of the patient to throw off the yoke of an unbearably punishing conscience, or a desperate attempt to ward off the throes of depression, or a symbolic effort to devour the environment so as to eliminate its threats or keep it under control. All of these explanations seem plausible, even probable, when one observes a manic patient in action.

The disturbances in feeling are demonstrated in the symptoms of elation and euphoria. Elation means transcending or exultant joy or happiness. The patient often finds everything uproariously funny, even the most serious or tragic of events, including those in his own life. His conversation and actions are often full of jokes, puns, witty sayings. Sometimes we see rhyming and neologisms (words, or combinations of words, that he makes up himself), word hash, or word salad. In some instances, it is difficult not to join him in his high good humor and thus stimulate him further. At other times, his laughter and boisterous hyperactivity are so inappropriate that they are sources of irritation and fatigue, and sometimes result in outright rejection or punishment from others.

The distortions in thinking are reflections of the disturbance in mood—delusions, illusions, flight of ideas. The patient has grandiose delusions that are often wish fulfillments meant to compensate for his failure and inadequacy. He has success and wealth and fame in abundance. He is not just rich, he is a billionaire. He is not just a successful businessman, he is the head of the biggest corporation in the world. He is not just well-known, he is constantly hounded for his picture, autograph, or endorsement.

Illusions are defined as misinterpreted sensory perceptions of external stimuli, based upon underlying emotions. We find illusions common in healthy as well as unhealthy behavior. For example, if a person is home alone at night and afraid of burglars or intruders breaking into the house, he may misinterpret the sounds of the night, or the house creaking, as the approaching steps of the expected burglar or intruder. He may misinterpret the changes in light as shadows of his unwanted guest. Optical illusions are common in healthy behavior and are the basis of a magician's success. "The hand is faster than the eye" and a person does not actually see what he thinks he does. The most common example of optical illusion is the sight of water on the highway ahead when there is none, a misinterpretation of external stimuli. Because of the angle at which the light rays strike the receptors in the eye, the sensation is incorrectly perceived. There are as many descriptions of an accident or crime as there are witnesses at the scene. People are influenced deeply and unconsciously by their emotions, which color all perceptions of reality so that each person experiences the same situation differently because his feelings are different.

The manic patient interprets all his sensory experiences in the light of his elated, euphoric mood. What he perceives is not only rose-colored but is related directly to himself. For example, he misperceives the friendliness of others and interprets it as adoration or love or adulation for him. He hears someone else being praised and assumes the conversation is about him.

Flight of ideas means moving so rapidly from one subject to another that one thought or sentence is not completed before going on to the next, so that communication may not make any sense at all. This may deteriorate into word hash or word salad—that is, words thrown together without any connection that is apparent to the outsider. Not only does a patient make rapid associations but he may also incorporate what he is receiving from his environment at the same time, so that there are often irrelevant references to people, objects, events around him interspersed in his conversation. In the thought process he may have difficulty attending to the business at hand and screening out extraneous stimuli. With such a limited attention span, it is often impossible for him to carry out or follow through with one activity or idea at a time. He may be bombarded with stimuli, internal and external, and unable to decide which to ignore and which to respond to. If he tries to respond to them all, the result will be that he responds to none adequately.

His overactivity may give rise to a number of symptoms and problems to be overcome in caring for him. He may rush headlong into his environment with little ability to control or direct his actions. As a result, we may see the direct expression of basic impulses which have not gone through the refining process of social acceptability. He may swear, use obscenities, express sexual desires and biological urges openly. His impulsiveness may become destructiveness with little provocation. He may tolerate restrictions poorly and become suddenly irritable, insulting, rebellious under imposed restraint. He may be into everything around him—including other people's possessions and conversations.

Because of his increased activity, inability to attend, little attention to reality, and the lack of ability to control and direct his own behavior, he may seriously neglect his personal hygiene. He may have to be fed, taken to the toilet, bathed, and put to bed like an infant. Food, fluids, and elimination may need particular nursing attention so as to prevent dehydration, loss of weight, and physical illness. Stimulation may have to be reduced, and sedation given to provide for adequate rest, because he can become exhausted easily from his increased activity level.

Depressed type. In the classical picture of depression, sometimes called retarded depression, a patient's functioning in all areas is below normal—thinking, feeling, and doing. The symptoms of the feeling disturbances are those of extreme sadness, despondency, despair, guilt, unworthiness, inadequacy, and inferiority. His self-punishment may be so severe that he cannot allow himself any pleasure or satisfaction, no matter how simple. Everything may appear black and bleak; he may feel hopeless and helpless, regardless of how near or far that perception is from reality. He may dread the punishment that he is sure he deserves and apologize repeatedly for causing others to suffer also or for even being alive. He may feel that he is a drag to his family, a millstone around his wife's neck, a bother to the nurses who care for him. He may feel that nobody likes him because he is not fit or deserving of the time, effort, or attention of other people.

As in manic behavior, the distortions in thinking are reflections of the disturbances in mood—delusions, illusions, or retardation. His delusions may also be grandiose, but they reflect the opposite feeling. He may be convinced that he is the worst sinner in the world or that nobody has ever done or thought or felt the terrible things he has, or that no one could be so bad or guilty or unworthy as he is, or that even his mother, wife, or dog cannot love him.

His illusions, too, reflect the depths of his despair. He may hear the steam pipes rattling in the night and he says, "Do you hear that, they're making a coffin for me in the basement." Another patient may become upset or distressed and he feels that he is the cause of it. He may see the nurse frown and thinks that she is angry with him. He may misinterpret everything around him in terms of himself and his own low mood.

His whole thought process may be so retarded, slowed down, that he is only able to manage the simplest of thoughts—this is called poverty of thought. It may take great effort for him to produce any verbal response, and then it may center around his hopeless, helpless feelings about himself. He may go over and over the sins of his life, his faults, his unworthiness, indulging in the process called rumination. (The ruminant animals such as the cow are so named because they chew their food over and over again. In a similar fashion a depressed patient may chew his hopeless ideas over and over.) He may not be able to attend to other things because he is so preoccupied with his own terrible thoughts. His delusions focus upon his extreme (grandiose*) worthlessness, and the malfunction of his body organs (somatic).

Again reflecting his depressed mood is the underactivity of the depressed person; all his actions may be slowed down. He may be so depressed that it is difficult for him to move. He may sit or stand or lie in his bed for hours, doing nothing, not moving or talking. He may look worried and worn out, sad and lonely, with everything sagging or hanging down. The physiological function of all body systems may be slowed down—digestion, circulation, respiration, elimination, body temperature, and so on, may all be affected. He may eat, sleep, and dress poorly, and need assistance with all the activities of daily living. The satisfaction of his physical needs is often seriously hindered because of his inability to take care of himself and because of his suicidal ideas. Despite his lack of activity, the continued strain of anxiety and tension may cause extreme fatigue and even exhaustion.

---

*Grandiose in the sense that he believes he is the greatest sinner, the worst person on earth, and his misdeeds are of great significance to others.

In agitated depression, the disturbances in feeling and thinking are similar, but the difference from retarded depression lies in the function of doing. Rather than being slowed down to a level of underactivity, his doing is increased to a level of overactivity. A patient may be restless, pacing up and down, wringing his hands, crying, picking at his fingers, and so on. Often a patient is in frantic, almost constant movement—hence the term agitated. He may be possessed by the feeling of impending doom or disaster and is close to panic, unreasonable terror impelling a person to blind, frantic action. He may be negativistic and hostile without provocation. It is this kind of depression that often ends with suicide.

Sometimes in the process of treating the patient with retarded depression, the first response we see is an increase in his activity level after only a few days of treatment. He may still have feelings of despondency and despair and delusions of worthlessness and guilt, but he may have enough initiative and motivation restored to successfully carry out a suicidal attempt. It is usually the threat of suicide and the helplessness and frustration of the family that bring this patient into treatment, particularly in the psychiatric hospital.

Usually in affective disorders the patient has recurrent episodes, particularly of depression. He may be treated psychiatrically either in the hospital or on an outpatient basis, or he may recover spontaneously without psychiatric treatment. His chances of recovery for the particular episode are good. However, the episodes tend to come with increasing frequency and duration, particularly if he does not receive psychiatric treatment. If he is treated just for the acute episode and has no followup care, he does not have an opportunity to work out the underlying problems and make the necessary corrections in his way of life.

Now let us look at some actual case histories of patients with manic-depressive psychosis which demonstrate the types, symptoms, process of development, and progression of the illness as we have discussed it.

Case Example No. 1

The patient is a 49-year-old married woman without children. She has displayed depressed, hypomanic, and manic behavior for years. She went on shopping sprees, buying expensive musical instruments and wigs, among other things, had a telephone answering service installed in her apartment, consulted real estate agents regarding the purchase of new houses. Her husband was unable to pursue his work because he had to stay home and look after his wife. He persuaded her to take a trip to the psychiatric hospital to look it over, and she entered the hospital voluntarily.

On admission she was dressed conspicuously, and as she was interviewed, she walked and gestured in a grandiose manner, her costume jewelry rattling. She appeared to be above average in intelligence, her memory was unimpaired, and she was well oriented. Her thought processes were accelerated, her mood was euphoric, and her speech and motor activities were increased. She denied being mentally ill and was somewhat reproachful of her husband for keeping her in mental hospitals; however, it was easy to persuade her to sign a voluntary admission. Physical and laboratory exams were negative.

The patient's mother apparently did not enjoy her domestic duties, including raising her children, with the result that her husband divorced her. The patient, her mother, brother, and sister lived with the maternal grandmother for some years. Mother worked during the day, and the patient was primarily responsible for herself and the other two children during that time.

Patient entered the university at age 17. She was financially unable to join a sorority and this made her feel inferior. To compensate for this, she started to date a man who provided her with a chance to take part in social activities off campus. She was given a conditional grade in English composition which had always been her best subject. This hurt her to the extent that she left the university and eloped with her boyfriend. They were married for about ten years. When she learned that he had been unfaithful, she left him and obtained a divorce.

She found a job as a clerk working for the government. After about six years at this job, she met her present husband who was still in the service. They were married for about two years when he got out of service; they both obtained government jobs and worked at the same installation for about six years. They asked for and obtained a transfer out of the country; however, they stayed for less than a year because the patient got sick, and it was necessary for them to return to this country.

According to the patient's husband, she had her first mental breakdown twenty years ago, shortly after the divorce from her first husband. Approximately fourteen years later, she had a depressive episode which necessitated their returning to this country. She has been in and out of private and state psychiatric hospitals ever since, that is, for the past six years. Her husband states that when the patient is in her manic stage, she is obsessed with the idea that she must become a business and financial success, and when she is in her depressed stage, she is helpless and clinging to him.

Diagnosis: Bipolar disorder, mixed type.

Case Example No. 2

Patient is a 35-year-old married man with no children. He was admitted to the psychiatric hospital following a period of disturbed behavior which seemed to develop after the death of his father four months ago.

On admission, the patient was described as a physically well, normally intelligent man, who throughout his life has tended to dramatize daily occurrences for the benefit of his wife and associates and has consciously nurtured the idea that he is a temperamental artist and genius. His goals have been high and inconstant, and few of them have been attained. Four months ago, under the stress of his father's death and plans for a new position, he developed euphoria, restlessness, mild overactivity, sleep disturbance, and distractability.

As a child, he had nightmares and was described as a daydreamer. He did not talk until age three and bladder control was not achieved until seven years of age. He completed high school and entered college with the intention of majoring in chemical engineering. He discontinued because of an asthmatic condition which was aggravated by his work in the lab. He later entered a school of music which he attended for three years. He did some postgraduate work in a conservatory of music. His work has been that of a musician, including orchestra leading, organizing, arranging, and teaching. He played in orchestras on various ships, and was the bandleader on a round-the-world cruise. He organized his own dance orchestra, and was, for a time, successful. He enjoyed and fostered the reputation in the community of the "mad maestro." In the years that followed, he suffered a number of reverses. Characteristic of his activities was that of surrounding himself with a group of novices, teaching them to play the necessary instruments, and with burning energy, molding them into a fairly respectable musical organization only to have the band disintegrate because of financial troubles.

He married his wife ten years ago and the union has been a fairly happy one despite his tendency to become infatuated with young female students. He even brought a number of them home with the idea of teaching them about life and thereby improving their musical artistry. His wife has always excused his actions on the basis of his musical genius and temperament and what she regarded as an instability beyond his control.

Two years ago he was forced to seek employment other than in the field of music. He got a job as a recreational supervisor working for the government and entered into this with characteristic drive and efficiency which ultimately exceeded the bounds of normal, just prior to admission. Following his father's death four months ago, he became overly religious and expressed the idea that he had some special mission to carry on for his father. He began to work day and night, often sleeping as little as two hours in twenty-four, and started a forty-day fast.

Diagnosis: Bipolar disorder, manic type.

Case Example No. 3

Patient is a 49-year-old married woman with no children who comes to the psychiatric hospital for the second time. She was first admitted three and a half years ago, and was hospitalized for about a month at that time. Her husband reports that she had been doing reasonably well since her discharge. However, during the last six weeks, she had been very agitated, excitable, and afraid of almost everything. She had obtained some medication from her physician and seemed to improve for about a month. The last few weeks she had been getting worse until she could no longer do her housework.

On admission, the patient was described as a very obese, white-haired lady who looked about 70 years old. She appeared bewildered, frightened, and spoke in a whispering, monotonous, little-girl voice. She was well-oriented but appeared to have difficulty concentrating. She constantly referred to numerous somatic complaints and body preoccupations. She expressed the desire to get rid of her fears so she could go home very soon. It was difficult to engage her on any other subject except her own preoccupations. She appeared to have poor judgment and no insight. Her affect was predominantly depressed. Physical exam showed ankle edema and mild shortness of breath on exertion. EKG revealed an incomplete right bundle branch block. Chest x-ray revealed moderate cardiomegaly without pulmonary congestion.

Little information is available concerning the details of the patient's early life. She was born in Norway, came to the United States as a child, and grew up on a farm. Her parents were hardworking and poor. During adolescence, she was described as shy, withdrawn, timid. She obtained an eighth-grade education, doing average work in school. Throughout her earlier life, the family maintained close social and personal ties with Norway; as a result, most of the people she came into contact with were of Norwegian descent.

She married her husband thirty years ago. He is also Norwegian and several years older than the patient. He is retired and financially independent, the landlord for several small apartments. He made his living before retirement as a fisherman. Throughout their marriage they have maintained many Norwegian customs within their home, had no close friends, and depended exclusively upon each other. The patient has always had a tendency to be nervous and tense, to worry excessively, to be introspective and self-observant. All of such behavior is described by her husband as being "normal." One of the mainstays of their relationship has been the patient's ability to keep a clean, neat house which lives up to the expectations of her husband. Over the past couple of years, because of her increasing age and fatigue, the patient has found housework more and more difficult. For this reason they moved recently into a trailer home.

About 28 years ago she was hospitalized in a private sanitarium for several weeks because of a "depression." At that time, she made a suicidal attempt, taking lysol, which she still feels guilty about. She described her symptoms as those of severe anxiety, fears, and feelings of sadness and hopelessness. She lost her appetite, could not sleep or concentrate on her housework. She became agitated and extremely worried. She recovered completely after two months and did well until three and a half years ago, when she was admitted to the psychiatric hospital because of insomnia, agitation, restlessness, confusion, and preoccupation with guilt feelings. She responded well to psychoactive drugs and after two weeks was discharged from the hospital to the community mental health center.

About six weeks ago they moved from their home into a newly purchased trailer home. She became increasingly irritable and agitated, a condition she described as "being excited." This hampered her attempts at housework, interfered with her sleeping pattern, and made it difficult for her to live up to the expectations she set for herself to be an adequate housekeeper and wife. Her inability to function adequately led to guilt feelings and ruminative preoccupation with feelings of dissatisfaction concerning their new trailer home. She began to spend long periods of time sitting and staring, feeling guilty over housework that needed to be done, and incessantly worrying over small details. Eventually, she was unable to talk rationally with her husband, and this resulted in the recommendation by the family physician that hospitalization be considered.

Diagnosis: Bipolar disorder, depressed type.

Case Example No. 4

Patient is a 51-year-old unmarried school teacher. This is her second admission to the psychiatric hospital, and she returned because of increased feelings of depression. A year ago she was discharged from the hospital to a nursing home, and after four months she went to work in a religious school. Apparently she did well until two or three months ago when she began to become depressed and would not eat or take fluids correctly. She returned to her brother and sister-in-law's and they brought her to the hospital.

Upon admission, the patient stated that she had lost hope and admitted suicidal thoughts and somatic delusions. She was fully oriented, with normal-to-above-average intelligence. Her attention span was decreased, memory slightly impaired. Her appearance and affect were those of depression, and she was negativistic and hostile. She had a fair amount of insight to come to the hospital voluntarily for treatment. She has had a colostomy for the past two years following surgery for cancer. Eye exam revealed glaucoma for which she has been taking medication for 15 years.

Patient was raised by what she described as God-fearing, hardworking parents. She has a brother eight years her senior. Her early childhood she described as pleasant. She was introduced very early to the idea that one didn't get any place without hard work. She made average grades in school, went on to college, and got her teaching certificate. She failed Latin in high school, but went on to become a language teacher and taught Latin. She held one teaching position for 17 years and another for 10 years. Her previous episodes of depression have occurred while she was in teaching positions in which she felt overworked and unable to cope with her classes.

This is her fourth depressive episode in the past ten years. The first time she became depressed in a stressful work situation she became insomniac, anorexic, and guilt-ridden. She felt there was no alternative but to take her own life, so she slashed her left wrist, which left her with a deformity. She was hospitalized, treated with antidepressant drugs, and did well following her discharge. She became depressed again approximately three years later, again in relationship to increased stress in her work situation. She was hospitalized again, treated with antidepressants, and returned to teaching. Three years ago she lost her job as a teacher, and went to live with some missionary friends in Mexico. She became increasingly tired, and it was discovered she had cancer of the colon. She returned to this country for surgery, and went to stay with her brother and his wife while she was recuperating. She felt she was a burden to them so she went to live with a friend, but she felt she didn't belong there either. She became increasingly depressed, with insomnia and anorexia, and worried about her ability to teach and her relationship with God. She was admitted to the psychiatric hospital and treated successfully with antidepressant drugs, discharged to a nursing home, and, four months later, went to work in a religious school. She was relieved from her position by a "better teacher" with more experience. She became increasingly depressed, returned to her brother and sister-in-law's home, and they brought her to the psychiatric hospital.

Diagnosis: Major depression, recurrent.

CARE AND TREATMENT

The treatment of the major affective disorders must be directed toward the cause of the feeling disturbance. It is, therefore, likely to be a combination of the physical, emotional, and social approaches that we discussed earlier in Chapter 7. To be effective, care and treatment must take into consideration the particular person and his individual reaction to the illness. In the emergency situation, somatic therapy may be the treatment of choice to provide immediate intervention and thus prevent the sick person's attack upon himself and others in his environment. However, unless the patient has emotional and social treatment as well, he is apt to suffer again and again from episodes of illness with the same symptoms. Very often the patient is treated for the acute attack in the hospital; he responds quickly, is discharged, and fails to follow through with the aftercare that has been recommended. As a result, he frequently returns to the hospital with a relapse, sometimes many relapses.

We will discuss the care and treatment of the depressed type of affective disorder, because it is the most common form of the illness in clinical practice and because it incorporates all the different kinds of care and treatment employed in treating the major affective disorders.

Physical. The physical care and treatment of the depressed patient are related first of all to the slowing down of all body processes. For example, satisfying his basic need for food may be a real problem because of the slowing down of his digestive system, his lack of exercise, and his suicidal ideas. It may be necessary to give him a stimulant such as Dexedrine, to increase his activity and also to elevate his mood. He may be so retarded and helpless that all of his physical needs have to be met for him, and he has to be cared for like a small child—fed, clothed, housed, and activated. He may require medication to aid in the elimination of waste products from the digestive tract in the form of a mild laxative such as milk of magnesia or Dulcolax, or a stool softener such as Colace. And he may also need additional vitamins, either by mouth or by injection, because of inadequate food intake, such as multi-vitamins or vitamin B complex, which also tend to increase his appetite and muscle tone. It is very important to force fluids in order to prevent dehydration, promote elimination, and reduce the possibility of physical illness. Sedation such as chloral hydrate is often indicated because of his poor sleep pattern, agitation, and possibility of suicide.

Physical treatment for the depressed patient usually combines the somatic types of therapy discussed in Chapter 7, particularly drug therapy. If ECT is given, it is usually in combination with drugs, or when the patient does not respond well to psychoactive drugs.

Emotional. The emotional care and treatment of the depressed patient are often omitted because the patient usually responds rapidly to somatic therapy. However, as has been pointed out, it is very important that the patient have an opportunity to work out better ways of resolving his problems in life than those which end up with recurrent episodes of depression.

Again, as for other patients, one of the common and current kinds of psychotherapy employed is that of counseling. The general goal of counseling for the depressed patient is to help him relieve his hostility by airing his resentment, learning to be more realistic and accepting about himself and others, and finding socially acceptable and constructive ways of expressing anger instead of turning it inward upon himself in the form of self-punishment. This may be done using the directive, permissive, or confrontation counseling techniques discussed in Chapter 11.

Often family therapy is employed, particularly with husband and wife, because of the need for the family to understand the illness and help the patient overcome his faulty method of handling hostility. Therapy may require changes in the family's way of doing things, and they often need help in making such changes. It may be necessary, for example, for other members of the family to assume more responsibility in the decision-making in order to reduce the load a patient is carrying for the entire family group.

Social. The social care and treatment of the depressed patient are aimed toward providing him with socially accepted, productive channels through which he may direct his hostility outward rather than inward. All of the activity therapies may be employed—O.T., R.T., and industrial therapy, particularly—to help him learn new and more successful ways of expressing his hostility. In O.T., pounding things, as in leather or copper work, carpentry or sculpting, helps the patient get rid of pent-up feelings and at the same time, produce something worthwhile which makes him feel adequate, important, and accepted. In R.T., active games like pingpong or basketball provide for the expression of hostile feelings and the exercise necessary to relieve physical tension and promote good health. In industrial therapy, jobs like washing dishes or scrubbing floors or cutting meat provide constructive ways of expressing one's feelings, and at the same time, get him the praise, recognition, and approval he needs so much.

The therapeutic environment of the depressed patient must not allow him to continue punishing himself. That means that people, routines, and activities must concentrate upon bringing the patient's hostility out into the open so that he may learn to deal with it more directly and in a healthier fashion. It is important to remember that when his hostility does come out in the form of a blast directed toward the hospital or nursing staff, he should meet with acceptance and approval, rather than rejection and disapproval which would serve only to increase his depression.

He must, in addition, have experiences of all kinds that help him correct the distorted picture he has of himself as inadequate, inferior, and unworthy. He should not be expected to achieve beyond his present physical and intellectual capacity. He needs to have all of the success that it is realistic to provide for him. For example, as we shall see in Case Example No. 4, for a depressed patient with a college degree to successfully manage a part-time job in the library may be a noteworthy achievement although it may not seem like much to us.

Let us look now at the care and treatment plans and progress for the last two case examples cited previously—No. 3 and No. 4.

Case Example No. 3 (See p. 211)

On admission the patient was given Asendin 300 mg. h.s. She was described as sitting on the edge of the bed, looking tense, and stating she was worried about everything. By the fourth day she started to relax, and on the sixth day she was well organized, shampooed her hair, washed her clothes, and stated she was most grateful for the help she was getting. She was assigned to a counselor and an activity group.

Patient was seen initially by her counselor three days later. She appeared to be a pleasant and cooperative but passive and dependent woman, who was unsure of herself and eager to please. She placed emphasis on her physical health and was preoccupied with numerous worries concerning minute details, such as what to talk about with her counselor, how to arrange the furniture in her trailer, what would be the best way to wax the floor, what her husband's reaction was to her coming to the hospital, and so on. From the outset in counseling the patient was insistent upon returning home; however, her ambivalence about doing so was marked. Emphasis was placed upon helping her sort out those aspects of living at home that she found annoying. She talked about her dissatisfaction with the trailer, her difficulty in living up to her own expectations as a housewife because of her obesity and excessive physical fatigue, her feelings of loneliness and isolation.

While the patient attempted to deal with these problems, her husband was seen on several occasions. He was reluctant to discuss his wife's condition, stating that she had no problems and was doing well. It became evident that the patient did not really wish to return home, but felt obligated to obey her husband's wishes. He was placing considerable pressure on her to do so. This denial of her illness on the part of the husband was an attempt on his part to have her home as soon as possible to relieve his own loneliness.

She continued to pressure to go home, although it was obvious she was not ready or willing to do so. This provided an excellent opportunity to explore with her in detail her feelings surrounding her current living situation. She began to show gradual improvement, demonstrating increased activity, alertness, and interest.

On a weekend visit home, she discovered her ability to do housework, and this further enhanced her self-worth. Her husband, pleased with her improvement, became quite helpful in his wife's treatment program. This amounted to transporting her for social visits, visiting her frequently at the hospital, and paying more attention to her needs when she was home.

Patient was discharged to the outpatient department, to be seen twice a week in counseling, and was referred to a community center where she would have increased social activity. She will continue to be seen on an outpatient basis at decreasing intervals, and will see her family physician concerning medication and her physical condition.

Case Example No. 4 (See p. 212)

On admission, the patient was started on lithium 300 mg. q.i.d., chloral hydrate 0.5 gm. h.s., thyroid gr. ii, and pilocarpine 1% gt. i to each eye b.i.d. She felt her head was detached from her body, and her sins were going to be reported to the whole world. After three weeks, she was still not sufficiently improved, so Haldol 10 mg. b.i.d. was added. She began to show improvement almost immediately.

She was assigned a counselor and an activity group to attend daily. When routine colostomy care was established, her depression markedly subsided.

Her family situation was not good. Although she received mail, she had no visitors and no place to go. Her family did not even come to visit her or take her out over the holidays. She did not feel very hopeful about the future, and was still worried about the colostomy. She did not want to return to teaching, and she was not prepared for anything else, so her financial worries were realistic.

Plans were made with the social worker. She went to a retirement home close to the hospital and came in twice a week for counseling. She has gained weight, is cheerful, and is satisfied with the living situation at this time. For recreation she grows vegetables and goes for walks with the other residents of the home.

NURSING CARE AND TREATMENT

Physical. As in schizophrenia, in meeting the physical needs of depressed patients, there are some common problems that deserve comment. The nursing care should do more than provide food, clothing, shelter, and activity. It should be given in such a way as to promote the patient's feeling of self-worth and interpersonal success. "I care for you, not just because you are a patient, but because you are a person of essential worth and dignity, and because you are important to me" characterizes the attitude which must underlie the nursing care that is given, and which the nurse must communicate to the patient by the way in which she gives that care. The revision of his distorted self-image can only take place through interactions with him, not in denying his delusions with words.

There are likely to be physical nursing care problems centering around the digestive system of a depressed patient. He may feel so unworthy, or suicidal or preoccupied, or anorexic that he does not eat or drink, so it is important for the nurse to see that he has sufficient food and fluid intake. This may be accomplished by frequent or interval feedings in liquid form, reenforced with proteins and vitamins. It may be necessary for him to be fed by hand or tube. Because of the slowing down of his body processes, his lack of exercise, and insufficient bulk or roughage in his diet, elimination of waste products, particularly from the digestive tract, may be a problem. He may be given foods which stimulate bowel function such as prune juice or whole-grain cereal, or it may be necessary to give him laxatives or enemas on a regular basis. It is important to try to help him establish regular bowel habits and he may have to be taken to the toilet on a regular schedule.

His preoccupation and concern with his terrible guilt make it necessary to observe him carefully for any sign of infection or injury which he may feel is his just punishment and therefore not report. He often must be protected from hazards in his environment, which he might use in some way in a suicidal attempt. However, the best suicidal precaution is the physical presence of the nurse. He may have to be checked for warmth also because often his circulation is slowed down so severely as to endanger the blood supply to his extremities.

Very often a depressed patient has delusions concerning his body functions, and he may have some strange somatic complaints like the patient who believed that his bowels hadn't moved for two years. It is important that the nurse neither corroborate nor deny the delusion; however, she must investigate the complaint sufficiently to know what the patient's physical status is and deal with it as matter-of-factly as possible. The somatic delusion may be an exaggerated or unhealthy way of expressing actual physical discomfort, malfunction, or pain, so it should not be dismissed as just a symptom of mental illness without knowing what the situation really is. Mentally ill patients can, and frequently do, become physically ill just like anyone else.

Another important aspect of the physical nursing care of a depressed patient is appropriate activity. Physical exercise will aid in maintaining or restoring a patient's physical health, increasing his appetite, digestion, elimination, circulation, muscle tone, and ability to sleep; this is much better for him than medication. The kind of activity is as important as the activity itself. It must fit the individual patient's physical, emotional, and social needs as well as his particular ability. For example, to expect him to participate in an activity that requires concentration and a long attention span such as a game of basketball may be more than he can manage, and will result in failure and further depression. However, getting him to throw the basketball to you may be a major accomplishment.

Emotional. The nurse's relationship with a depressed patient must be one which avoids as much as possible any reenforcement of his distorted picture of himself as unworthy, inadequate, and inferior, and of his pattern of failure, rejection, hostility, guilt, and self-punishment. He may learn from his interactions with the nurse to correct his misperceptions about himself. He must be encouraged first of all to direct his hostility outward. The process of self-punishment must be relieved before he hurts himself further or irreparably. If the patient can get angry at the nurse, and she can accept that anger, he may begin to reassess the picture he has of himself and change it accordingly. The first approach of the nurse, then, may be aimed toward provoking the patient's anger toward her or drawing his fire, so to speak. It doesn't help to increase his anger if he continues to introject it, or if the nurse is not able to accept it and thus rejects the patient for it. Both kinds of interaction will only deepen his depression. Once a patient is able to direct his hostility outward, then the nurse may help him find acceptable ways of channeling it.

Some nurses prefer to reverse these steps and provide the acceptable channels before encouraging a patient to express his feelings of hostility and aggression. Both methods are effective; the second one has some advantages of setting the limits for the patient in advance so that he knows how to proceed safely without risking the possibility of rejection and intolerable hurt.

It is very important that the nurse not further insult or reject a patient by denying his symptoms or making light of them. It is often a temptation to try to cheer up a depressed patient, or point out to him how foolish his notions are, or jolt him out of his self-pity. Any such approach may be risky and can be very harmful, indeed. If a patient is feeling down at the bottom of the pit, it doesn't help to stand up above and shout at him, "It's a beautiful day up here." Neither does it help someone who feels as terribly inadequate as he does to tell him how capable he is. It does not help him feel better when you disagree with his conviction that he is the worst person in the world. Those are his feelings, the basis of his illness, and the nurse must accept them as being very real to him. To deny or disapprove of those feelings is to make him feel angry or hurt or sad, convincing him that you do not understand how he feels and furthering his feelings of loneliness and despair.

The nurse must begin by accepting how the patient says he feels as being exactly how he feels, requiring no denial or corroboration on her part. It is much more therapeutic to make a simple statement that conveys that you understand and accept how he feels such as "That must be very distressing to you," "I can understand how that would make you very uncomfortable," or "It must be difficult for you to eat under those circumstances."

It doesn't help, either, to get down in the pit with him—then neither of you may get out to the daylight. To focus upon a patient's disability is to disable him even further. The nurse must reach out for the patient and say, in effect, "I know it's hard for you, but here's my hand; try to climb up here with me." It doesn't help to agree with a depressed patient that he isn't capable of handling the job; instead the nurse tries to appeal to his fighting spirit. She might say, "I can understand how you feel, but it doesn't seem right to let someone else take over." It doesn't help, either, to agree with a patient that he's the worst person in the world, but the nurse can certainly understand how he might feel that way. She might say, "It must be awful to feel like that. Let's do something together to make it a little easier for you."

Social. If a patient is provided with productive as well as acceptable channels for directing his hostility outward, then more than one therapeutic goal is achieved. If the patient can produce something worthwhile from his harnessed anger, then he not only gets rid of his anger but relieves the accumulated tension, gets the much-needed physical exercise, and gets the satisfaction he needs as well—the feeling of acceptance, importance, adequacy, and productivity. These channels or activities have been called "hostility outlets." Activities that include such actions as tearing, cutting, chopping, pounding, slapping, scrubbing, burning, digging all help express destructive impulses and feelings in constructive ways. Tearing up rags to make rag rugs, cutting out patterns or decorations for the ward, sawing or chopping wood for kindling, raking and burning leaves, pulling weeds in the garden, mowing the grass, digging ditches are some of the ways people relieve anger and tension constructively. All kinds of household chores offer such an opportunity—scrubbing the floors, cleaning windows, slicing and chopping food, washing dishes, scrubbing pots and pans. All kinds of jobs related to carpentry offer such an opportunity—sanding, sawing, pounding nails, painting. Jobs on and off the ward that include some kind of service to others offer such an opportunity—nursing aide, food service, maintenance work.

Usually, the best kind of hostility outlet for a depressed patient is some kind of work rather than some kind of recreation because of his need to atone for his sins, pay for his misdeeds, earn his way. Recreation is usually associated with some form of fun or pleasure which may add to his need for self-punishment rather than relieve it. However, recreational activities where he provides some kind of service to others may be helpful. Recreational activities where the product is shared with others may be used, such as cookie or candy making, making toys for children, knitting things for others, entertaining others with music or singing, teaching others how to knit or play cards or dance.

As with other kinds of care and treatment, whatever the activity, it must be appropriate for the particular person, and it must be aimed toward directing his hostility outward into productive channels, relieving his tension and self-punishment, and correcting his distorted picture of himself. It is important, therefore, in group activities that he not become the target of other people's anger and rejection. He must be encouraged to be with other people, allowed to participate at whatever level he can, and progress at his own rate. If he feels safe and secure in his environment, he will reach out for more responsibility and greater independence when he is capable of doing so.

The major affective disorders are the second most common kind of functional psychoses. The most common form that these illnesses take is that of depression.

Depression is a primary mood disorder, in which the characteristic disturbances in feeling are the symptoms of despondency, despair, and melancholia. The accompanying disturbances in thinking are delusions associated with guilt or body function, slowing down of the thought process, and preoccupation with ideas of unworthiness and suicide. The disturbances in activity are underactivity in retarded depression and overactivity in agitated depression.

The illness stems from turning feelings of hostility in reaction to stress inward upon the self in a destructive manner, using the coping method of introjection. Any threat to the survival or security of the person sets off the sequence of failure, rejection, hostility, guilt, self-punishment, and depression. The depressed patient is reduced to a state of helplessness and hopelessness.

Each care and treatment plan must be geared to the needs and abilities of the individual patient and aimed toward the resolution of the core problem of the illness: to reduce the hostility, turn it outward, and relieve the self-punishment. This is accomplished by the use of ECT, antidepressants, and tranquilizers in somatic therapy. Psychotherapy or counseling and therapeutic relationships are aimed toward helping the patient correct his own distorted picture of himself as unworthy, inadequate, inferior. Social therapy is aimed toward helping the patient find more acceptable and constructive channels through which to express his destructive impulses and feelings.

REFERENCES

Arieti, Silvano: *Severe and Mild Depression,* Basic Books, New York, 1978.

Dobihal, Shirley V.: "Hospice: enabling the patient to die at home," *American Journal of Nursing, 80* (August, 1980) pp. 1448–1451.

Dubree, Marilyn, and Ruth Vogelpohl: "When hope dies—so might the patient," *American Journal of Nursing,* 80 (November, 1980) pp. 2046–2049.

Hankoff, L.D., and Bernice Einsidler: *Suicide Theory and Clinical Aspects*, PSG Publishing Company, Littleton, Massachusetts, 1979.
Hendrix, Melva Jo, et al.: "The battered wife," *American Journal of Nursing, 78* (April, 1978) pp. 650–653.
Knowles, Ruth Dailey: "Dealing with feelings: handling depression by identifying anger," *American Journal of Nursing, 81* (May, 1981) p. 968.
Knowles, Ruth Dailey: "Handling depression through activity," *American Journal of Nursing, 81* (June, 1981) p. 1187.
Knowles, Ruth Dailey: "Handling depression through positive reinforcement," *American Journal of Nursing, 81* (July, 81) p. 1353.
Limandri, Barbara J., and Diana W. Boyle: "Instilling hope," *American Journal of Nursing, 78* (January, 1978) pp. 79–80.
Mandel, Henry: "Nurses' feelings about working with the dying patient," *American Journal of Nursing, 81* (June, 1981) pp. 1194–1197.
McLaughlin, Mary: "Who helps the living?" *American Journal of Nursing, 78* (March, 1978) pp. 422–423.
Miller, Arthur: *Death of a Salesman*, Penguin Books, New York, 1976.
Toth, Susan B., and Andre Toth: "Empathic intervention with the widow," *American Journal of Nursing, 80* (September, 1980) pp. 1652–1654.
White, Cheryl Lynne: "Nurse counseling with a depressed patient," *American Journal of Nursing, 78* (March, 1978) pp. 436–439.

Chapter 13

Psychotic Reactions to the Stress of Aging

Organic mental disorders are those in which there are behavioral or psychological disturbances due to transient or permanent dysfunction of the brain. They include (1) primary degenerative dementia, senile onset, with delirium, delusions, or depression or uncomplicated; (2) primary degenerative dementia, pre-senile onset; (3) multi-infarct dementia; and (4) substance-induced, including those caused by alcohol and drugs (see Appendix B).

The resulting symptoms are of two kinds—those due directly to the CNS dysfunction and those due to the individual's psychological reaction to the additional stress. For example, the aging process is likely to be stressful for most people; most people adjust to it, but some develop the physical and psychological symptoms of senile dementia. It is often difficult to determine whether the symptoms are a direct result of damage to the brain or a psychological reaction to the loss of intellectual or physical ability.

A person reacts to his life situation as a total entity so that physical, emotional, and social factors blend together and often become indistinguishable. Most illness, then, is a combination of these same factors so that all people do not experience the same illness in the same way, with exactly the same symptoms. People who drink or have epilepsy or a brain tumor or get old do not all react in the same way physically or emotionally or socially. Some people adjust in a healthy way and there is no handicap or disease, some develop physical symptoms or disease, others act out their hostility in antisocial ways, and some people develop psychotic reactions.

Psychotic reactions in elderly people—that is, 65 years of age or over—account for over one-third of the patients in mental hospitals across the country. It is probably fairly accurate to estimate that half of the resident patients in mental hospitals fit into the category of geriatric patients. Geriatrics means the treatment of diseases of the aged, and gerontology means the science and study of old age. Included in the large group of geriatric patients in mental hospitals are (1) those who have been mentally ill for a long time, and grow old in the mental hospital; (2) those who have had recurrent mental disorders in reaction to the stress of living, including an episode in later life; (3) those who have become acutely ill for the first time as a reaction to the stress of aging.

Not only are there a large number of elderly patients in mental hospitals, but there are also many geriatric patients being cared for in nursing homes, extended care facilities, general hospitals, rehabilitation centers, day care centers, and other community facilities. There are, in fact, so many elderly people being treated in the modern practice of medicine that it has become a clinical specialty, geriatrics, like pediatrics, orthopedics, gynecology, obstetrics. People are also beginning to distinguish the study and treatment of mental illness in the elderly as geriatric psychiatry. It is this group of mental disorders that we will focus upon in our discussion of the organic psychoses.

DEFINITION

The organic psychoses which occur as reactions to the process of aging result from the failure of the individual to cope effectively with the stresses of later life. He becomes unable to meet the demands of life or to satisfy his needs in ways that are acceptable to himself and others. These psychotic disorders are characterized by (1) serious disturbances in the thinking, feeling, and doing of the individual; (2) marked interference in his ability to distinguish between reality and his own subjective experiences; (3) severe disruption in his relationships with other people and his environment; (4) pathological physical conditions which add to his general lack of well-being.

We are not talking here just about old people or that process in life we refer to as "getting old." We are talking, rather, about people with the kind of behavior, understandable as it is, which represents the abnormal, the deviation from health, the failure on the part of the individual to behave in accord with expectations. Everyone who lives long enough gets old. Most people adjust to the changes in expectations, abilities, capacities, and stresses in the last stage of the life cycle. They manage to enjoy later life in peace and tranquility, with the sense of integrity which climaxes a successful life.

However, many people suffer from the physical and mental infirmities of the aged, which we have come to refer to as senility. Senile actually means having the characteristics of old age. Senility means the senile state or old age. Senescence means the process of growing old, or the aging process. We have, however, come to attach a special meaning to these terms. When we use the common expression, "Oh, he's just senile," we commonly mean that the person is childish, dependent, irritable, demanding, forgetful, or feeble, with physical and mental weaknesses. However, he is not necessarily psychotic and does not usually need psychiatric treatment. Most often he is cared for at home, in a nursing home, or in an extended care facility in the community.

Some people succumb to the stresses of this stage in life and lose their ability to behave appropriately. A few develop the psychotic symptoms of paranoid schizophrenia or depression, and it is that comparative few we are discussing here. A patient is not put in a mental hospital because he is old or feeble or senile, but because he is no longer able to master the stress in his life, whether it be physical, emotional, or social in nature, and because his condition requires psychiatric care and treatment.

TYPES

The most frequent diagnoses of psychotic disorders associated with organic brain syndromes in the elderly are primary degenerative dementia, senile onset, and multi-infarct dementia.

Senile dementia or psychosis occurs with senile brain disease, the causes of which are largely unknown. It generally includes loss of intellectual abilities, memory impairment, impairment of abstract thinking, impaired judgment, sometimes aphasia or other language difficulty, and some specific or presumed organic factor related to the disturbance. In senile dementia with delirium, the essential symptoms include clouding of consciousness, difficulty focusing attention, perceptual disturbances, difficulty thinking and speaking, often restlessness and hyperactivity, disorientation, and memory impairment. In senile dementia with delusions, the predominant symptoms include delusions without clouding of consciousness or hallucinations. In senile dementia with depression, the essential symptom is depression, without clouding of consciousness or hallucinations. In multi-infarct dementia, the symptoms are patchy intellectual deficits and neurological signs and symptoms of cerebrovascular disease, such as reflex response, palsy, faulty gait, weakness of extremity. We will discuss the psychotic disorders associated with the aging process in terms of their common clinical symptoms or syndromes rather than trying to fit them into a specific diagnostic category.

THE PROCESS OF DEVELOPMENT

Aging is a normal process which, in general terms, begins at birth, even though most people think of the aging process as being associated with the last half of life—from age fifty onward. From birth through adolescence to early adulthood, age 18 to 21, there is a tremendous growth curve that goes practically straight up on all of the graphs. However, once an individual has reached adulthood or maturity, his growth tapers off or starts downhill.

For many people the aging process has less to do with physical or chronological age than with life experiences and how to resolve the problems of living. Some people get old early in life, and others stay young all their lives. This is dependent to some extent upon how open, receptive, and competent a person is in reacting to change and learning new ways of functioning that continue to contribute to his successful living. Once a person becomes rigid, set in his ways, unable to change with the times or the expectations of the stages of life, then he tends to grow old faster and sooner than others.

As a rule, the first twenty-five years of an individual's life is made up of tremendous growth in every aspect of his functioning —thinking, feeling, doing—and in all parts of his being—physical, emotional, social. The next quarter of his life is focused upon translating the results of that growth into operational rewards. The third quarter is taken up with broadening, deepening, consolidating his gains. The last quarter of his life should be concerned with the refinement and enjoyment of what he has accomplished before, is accomplishing now, and has yet to accomplish in his lifetime.

Some people give up the ghost after the first quarter and settle down into a life of boredom or misery. Some stick it out to the midway point in life and then retire into seclusion or ill health. Some manage to live successfully until the end of the third quarter and then throw in the sponge, while others finish out their century with health, enthusiasm, good humor, and a sense of well-being.

Each stage in the life cycle has its own peculiar stress to be mastered, and for each individual his particular life experiences add special kinds of stress. At any stage in his life he may be beseiged by one or a combination of the enemies of health—infection, injury, malfunction or malformation, and stress. In succeeding stages of life, unmastered stress or unresolved problems in living add to the load that an individual carries. A person's success as an adult is built upon his adjustment as a child and adolescent. Peace and security in later life rest upon his achievement during the productive years of adulthood. The competence of a parent is based upon his ability to learn how to be one as a son or daughter. To be successful in retirement, a person must have been successful in work. The foundation for success in each stage is laid in the preceding stages, just as the strength of the staircase rests upon the first step as well as the last.

If a person is healthy and comes through life with a sufficient degree of success, then he is in fairly good shape for the last stage of his life. If he is not healthy, and has not been sufficiently successful in his life so far, he is likely to have increasing difficulty in the last stage of his life. Psychotic behavior occurs when the person's ability to master stress has not been satisfactory, or when the stress is sufficiently prolonged, widespread, and intense as to be overwhelming, or when his life situation is so altered as to leave him more exposed with fewer resources within himself and his environment. Psychotic behavior in reaction to the aging process results often from a combination of these factors when the individual finds he cannot resolve the crisis in his life by himself.

FACTORS IN THE STRESS OF AGING

Decrease in Status. Let us look first at the sources of stress common to the aging process. The first one is the *decrease in the elderly person's personal and social status.* An individual's attitude toward aging is determined to some extent by the culture. If older people are held in high esteem, thought to be important and useful, then a person may look forward to later life. However, if the general attitude is the opposite, the individual tends to look upon this period with dread and anticipated doom. Some people go so far as to deny or distort the whole situation.

In this country, great value is placed upon youth and little upon age. In fact, the elderly person is stripped of his dignity and worth in many ways. He is laughed at for his effort to remain young. He is ridiculed for his old-fashioned ways, ideas, and clothes. Fun is poked at him for his ideals, morals, and sentiments. His contribution is dismissed with a joke or an insult, or by calling him names like "old fogey." This is not true of other cultures. For example, Oriental people revere and respect the old.

In the United States, we carry this disregard or disrespect for the old into the field of ideas, events, and objects as well as people. There are comparatively few landmarks left standing in this country. We tear down the old to build something new, and even before it is finished, it may already be obsolete because it does not meet our desire for the latest, most modern and fashionable object possible. Often we seem bent upon destroying the heritage and tradition of past and present by looking always to the future, forgetting that the future is a culmination of the past and present. We might well pay heed to the advice of Alexander Pope in his Essay on Criticism, "Be not the first by whom the new are tried, Nor yet the last to lay the old aside."

Retirement. The elderly person's feelings of importance, usefulness, and self-esteem are lessened by *forced retirement.* At an arbitrary age, 65 or 70, he is told he must retire from his position whether he wants to or not, whether he is still capable or not, and whether he can afford to or not. At a certain age he is told that he is no longer needed or wanted or competent in his work. If there is no alternative for forced retirement in this technological age, in which we must make way for the younger generation, then we should explore new avenues of productivity and contribution for the elderly. We have created an area of primary social conflict for ourselves and our children. We have lengthened man's life span with all kinds of scientific and technological progress without providing for the necessary sources of satisfaction. What advantage is there, if we live to be 100 (scientists tell us the time will come when it will be 200 or 300), if in the last quarter of our lives we are good for nothing? Who wants to live longer when there is nothing to live for?

Very often, the elderly person is *unprepared for retirement,* financially or emotionally. If he has not been able to put some money away during his productive years on the job, for whatever reasons, he will be dependent upon others for his very existence. He may become dependent upon his children or upon public assistance or some other kind of social welfare, all of which are notoriously ungenerous in their contributions to his subsistence. Many, many elderly people live in the most miserable life conditions imaginable without the necessities basic to survival. Because they have not been thrifty (and there may be many good reasons why they could not save money), they are rejected, punished, and degraded by those who are in a position to help them—paid workers or unpaid volunteers or inconsiderate children.

It is not unusual for people to die shortly after retirement and this is not accidental or coincidental to the trauma associated with giving up a part of one's life that has been an *important source of satisfaction.* In fact, their work may have been a major or single source of satisfaction for most of their lives. Unless a person has developed other resources so that his needs may be satisfied by other people, activities, or kinds of production, he is apt to suffer severe stress from the resulting deprivation.

Role Reversal. Often associated with the aging process is a *role reversal* for the elderly individual. A competent, successful, independent person may become dependent, helpless, infantile in his relationship with society and family. He may have been the head of the household in his prime, lord and master of all he surveyed, but as an unproductive, unwanted, dependent old man he is a different person. It is as difficult for the children as it is for the elderly parent to have to switch roles. It's pretty hard for a son or daughter to restrict the activities of an elderly mother in the kitchen when they have enjoyed her cooking most of their lives. It is difficult for all concerned when the children have to assume more responsibility in the decisions that once were the prerogative of the elderly parent alone. It is difficult for children and parents to accept circumstances which require that the nature of their lifelong relationships change.

Loss of Significant People and Objects. Another factor contributing to the stress of aging is the *loss of significant people and objects* that have been major sources of satisfaction. Children grow up, leave home, and establish their own families and lives, separate and apart from their parents. Sometimes they become so involved with their own lives that the communication between parents and grown children may be nonexistent. Further, if the communication stems from a feeling of duty or obligation, rather than from genuine affection or concern, it is likely to do more harm than good. As William Shakespeare says in his classic tragedy, *King Lear,*

> How sharper than a serpent's tooth it is
> To have a thankless child!

The loss of significant people includes wife, husband, close friend, ally, associate, or peer. Often during this period, the elderly person loses one contemporary after another, and the mounting stress can be overwhelming as the hand of death strikes closer and closer to him. A person suffers losses all during his life, but the elderly person's losses are greater because of his lack of sources of satisfaction from which to draw security and strength. A person can endure great hardship and even deprivation if he has people close to him whom he loves and who in turn love him. However, the elderly person is often left in isolation by friends and family and lives out his life alone.

Sometimes it is necessary for the elderly person to *give up his own home* and move in with his children or enter a foster home, nursing home, retirement home, or extended care facility. This is a particularly traumatic move for an elderly woman who has managed her own home successfully for years and then has to give it up along with everything in it and all that it stands for. A favorite chair or cooking utensil or hand-crocheted afghan, or one's own bed becomes an extension of the person, and to be separated from it is like losing a piece of one's self. Often, the elderly person tries to crowd his most prized possessions into the small apartment or room in an attempt to preserve something of himself and his life.

Decrease in Physical Ability. Another major source of stress in the aging process is the decrease in physical ability. There is a general *slowing down of all body systems and physical functioning.* The elderly person's process of digestion and elimination often does not work as well as it used to, and he may have to change his eating and toilet habits. He may worry about these changes, often resists them, and sometimes refuses to make the necessary alterations with resulting physical problems of a more serious nature. For example, the lack of proper nutrient intake or the lack of proper processing of the intake may result in protein deficiencies which contribute to the possibility of fracture. Vitamin deficiencies may contribute to skin disorders in the form of the decubitus ulcer, or bedsore, which often plagues elderly people, particularly if they must be hospitalized.

A decline in his physical functioning may result in a person having to *give up activities* that have been a great source of satisfaction for him. His inability to accomplish what he once could may be a constant source of irritation. Often elderly people reminisce about the things they used to do in order to compensate for their inability to do them now. An elderly gentleman tells anyone who will listen about the number of miles he walked to school as a boy, implying that modern youth would come off second best if such physical accomplishments were expected of them. An elderly lady tells of the many times she did a whole family wash by hand on a tin washboard, and hung the clothes out to freeze dry, all the while insisting that freshly washed clothes these days don't smell nearly as good.

Not only do body processes in general slow down with aging, but also the *vital parts wear out,* seriously interfering with physical functioning and even interrupting life. The heart and blood vessels, the lungs and bronchi, the kidneys and bladder, the uterus and prostate, the pancreas and thyroid, the joints and sockets, any of the muscles, the stomach and intestines, sensory and motor nerves—all may be subjected to particular wear and tear, stress and strain in the process of aging.

The wearing out of the special sense organs presents great stress to many elderly people. For example, defects in vision such as presbyopia (sometimes called "old eyes") or cataracts are often a great handicap to an elderly person. The condition may be severe enough to make it difficult to find ways of correcting the defect, or ways of compensating for it. He may not be able to see well enough to get around by himself, read, watch TV, or participate in the usual activities which give him satisfaction and pleasure. It is often difficult to find substitute activities because the choice is so restricted by his limitations.

The elderly person may be further handicapped by a hearing deficit. Likewise, his senses of touch, taste, smell, and motion may be diminished. If his special senses are thus affected, it becomes increasingly difficult for him to find satisfaction in interaction with the world he lives in. Thus, he may withdraw from it, or fight with it, or distort it, in an attempt to lessen the threat of his inability to cope with it successfully.

There are also an *increased incidence of illness, a slower rate of recovery, and a greater possibility of residual impairment in the functioning of the elderly.* For example, an elderly person is much more likely to have recurrent upper respiratory infection with a greater chance of developing pneumonia and the possible complication of emphysema, which may leave him with the symptoms of chronic bronchitis. If an elderly person suffers a fall or other accident, the injury may take a greater toll than just the affected part; he may be shaken up all over and may not recover from the broken arm or hip or shoulder. He is generally likely, then, to have some evidence of physical disease, handicap, or impairment which may result either from the aging process itself or from prior infection, injury, malfunction, malformation, or stress. For example, he may have diabetes which develops later in life in association with the aging process, or he may have diabetes in later life because he has had it all his life.

Finally, the elderly person lives with the constant threat of *approaching death.* He may suffer recurrent and frequent bouts of serious illness which bring him again and again in close contact with death. For some people, death is less terrifying than for others, but as a threat to survival, it is always anxiety-provoking. If a person has lived successfully and happily, he is more likely to accept the fact that his life must end. If he feels he will be rewarded in some kind of happy afterlife, he may seem to look forward to the end of his life on earth. If he is tired or worn out or disappointed from his life, he may surrender it more willingly and with resignation. But most people, when the time arrives, struggle instinctively to survive.

Decrease in Intellectual Capacity. It is fairly well accepted that as a person grows older, it becomes *increasingly difficult for him to learn new things.* He tends to settle for the old ways of doing things that have worked for him in the past and with which he is familiar, and that makes him *increasingly resistant to change.* The more resistant to change he becomes and the more set in his ways, the more difficult it is for him to learn, and the vicious circle is formed. He often has less enthusiasm or zest for life, and is *slower to respond to challenge.* He may be more interested in what he has already experienced than in what he is now experiencing or what he may yet experience. Thus, he develops the "good old days" attitude toward life, becomes less involved with the world happenings, and *does less planning for the future.* Of course, he has less future to plan for and his daydreams most often deal with the past. It becomes *increasingly difficult for him to retain information,* particularly newly acquired information, and this may be due at least in part to his lack of attention to the present or increasing difficulty in dealing with the world around him. His *lack of adequate sensory perception* alone may result in impairment of his judgment. If he does not correctly perceive events, objects, or people around him, then the conclusions that he draws, the decisions that he makes, and the actions that he takes may all be faulty or impaired or inappropriate. For example, if an elderly person believes that the black object he sees in the corner is his cat instead of the black purse that it actually is, his behavior might be described as inappropriate, ridiculous, or senile, depending upon the knowledge and understanding of the observer. It is likely, then, that others around the elderly person may interact with him on the basis of their own distorted perceptions. Accordingly, they may scold him, or laugh at him, or humor him.

An elderly person may sustain combined losses in personal and social status, significant people and objects, physical ability, and intellectual capacity. If he does, he is likely to experience severe interference in the satisfaction of his needs, or *deprivation.* How he handles the core problem of deprivation may result in a variety of reactions. First, he may withdraw from the world of reality, and turn to his own world of fantasy. Second, he may become increasingly irritable and fight with those around him for no other reason than to relieve his misery. This kind of behavior is often called cantankerous, and is associated almost exclusively with the elderly. Third, he may become sad, lonely, tearful in his terrible isolation, and pose a serious suicidal threat. Fourth, he may distort what goes on around him, and become suspicious, distrustful, hostile. These are the ways the elderly person uses to effect adjustment to his failing competence as a person. If these ways help to satisfy his needs, if he still remains within the boundaries of acceptability, and if his life situation is such as to tolerate his idiosyncrasies, then he remains within the dimensions of health. However, if any one of these conditions is not present, then we may see the appearance of unhealthy behavior in the form of psychotic symptoms.

SYMPTOMS

The psychotic behavior syndromes that we see in elderly patients are similar to those we have already discussed under paranoid schizophrenia and psychotic depression. However, there are some characteristic symptoms of the psychoses associated with the aging process that are not commonly seen in younger patients. We will focus our discussion upon these differentiating symptoms, and try to eliminate as much repetition as possible. It might be worthwhile here for the student to review the previous Chapters, 11 and 12.

First of all, disturbances in sensorium, or conscious awareness, commonly associated with organic brain syndromes, result in the following symptoms:

(1) Impairment of orientation

(2) Impairment of memory

(3) Impairment of all intellectual functions such as comprehension, calculation, knowledge, learning, and so on

(4) Impairment of judgment

(5) Childish responses in affect and action

The common distortions in thinking in the elderly psychotic patient include disorientation, confusion, and memory loss. Orientation refers to the degree of awareness of person, place, and time. If the patient knows who he is, where he is, and the date, we say he is oriented in all three spheres. If he does not know who he is or where he is or what date it is, we say he is disoriented as to time, place, and person. Often accompanying disorientation is confusion, a state characterized by bewilderment, lack of clear thinking, and clouding of conscious awareness, all of which interfere with a person's ability to distinguish, recognize, or restore order to his surroundings. He may be unable to identify people, misinterpret sounds he hears or things he sees, or be unable to comprehend the events going on around him. The result is often very disturbed behavior, in the form of agitation, panic, hyperactivity. For example, if you have ever awakened in a strange bedroom, you know there is a moment of bewilderment and sometimes panic before you are able to put things into their proper focus and order—before you know where you are, how you got there, who you are with, and so on. Disorientation and confusion are often accompanied by the third symptom of amnesia (memory loss), which makes figuring things out in a logical fashion difficult, if not impossible, for the elderly psychotic patient. The anxiety that is provoked by such distortions in thinking is easily understood, and accounts for additional distortions in thinking, feeling, and doing. The elderly person may try to cover his lack of memory with the additional symptoms of retrospective falsification or confabulation. Retrospective falsification means distortions in remembering and reporting past experiences based upon emotional needs. Confabulation means falsification of memory, replacing memory loss by fantasy or by reality that is not true for the occasion.

An elderly person may react to the stress of his life by resorting to withdrawal from reality, and then we see the additional symptoms of distorted thinking of the schizophrenic patient—hallucinations, delusions, and blocking. He may react by turning his hostile feelings inward upon himself in a punishing way, and then we see the symptoms of blocking, illusions, and retardation. Or he may react by doing both, and then we see the whole gamut of symptoms of distorted thinking—disorientation, confusion, memory loss, hallucinations, delusions, blocking, illusions, and retardation.

The accompanying disturbances in feeling in the elderly psychotic patient may be similar to those of the schizophrenic reaction—ambivalence, sensitivity, fearfulness, distrust, loneliness, shallow or inappropriate affect, or apathy. They may be similar to those of the depressive reaction—sadness, despondency, despair, guilt, unworthiness, inadequacy, and inferiority. They may be a combination of the symptoms of the two.

The disturbances in doing may be similar to those of the schizophrenic reaction—autistic, regressed, negativistic, inappropriate, impulsive, unpredictable, or ritualistic behavior. They may be similar to those of the depressive reaction—underactivity as in retarded depression, or overactivity as in agitated depression. They may be a combination of the symptoms of the two.

An elderly individual may react to stress with a passive behavior pattern, and we might see withdrawn or regressed behavior. He may react with an aggressive behavior pattern, and we might see self-punishment or antisocial behavior. He may react with a paradoxical behavior pattern, and we might see suspiciousness or physical symptoms.

Physically, we will see the symptoms of whatever pathological organic condition exists, and there are some that occur more commonly than others. Often these physical symptoms or conditions are directly related to the psychotic symptoms we have just discussed, so that treating the physical condition will also relieve the psychotic condition and vice versa.

In the circulatory system, we often see symptoms of cardiovascular dysfunction. A common pathological condition in the elderly patient is arteriosclerosis, including arteriosclerosis of the arteries supplying food and oxygen to the brain, resulting in the symptoms of organic brain syndrome which we have already discussed. Sometimes there is evidence of ischemic attacks or small strokes, or a CVA, that have left some residual paralysis or dysfunction of the extremities or muscles of the face. There are often symptoms of poor circulation to the extremities, the skin, hands and arms, feet and legs, such as cyanosis or edema. Sometimes the heart itself or the coronary vessels have suffered damage from use over the years, and we may see hypotension or hypertension, or congestive heart failure.

In the musculoskeletal systems, we often find arthritis, deformities of the joints, deterioration of the bony structures, and resulting fractures. In the urinary system there are often symptoms of urinary retention, or urgency and frequency, or uncontrollable dribbling because the muscular sphincters do not work properly or have lost their elasticity. In elderly male patients we often see hypertrophy of the prostate which interferes further with urinary function. In elderly female patients, prolapse of the uterus is not uncommon, or there may be other dysfunctions of the reproductive system. In the endocrine system, there are two rather common diseases observed in the elderly—diabetes and hypothyroidism. Diseases of the respiratory system include chronic bronchitis and emphysema. The nervous system is affected by the organic conditions leading to defective sensory-motor perception—loss of sight, hearing, touch, taste, smell, motion. We will not discuss each of these physical conditions in detail so the student may want to take advantage of the reference reading related to geriatric nursing.

Now let us look at three actual case histories of elderly psychotic patients which will demonstrate the types, symptoms, process of development, and progression of illnesses as we have discussed them.

Case Example No. 1

Patient is a 61-year-old divorced woman who has been a telephone operator most of her life. She has worked for the same firm for the past 21 years until about a year ago when she lost her job. Since then she has become increasingly agitated and suspicious. She was committed to the psychiatric hospital by her sister.

On admission she was described as restless and uncooperative, and when an attempt was made to talk with her, she would just say "thank you" and walk by. She was fully oriented, of average intelligence, and her memory was intact. She was extremely guarded, and would not speak of her auditory hallucinations except when asked about their contents. She stated that they did not let her sleep, consisted of high-volume voices that were so derogatory that they would not give her any peace. Her guarded, suspicious behavior made the exam procedures quite difficult. She showed a certain degree of insight and recognized that her hallucinatory state was a sign of mental disturbance. Physical and laboratory examinations were essentially negative.

She was born and lived in the same state all of her life. She has two sisters. Her education stopped at the eighth grade. She married at age 22, was divorced after eight years. She got a job as a telephone operator in a large hotel in the city, and has lived a more-or-less lonely life ever since. She has lived alone in an apartment for the past six years.

About two months ago she began hearing voices, mostly at night.

They were soft-spoken voices that would sometimes be very vulgar, and seemed to be coming from within her stomach. At other times she felt that someone was pulling from the left side of her stomach to the right side. Often she would be startled by the vibration of the house, and sometimes she would see lights switching off and on all day.

Diagnosis: Schizophrenia, paranoid, chronic.

Case Example No. 2

Patient is a 63-year-old music teacher, married, with two daughters and a teen-age son, who came to the hospital for the second time as a voluntary patient. He was discharged from the hospital a year ago; however, he did not follow the post-hospitalization plan recommended for him. He admits to a distrust of doctors in general, psychiatrists in particular. He got along fairly well for a time, but in recent weeks had a return of his depressive symptoms. He presented himself as a glum, unspontaneous, rigid man, appearing younger than his stated age, who somewhat grudgingly acknowledged his need for help.

On admission the patient was alert, fully oriented, and grudgingly cooperative. His mood was markedly depressed. His thought content was marked by preoccupation with feelings of despondency, helplessness, and hopelessness. He has some insight, but his judgment is difficult to evaluate. Physical and laboratory examinations were within normal limits.

He is described as a rather shy, sensitive person who has been extremely self-conscious all of his life. Apparently, he had a tendency early in life to stutter occasionally, and for many years has been unduly concerned with this speech problem. Despite this concern, he has been a competent teacher for the last twenty years, well-accepted by faculty and students. One younger brother suffered from severe, prolonged mental illness and committed suicide. One of the patient's daughters has been admitted several times to the psychiatric hospital for the treatment of schizophrenia.

His severe depression began approximately three months prior to his first admission to the hospital. At that time he was the director of a school choir which he took on tour. On the tour he developed the fear that he would be unable to speak in public because of possible stuttering. This obsession became exaggerated until it finally assumed delusional proportions, and it made him extremely apprehensive. He returned from the tour exhausted and deeply depressed. He developed insomnia and severe feelings of depression, rejection, and hopelessness. He lost weight and ruminated about suicide. He sought psychiatric help from a private psychiatrist who treated him with psychotherapy, antidepressants, and tranquilizers. The patient did not improve; in fact, his depression became gradually worse, and his symptoms so severe that his psychiatrist felt intensive inpatient therapy was indicated and he was admitted to the psychiatric hospital.

He was described as profoundly depressed, with motor retardation, lethargy, insomnia, and loss of appetite. He felt hopeless and despondent, was preoccupied with suicidal ideas. He was overly concerned about what he called "blocking of speech"; however, he showed no speech difficulty throughout his hospital stay. He responded well to psychoactive drugs, and actually stayed in the hospital only 13 days.

His condition was discussed with his private psychiatrist and he was referred to the psychiatrist for followup therapy. He was encouraged to continue on Tofranil 25 mg. t.i.d. and Mellaril 25 mg. t.i.d. He failed to report his progress to the hospital as he had been asked to do but it was learned that he continued to feel well and seemed to be in excellent spirits following his discharge. He did not contact his psychiatrist again until the symptoms returned.

Diagnosis: Major depression, recurrent.

Case Example No. 3

Patient is a 67-year-old married woman, with one daughter, committed to the psychiatric hospital for the first time. She was agitated, confused, unable to function at home. She thought the neighbors were after her and something terrible was about to happen to her family. She expressed feelings of guilt, unworthiness, and hopelessness. She did not think she was mentally ill, and said her husband was calling to her to go home.

On admission she was described as an obese, pale, gray-haired woman, unkempt in appearance. She was oriented to place and person but not to date. Memory was fairly good for remote but somewhat confused for recent events. Retention and recall were poor. She gave the impression of normal intelligence but poor judgment, and lacked insight regarding her illness. She stated, "There is no future in me, everything is hopeless, the world is going to end, because we are under the evil spirit's influence." Physical and laboratory exams were negative.

Patient is the oldest of seven children, and described herself as shy and seclusive as a child. Her father was a machinist, very interested in politics, and gone from home a lot attending meetings. Her mother was a moody, nervous woman, depressed at times. Relations between parents were cool, and the mother was unhappy in her marital life. Patient's attitude toward parents and sisters was mostly cool and tense. She loved her only brother more than the other members of the family. She was separated from the family in early adolescence and does not know much about them.

She went through the seventh grade in school and had many friends. She worked as a milliner for four or five years, and quit after she was married to devote full time to the household. She was married at age 23, a "love match," and has one child, a daughter. She is a neat and conscientious housekeeper, works in her garden and home, and reads good books, mostly of an abstract, philosophical and religious nature.

Her husband and daughter state that all of her life she has been high-strung, domineering, and stubborn. At times she was hyperactive and argumentative, and never wanted to accept other people's opinions. She often had difficulties because of her argumentative, superior attitude. She was not overly religious, but recently she has become increasingly interested in religious problems, started arguments and got upset about religious questions. She felt she was a criminal and not worthy of food or clothing. As a result, she did not eat very well and became dehydrated. She felt the neighbor women were after her, spying on her, tapping her telephone, and were responsible for her being admitted to the hospital.

Diagnosis: Primary degenerative dementia, senile onset, with delusions and depression.

Case Example No. 4

Patient is a 73-year-old widow with five children who came to the hospital as a voluntary patient because of "exhaustion." She has been living and working in another state for the past three years. She returned to live with her sister because she was exhausted, confused, and unable to care for herself any longer.

She was employed for 17 years as a practical nurse at the same hospital where she was admitted. She was described as a conscientious and dependable employee and her reason for leaving is not clear. Her husband of 30 years died three years after she left the hospital's employment; according to the patient's relatives, her husband's death did not seem to have any effect upon her. However, she left the state shortly after his death and little is known about her life since then. The patient's memory seems to be very inaccurate for that period of time. She recollects leaving the state and describes her feelings as those of anxiety, despondency, and exhaustion. She does not remember how she found her way to her sister's place.

Upon admission she was described as an obese, gray-haired, pleasant old lady who was disoriented as to time and confused about her surroundings. Her facial expression was that of bewilderment and apathy. Her speech was rambling, circumstantial, incoherent, and retarded. Her mood showed signs of despondency and her thought content showed preoccupation with events of the last three years in an attempt to determine what was true and what was fictional. Her remote and recent memory was very poor. Her abstractions, conceptual thinking, concentration, and attention span were grossly disturbed.

The medical workup showed a mild diabetes. There was also neurological deficit on the left side consisting of absence of deep tendon reflexes and some rigidity of the left upper extremity suggesting the possibility of an organic lesion. Patient's sleeping and eating patterns were regular. Personal hygiene and appearance showed marked deterioration.

Diagnosis: Primary degenerative dementia, senile onset, with depression.

CARE AND TREATMENT

The goal of care and treatment of elderly psychotic patients is the restoration of optimum functioning in the individual. Thus, care and treatment are aimed toward treating the reversible disease process, medical and psychiatric, and manipulating the environment to accommodate for irreversible deficit. The treatment program is based upon the individual patient's reaction to the process of aging—physical, emotional, and social.

Physical. Often the care and treatment are focused upon the physical aspects because the way in which the elderly patient's physical needs are met, the way in which he is treated medically for his organic disease, and the way in which he is treated somatically for his mental disorder all provide emotional and social treatment as well.

Intake-Output. The elderly patient's intake and output are of particular importance to his physical and mental health. Often he does not eat and drink properly to maintain good nutrition, or his body processes do not provide for adequate assimilation, or his physical functioning interferes with healthy metabolism. His diet should be planned to fit his particular physical needs and condition.

It may be a diet high in protein, vitamin and mineral content, because these are often lacking in the diet of the elderly person. In fact, elderly patients often need more of these essential nutrients to make up for degenerative processes involving bone, muscle, and blood.

Elderly patients have often been on inadequate diets prior to acute illness, or have established poor eating habits. It may be necessary to provide dietary supplements high in these essential nutrients, or medication in cases where necessity demands it, such as multivitamins; vitamins A, B complex, C, and D; and potassium, iron, and calcium.

It is important, too, that the diet be easily digested. It is estimated that half of all Americans have lost their teeth by the age of 65, and more than two-thirds by the age of 75. Many elderly people, because of bone and tissue changes in the mouth, find that dentures are ill-fitting and even painful, so even if they have them, they may not use them, especially to eat. If the edentulous patient cannot be properly fitted with dentures, then the diet will have to be altered to make up for the deficit. Also, the diet should be in the form of frequent, small meals as an aid to digestion and cardiovascular problems. It is thought that infrequent, large meals, such as one meal a day in the form of a heavy dinner at night, add to the fatty deposits and cholesterol supply in the body, thus increasing the possibility of cardiovascular disease including obesity, arteriosclerosis, and ischemic attacks.

It may be necessary to give the patient some medication in order to increase his appetite. This can be done with small amounts of an alcoholic beverage before meals that serve also to promote circulation and relax tension. It can also be accomplished with vitamins, particularly vitamin B complex, which serves to promote muscle tone and general health as well. Occasionally, small doses of insulin, given before meals, may also serve to provide for diabetic control. It may be necessary to decrease or control appetite, for which the amphetamines such as Dexedrine may be used; this also helps to increase the activity level of the patient. Obviously, when a medication can be used that will serve more than one purpose, it is to the patient's advantage to use it.

It is important that the elderly patient have sufficient intake to maintain fluid balance and that may necessitate either forcing fluids or restricting them. For example, it might be desirable to force fluids on a patient with urinary problems, while for another patient with cardiac problems, the fluids might be restricted.

The problem of elimination is a common one in the elderly patient. The most desirable method of correcting this problem is with a proper diet, such as roughage, bulk foods with laxative action, and sufficient fluids. Sometimes the establishment of regular toilet habits is sufficient to eliminate the problem. Sometimes it is necessary to use medications such as Metamucil, which provides bulk, or Colace, which is a stool softener. It is better not to use harsh cathartics or enemas unless the situation demands it, and then they should be used only as a temporary and specific measure, for example, to rid the lower bowel of accumulated or impacted fecal matter.

Activity Level. Another major aspect in meeting the physical needs of elderly psychotic patients involves their level of activity. It is extremely important to get the elderly patient ambulatory as soon as possible. First of all, it is important to his general physical health—appetite, digestion, elimination, circulation, muscle tone, warmth—that his level of activity be sufficiently high. Second, it is important to make the necessary compensation for irreversible handicap on the part of the patient. The use of a cane or walker or wheelchair may facilitate the individual's ability to ambulate despite his handicap. Third, it is necessary to interrupt the isolated, lonely, withdrawn, or regressed pattern of existence of the elderly person. He will not be able to interact unless he is where the action is, and that means he must be able to move about, even if in a limited way.

Treatment of Disease. Another aspect of physical care and treatment of the elderly psychotic patient involves the medical treatment of organic disease. Treatment for cardiovascular disease commonly includes the use of vasodilators to lower blood pressure and relieve the resistance to circulation. For example, tranquilizing drugs may be used not only to provide relief from anxiety or psychotic symptoms but also to reduce the hypertension that often accompanies old age. Digoxin may be used to regulate and strengthen the heart muscle. The treatment of arthritis includes the use of physical therapy and rehabilitative techniques to restore range of motion, and drugs to relieve tension and pain. Sometimes a diuretic, such as Hydrodiuril, is used to relieve the retention of fluids in the bladder and tissues. Surgery may be necessary in severe or suspect cases of hypertrophy of the prostate or prolapse of the uterus. The most common treatment of diabetes in the elderly is an oral medication such as Diabinese and diet. Aminophylline may be used to control chronic bronchitis; it is also a diuretic, myocardial stimulant, and mild respiratory relaxant. Quadrinal is frequently used to relieve the symptoms of emphysema and asthma.

In the treatment of sensory and motor disturbances a minor tranquilizer such as Librium or Mellaril is often used to relieve the anxiety that results from a lack of understanding and ability to cope with the environment. There are many ways of correcting sensory and motor deficits or compensating for the deficits by making environmental changes or using environmental aids. A patient needs to have an eye examination to determine exactly what his problem is. He may need to be fitted with proper eyeglasses, or he may need a magnifying glass for reading fine print. Surgery may be required for cataracts, or pilocarpine for glaucoma, or Prostigmin for ptosis of the eyelids.

A hearing test should be given the elderly patient to determine the degree of dysfunction. He may need a hearing aid or to have the wax removed from the auditory canal periodically. He may need to have surgery to increase the conduction of sound. Often it is necessary for people to stand in front of him and address him directly and speak distinctly.

There are many other ways of compensating for deficits by environmental changes and aids, and we will discuss more of them in the section on nursing care and treatment.

The psychiatric treatment of the elderly psychotic patient is similar to that already outlined for schizophrenia and depression, depending upon the nature of the individual's reaction. Most often the treatment consists of a combination of antipsychotic and antianxiety tranquilizers such as Thorazine, Stelazine, and Librium, and an antidepressant such as Elavil, if it is indicated. It is very important that the elderly patient have a thorough physical examination including EEG, EKG, chest and spine x-rays, and blood and urine analysis to make sure there are no contraindications to somatic therapy.

The dosage of the psychoactive drugs is generally less than for acutely ill younger patients. For example, Thorazine may be given 10 to 75 mg. q.i.d., depending upon the degree of agitation. Thorazine spansules are often used 30 to 150 mg. q. 12 h. Sometimes Thorazine or Compazine spansules are used for sleep, as well as during the day for their tranquilizing effects. If sedatives are given, they are generally of the type that are readily excreted, such as chloral hydrate, and may be given in small amounts.

Acutely ill elderly psychotic patients are generally treated in the psychiatric hospital. However, they may be treated at home or in a nursing home or some other extended care facility. Usually there is an intensive treatment period followed by a period of readjustment; however, large doses of phenothiazines are generally not used because of the physical condition of the elderly patient. Sometimes the patient is treated for the acute illness and recuperates outside the hospital rather than in it. In other cases it is necessary for the patient to have an extended period of care in the hospital, or a protracted readjustment period. Sometimes it is not possible for the elderly patient to leave the hospital because of lack of adequate response on his part or lack of adequate placement in the community.

Emotional. Psychotherapy or counseling of elderly psychotic patients is generally directed toward helping the patient (1) assume as much responsibility for himself as possible; (2) cope more successfully with the problems he faces; and (3) accept more realistically the aging process. It is generally not related to changing the life style of the individual, but rather helping him live more effectively within his particular pattern. There is no effort to change the kind of person he is but rather to help him live out his life with some degree of peace and harmony. The idea is not to make his life situation different, but rather to help him manage it more successfully.

The attitude of the patient toward life and death has a great deal of influence upon the state of his health and his response to treatment. Thus, sometimes the counseling is directed toward helping a patient develop a more accepting or hopeful or positive attitude. Increasing his physical health, manipulating his environment so that he can negotiate it with some degree of success, fostering maximum personal independence, all help to change the patient's attitude.

It is extremely important that the patient maintain relationships with his family and friends—that the doors of the hospital or nursing home do not close behind him. He needs people now as he never did before, and he particularly needs those upon whom he depends for love, approval, respect. Families often need help in understanding the negative behavior of an elderly relative to prevent his being further isolated and deprived, and family therapy can help in this regard. Frequent visits from friends and family, home visits, and visits to community activities may be encouraged so as to help the patient keep in touch with the world around him.

Social. Everything in the patient's environment should be used in such a way as to promote the restoration of function—physical, emotional, social. For example, mealtime may be a big social event in the life of an elderly patient. Patients may dress for dinner, and men and women join together for the evening meal. They may share common living quarters as well as dining facilities where they all eat their meals together. They may go to a central dining room used by all of the patients and staff in the hospital.

Elderly patients may be given maximum responsibility for themselves and other patients in the readjustment period of treatment. They may live on an open ward, much like a dormitory, where they come and go pretty much as they please, make their own appointments, take their own medications, take care of themselves and their living quarters, and plan their own recreational activities. They may have patient meetings where problems in group living are discussed and resolved, and plans are made for participation in various activities and events in the hospital and community.

Environmental prescriptions may be written for individual patients. These prescriptions identify the kind and amount of environmental support that is required by an individual patient in order for his needs to be met. Such support may include anything from specific devices which assist him in mastering his environment to attitudes that staff should use in interaction with him. Environmental support is a kind of replacement therapy designed to compensate for the individual patient's deficits. It should include detailed observation of the patient's level of functioning in the activities of daily living, arranging the physical environment to suit the needs of small groups of patients, adapting routines and activities to the changing levels of functioning throughout the day, simplifying the environment as much as possible so that the patient may more easily master it. Since these are generally seen as nursing functions, we will discuss them further under nursing care and treatment.

R.T., O.T., and industrial activities should be geared toward the level of functioning of a particular patient or group of patients. These activities must fit within the individual life style of a patient and his particular physical condition. It is important that the activities also be planned to enhance the patient's feelings of self-esteem, usefulness, and importance. Most elderly patients are not in the habit of playing childish games like throwing beanbags at targets or dancing the heel-and-toe. Cards, bingo, and social dancing are generally more appropriate for recreation. Productive activities such as knitting, crocheting, leather work, and carpentry provide for greater satisfaction of elderly patients. Work assignments that provide some kind of meaningful service to others or to the community at large are particularly helpful to elderly patients. Just sitting and visiting, or group sings, are often enjoyable social activities for elderly patients. A good source of satisfaction for those who like to read but can no longer do so are the Talking Books made available through the Library for the Blind. Listening in a group and then discussing the stories create all sorts of opportunity for social exchange.

Case Example No. 1 (See p. 235)

The patient was admitted to the hospital and put on Taractan 25 mg. t.i.d., Kemadrin 5 mg. t.i.d. For the weight loss and poor appetite she was also given vitamins in the form of vitamin B intramuscularly. For her persistent cough she received liquifying expectorants in the form of potassium iodide and later Quadrinal 1 tab. t.i.d. and h.s., which relieved her greatly. She was seen in a medical clinic regarding her cardiac and respiratory status because of her chronic cough and constant expectoration. The medical consultant found her chest condition compatible with mild early emphysema and suggested she stop smoking. In the course of drug therapy, the patient developed a rash, which responded to Cholor-Trimeton 12 mg. q. 12 h.

It took approximately 12 days for the voices to become fainter and less frequent. She learned not to be frightened by them anymore, and she did not act upon them. In approximately one month, the patient improved considerably. The hallucinations completely subsided and her suspicious attitude disappeared.

Because of her history of unreliability in taking medication, she was thought to be a good candidate for Prolixin. She was given oral Prolixin 5 mg. b.i.d. for 5 days, and then started on Prolixin Decanoate 25 mg. I.M. q. 2 wks. At the same time she received antiparkinsonism medication in the form of Artane 5 mg. at 8 a.m.; to help her sleep, she received Thorazine 75 mg. spansule h.s. She was discharged to her sister and arrangements were made for her to return to the outpatient department every two weeks for counseling and I.M. injections of Prolixin Decanoate. Follow-up medical care was turned over to her family physician.

Case Example No. 2 (See p. 236)

The patient was admitted to the hospital and put on lithium 600 mg. daily, Thorazine 50 mg. h.s. He was assigned a counselor and an activity group to attend daily.

The course of treatment was marked by continual efforts on the part of the patient to dictate his own regimen, including his level of medication and projected date of discharge. In this, the patient was supported by his wife, who seemed to think the treatment program should fit into the academic calendar rather than the patient's rate of recovery, so that he should be well by the end of fall quarter. The patient and his wife were seen in family therapy and after about six weeks, the patient had begun to appear, at least, to accept the idea that the recommendations of the hospital staff were made in his own best interests. This was regarded as the development of some insight on his part and he was discharged with the recommendation that he receive private psychiatric help.

The prognosis in this case would appear to depend in great degree upon the willingness of the patient to cooperate in followup care. If the patient will continue (as was strongly recommended) to remain under professional care (and he has stated that he will do so), the prognosis may be favorable. The previous history of dropping out of followup care, however, together with the patient's admitted distrust of doctors and medications, make it appear that the prognosis may actually be no better than guarded.

Case Example No. 3 (See p. 237)

The patient was admitted to the hospital and placed on Haldol 10 mg. h.s., and Thorazine 25 mg. p.r.n. She was assigned to a counselor and a daily activity group. She regularly attended O.T. and R.T. After a two week stay in the psychiatric hospital, she was discharged to the outpatient department. She comes in every two weeks for her counseling session. She is living with her daughter and keeping house for her, and apparently she is getting along all right, although she still has delusional ideas and tends to be overly religious.

Case Example No. 4 (See p. 238)

Patient was placed on 100 mg. Diabinese once a day to control diabetes, Haldol 1 mg. b.i.d., chloral hydrate 0.5 gm. h.s. for sleep, and vitamin B complex injection 2 cc. 3 times a week to increase general health.

During the first four hospital days, she remained inactive, sat in a chair, and did not socialize. She was assigned a counselor and an activity group to meet daily. After about ten days, she began to show more interest in her surroundings and took an active part in O.T. Her sleeping and eating patterns improved. She became oriented, her speech was free-flowing and appropriate, her mood and energy level were about normal. Her memory of events for the past three or four years remained poor.

Because of her rapid response to treatment, patient was discharged to the outpatient department and took a job as a part-time housekeeper. However, her prior symptoms returned and she was unable to carry out the job successfully. She went for a walk and became lost three miles from home, left her purse in a store, and in general tried to do more than she was capable of in her desire to succeed.

She was depressed over having to return to the hospital but adjusted well to this. She was placed on Haldol 1 mg. b.i.d. Prognosis is for a limited recovery and she will probably be a nursing home candidate.

NURSING CARE AND TREATMENT

The care and treatment of elderly psychotic patients have some specific applications for nurses that need to be emphasized.

First of all, the observations of the nurses are extremely important because they determine the course of action to be taken in care and treatment. Therefore, the observations should be detailed and precise, identifying what a patient can do for himself, under what circumstances, at what time of day, and with what amount of help. For example, it may be possible for a patient to dress himself if his clothes are laid out for him in the order in which he puts them on. It may be possible for still another patient to pick out his own clothes and put them on without assistance.

It is important, too, for the nurse to share her observations with others in such a way as to aid in the establishment of an effective care and treatment program. For example, she may report that a particular patient is too confused to dress himself. The general conclusion would then be that he must be dressed by someone else. She may, however, report that this patient can dress himself after he has had his bath in the morning if his clothes are laid out for him in the order in which they are to be put on. Then the appropriate nursing action would be to see that he has his bath in the morning, and that his clothes are laid out for him afterward so that he may dress himself. The difference between the two observations, reports, and resulting actions is the difference between effective and ineffective care.

The nursing observations of physical signs and symptoms are also extremely important because patients' behavior may vary from not communicating verbally at all, to numerous somatic complaints. The nurse, then, must be especially alert and aware in order to correctly observe, interpret, and determine the physical condition of the patient. It is much better for her to be cautious and conservative in her estimate of the patient than to jump to conclusions, take his inabilities for granted, or be overly optimistic. With the elderly patient, it is not advisable to rely upon time and his own recuperative powers to take care of his symptoms. When he needs medical help, he generally needs it now—not next week or even tomorrow.

To create a therapeutic environment for elderly patients, the nurse must be able to manipulate the physical arrangement of the ward as well as the routines and activities so as to best suit individuals and groups of patients. The environment must provide for the safety, comfort, rehabilitation, and optimum functioning of the patients. Safety includes replacing any hazardous furnishings or equipment in the environment with whatever is safest for elderly patients. For example, it may be necessary to control the faucets in the lavatory so that water hot enough to burn the patient cannot be accidentally turned on. It may be necessary to cover radiators or registers so that the patient will not be accidentally burned on them. Hand railings along walkways and hallways and grab bars in the bathroom may be installed to protect the patient from falling as well as to enable him to move about more freely and independently. Throw rugs or cords on the floor should be eliminated in order to avoid tripping over them. It is often necessary to have the temperature higher for elderly patients. They may need a sweater and warmer clothing, and an extra blanket and warmer bedding because of their poor circulation and ineffective heat regulating mechanism. It is desirable to arrange sleeping accommodations so that the patient who needs a quiet environment is farther away from the center of activity at night. However, the patient who needs the security of people around him should be put closer to the center of activity. Patients who become confused, particularly at night, need to be closer to the bathroom facility so as to avoid incontinence.

To compensate for the patient's poor vision and to enhance his ability to master his environment, various kinds of visual aids may be introduced. The bathroom door may be painted a special color, or the figure of a man or woman may cover the door to help distinguish its use. Calendars with large letters and numbers or blackboards with large lettering may help to orient the patient to the date or important events of the day. Color coding may be used to help patients find their way about the ward more easily and be more independent as a result. Arm bracelets, bed cards, tablecloths, and towels of the same color may help a patient determine where he is to sleep, eat, and wash his hands and face. Installing Dutch doors will help the patient see into rooms and more readily identify where he is and where other people are.

It may be necessary to plan the day's schedule so that a rest period is included, because elderly patients often tire easily. Activities should be planned so that they come at the time of day when the patients are most capable of activity, such as mid-morning, mid-afternoon, or early evening. Mealtimes should be arranged so as to accommodate the needs of the elderly patients. This may mean providing five small meals a day instead of the usual three. It may mean mid-morning, mid-afternoon, and bedtime snacks so as to provide adequate nourishment, fluid intake, and pleasure for the elderly patients.

Probably the most important environmental factor is the attitude of the people surrounding the patient. The general atmosphere must be accepting, hopeful, realistic, encouraging, and relaxed if it is to be helpful. Often young people get along better with elderly patients than do middle-aged, perhaps because there is more distance between them and less of a parent-child relationship or role reversal. It is very important that the nurse care for an elderly patient with respect, regardless of his level of competence, physical condition, or behavior. I heard an elderly patient say the other day, "It's pretty upsetting when you've taken care of yourself for sixty years, to have some snip of a nurse come along and tell you what to do." If it is necessary to give instructions to an elderly patient, it should be done with all due consideration for the individual. It may help the nurse to keep in mind that the patient is not a child, nor feeble-minded, nor her grandpa. He is a person whom she is there to serve in the best way she knows how.

Rehabilitation begins with the onset of illness and the initiation of treatment, so that the nurse's role changes during the various stages of treatment. In acute illness, the patient usually goes through two stages of treatment—intensive care and readjustment. The elderly psychotic patient is treated as a medical emergency in the intensive phase, and nurses usually have less difficulty with this role than in the readjustment phase. However, even in the intensive care phase, the nurse must apply the principles of rehabilitation, and keep the patient as self-sufficient as possible. The nurse's role may include that of counselor, housemother, socializing agent, recreation director, companion, and friend. It is important that she not supply any more help than the patient requires because to do so undermines his self-esteem, confidence, and independence. She must be able to decide what kind of help he needs and when he needs it so as to avoid intervening when it is to the patient's advantage to rely upon resources within himself and his environment rather than depending upon her. It is rather like the good mother who allows her children to work out things for themselves, and interferes only when they need her advice or help. This does not imply neglecting or ignoring the patient. It actually requires that the nurse be more alert, observant, and knowledgeable about her patient than if she were giving him complete care because she must decide upon a course of action based upon inference rather than direct observation. Unfortunately, many people find it easier to take care of a patient themselves than to help him take care of himself.

If the patient is chronically ill or needs extended care, he should not be left to care for himself or punished because he cannot do so. It takes a healthy, secure, patient, and compassionate person to give complete care to an elderly brain-damaged patient who is not likely to recover. Sometimes patients are scolded or ridiculed or ignored because they are incontinent or messy eaters or noisy or otherwise unable to care for themselves. Well, if the patient could take care of himself, he wouldn't need the nurse, would he? If he could be well, he wouldn't be sick, in other words, and would not come under the care of the nurse at all. Again, it may help the nurse to remember that she is there to serve the patient like any other customer, and it is up to her to provide whatever she can to add to his comfort and pleasure. Many times elderly patients are made to feel that they are a nuisance or a burden to those who are entrusted with (and paid for) their care. This adds to their negative feelings about themselves and life in general and makes them behave in ways that pose further problems to those caring for them. It is no small accomplishment to be able to say you have made someone happier or more comfortable because your paths in life have happened to cross.

The nursing care and treatment should also be appropriate to existing physical diseases, the most common of which are cardiovascular disturbances, arthritis, defective sensory-motor perception, and fracture. We will not discuss these here, but the student is referred to Wells's *Problems in Geriatric Nursing Care* and Christopherson's *Rehabilitation Nursing* (see Chapter References).

The organic psychoses are those accompanied by organic pathology and dysfunction of the central nervous system. The symptoms we see are a combination of the individual's behavioral reaction to stress and the symptoms associated with impairment of brain or nervous system functions. The most common of these psychotic conditions are those which result from the individual's physical, emotional, and social reaction to the aging process, and are similar to the syndromes of schizophrenia and manic-depressive psychosis.

The last stage of the life cycle for many elderly people means not only great stress but a reduced personal capacity within the individual to master the stress, and critical changes in his life situation that further deplete his resources. The areas of stress which accompany the aging process include decrease in personal and social status, decrease in physical ability, decrease in intellectual capacity, and deprivation resulting from serious interference in the satisfaction of basic needs.

Treatment consists of treating the reversible medical and psychiatric disease and manipulating the environment to compensate for the irreversible deficits. This is accomplished by drug therapy, surgical procedures, the use of environmental aids, and surrounding the patient with a healing atmosphere. The aim is to restore optimum functioning in the individual, even in the face of permanent deficit, and foster maximum personal independence.

Nursing care and treatment consist of careful assessment of the individual's needs and his level of competence in meeting them so that only the help that is required is provided by the nurse. The nurse's role and function depend upon the outcome of this formula for nursing action. It may vary from providing complete nursing care to acting in a capacity similar to that of housemother. Whatever the care and treatment program, it is effective if it increases the patient's feelings of self-esteem, usefulness, and importance.

REFERENCES

Allen, Marcia D.: "Drug therapy in the elderly," *American Journal of Nursing, 80* (August, 1980) pp. 1474–1475.

Brink, Terry: *Geriatric Psychotherapy,* Human Sciences Press, New York, 1979.

Burnside, Irene Mortenson: "Eulogy for Mrs. Hogue," *American Journal of Nursing, 78* (April, 1978) pp. 624–626.

Burnside, Irene Mortenson: *Psychosocial Nursing Care of the Aged,* 2nd Edition, McGraw-Hill, New York, 1980.

Butler, Robert: *Aging and Mental Health,* 2nd Edition, C. V. Mosby, St. Louis, 1977.

Chamberlin, Adaline Boardman: "Providing motivation," *American Journal of Nursing, 78* (January, 1978) p. 80.

Christopherson, Victor, et al.: *Rehabilitation Nursing: Perspectives and Applications,* McGraw-Hill, New York, 1973.

Combs, Karen L.: "Preventive health care," *American Journal of Nursing, 78* (August, 1978) pp. 1339–1341.

Eliopolous, Charlotte: *Geriatric Nursing,* Harper & Row, New York, 1980.

Hogstel, Mildred O: "How do the elderly view their world?" *American Journal of Nursing*, *78* (August, 1978) pp. 1335–1336.
Lore, Ann: "Supporting the hospitalized elderly person," *American Journal of Nursing*, *79* (March, 1979) pp. 496–499.
Robb, Susanne S.: "Advocacy for the aged," *American Journal of Nursing*, *79* (October, 1979) pp. 1736–1738.
Storandt, Martha, et al.: *Clinical Psychology of Aging*, Plenum Press, New York, 1978.
Wells, Thelma: *Problems in Geriatric Nursing Care*, Churchill Livingstone, New York, 1980.

Chapter 14

Sociopathic Reactions to Stress

Some individuals adjust to the demands of life, and we call that healthy behavior. Some people develop distorted thinking, or profound mood and motor disturbances, and we call that psychotic behavior. Some people act out their conflicts with society, and we call that sociopathic behavior. Psychotic disorders represent basic disturbances in all areas of the person's functioning—thinking, feeling, and doing. Sociopathic disorders represent basic disturbances in a person's interaction with society. Such disturbances in social behavior are also referred to by other names, including behavior disorders, character neurosis, character disorders, psychopathic personality, or personality disorders. In general, all these terms refer to a severe disruption in the individual's social exchange. The names reflect the different theories explaining this type of reaction to stress, and they point up the controversy surrounding this kind of behavior.

Sociopathic behavior is probably the least understood of all the categories of mental illness. Despite the complexity of schizophrenia, for example, it is easier for most people to accept and deal constructively with schizophrenic behavior in others than with sociopathic behavior. In the first place, sociopathic behavior is either a direct or indirect attack upon society and what it stands for. This represents a threat to the security of the group and the members of that group, which includes all of us. Sociopathic behavior generally provokes defensive reactions in others which tend to reflect their prejudices about such behavior. Social and personal attitudes toward the use of alcohol and drugs, deviant ways of obtaining sexual gratification, and criminal acts perpetrated against society may cause people to react with fear, anger, distrust, revulsion, or vengeance. It is difficult for most people to even discuss such behavior, let alone accept, understand, and treat it therapeutically. It is probably the most misunderstood of all disorders because it involves actions that are contrary to and often in direct conflict with accepted social values. Therefore, the behavior is likely to be seen as immoral rather than sick, or it is seen as weakness, so that all the person needs is greater willpower to overcome it rather than assistance in the form of treatment.

Furthermore, sociopathic behavior involves the outward expression of aggressive and sexual impulses, which most of us spend our lives covering up. No other areas of human feeling or expression are so carefully and minutely governed, controlled, or guarded by social dictates as those of sex and aggression. Most people have worked hard to control and channel their feelings of anger and aggression, of sexual desire and passion, in accord with society's teachings. To see lack of control and the direct expression of primitive impulses in people who are supposed to be responsible adults, arouses feelings of resentment and sometimes envy in others. Most people have felt like cutting loose with negative feelings or primitive impulses at some time or another, but they have struggled to keep them in check. So if another individual behaves in ways we struggle to control or deny or even punish ourselves for, we may want to see that he pays for it.

Most people manage to incorporate the standards for behavior that their society dictates in the form of individual conscience. If a person does not conform to these standards, indeed flaunts them, he is thought to be guilty of wrongdoing and deserving of punishment. From the history of different cultures, one learns that mankind traditionally deals harshly with the nonconformist, particularly the antisocial person. Quotations from the Bible reflect the social attitude of retaliation and retribution for one's sins: "An eye for an eye, and a tooth for a tooth," and "If thy right eye offends thee, pluck it out."

There are many different kinds of sociopathic behavior and many different explanations as to why a person behaves in such a way. For example, people who drink do so for a variety of reasons: one to overcome his shyness, another to feel more confident, another to drown his sorrows. In fact, sociopathic behavior may range from almost healthy to psychotic, depending upon the degree of disturbance in the individual's functioning. Furthermore, the various kinds of behavior that are described as sociopathic may, instead, be symptoms of other underlying disorders. A person may drink to avoid the profound feelings of depression. A person may resort to sexual promiscuity, prostitution, or homosexuality in a schizophrenic effort to establish his own identity and some kind of interpersonal contact with others. A person may come to rely upon the effect of drugs to compensate for a life of deprivation.

Or he may use LSD or marihuana in a desire to experiment, rebel against authority, or simply belong to his peer group. A man may commit criminal acts against society because he thinks people are out to get him and he must strike first, as in paranoid schizophrenia, or because he feels he is no good and should be punished severely, as in depression.

At the risk of oversimplifying a very complex group of mental disorders, we are going to discuss some of the common features in the development, symptoms, and treatment of sociopathic behavior. But let us keep in mind that what is discussed here does not necessarily apply to all kinds of sociopathic behavior, and some kinds will not be discussed here at all.

DEFINITION OF TYPES

Personality disorders are deeply ingrained maladaptive patterns of behavior, with symptoms different from, yet similar to, those of psychotic and neurotic disorders. They are lifelong patterns, sometimes recognizable in adolescence and even earlier (see Appendix B). These disorders represent a marginal kind of adjustment which generally does not disrupt an individual's functioning to the extent that he sees himself, or is seen by others, as mentally ill. Therefore, he does not often receive treatment, especially in a psychiatric hospital, unless there are complicating features to his illness such as accompanying distortions in thinking as seen in schizophrenia, or disturbances in mood as seen in depression. Sometimes his physical condition, such as a severe toxic reaction to alcohol or drugs, may necessitate treatment in a general hospital. Illegal or criminal activities may bring him into conflict with the law, and then he may be treated psychiatrically as a part of the rehabilitation program of a correctional institution. Most often he sees himself, and is seen by others, as peculiar, eccentric, different, a social misfit, who should be punished rather than cared for.

The more common forms of sociopathic behavior are antisocial personality, psychosocial disorders, drug addiction, and alcoholism. Antisocial personality refers to that kind of behavior which brings an individual into repeated conflict with society and with the law. It includes such antisocial acts as burglary, theft, arson, assault, rape, and murder.

Psychosocial disorders include gender identity disorders, paraphilias, and psychosocial dysfunction (see Appendix B). The more common examples of sexually deviant behavior include pedophilia, exhibitionism, prostitution, sadism, and masochism.

Pedophilia refers to the pathological love of children by an adult that results in sexual gratification. Exhibitionism means exposing one's self, usually the genitals, to members of the opposite sex and usually in public places. Prostitution means resorting to sexual intercourse for money, livelihood, or favors. Sadism means deriving sexual satisfaction from torturing others by inflicting pain, ill-treatment, or humiliation upon them. Masochism means deriving sexual satisfaction from suffering pain, ill-treatment, or humiliation.

Drug addiction refers to physiological and emotional dependence upon a drug. The individual develops a typical withdrawal syndrome of organic origin when the drug is taken away. The symptoms include tremor, irritability, nausea, vomiting, profuse perspiration, hallucinations, and convulsions. It is thought by many that the use of addictive drugs changes the structure of cells in the body so that the presence of the drug is necessary in order to maintain normal cellular function. The majority of drugs upon which people develop a dependence fall into one of four categories: (1) opium and its derivatives, such as morphine, codeine, heroin, Dilaudid; (2) synthetic analgesics, such as methadone, meperidine; (3) sedatives and hypnotics, such as barbiturates, paraldehyde, chloral hydrate; (4) miscellaneous drugs, such as marihuana, mescaline, amphetamines, LSD, cocaine, and alcohol.

Alcoholism is a special kind of drug addiction, and because of its prevalence and severity as a health problem in the United States, it is usually considered a separate category of illness. Alcoholism refers to an intake of alcohol in sufficient amounts to damage the individual's health or personal or social functioning, or when it becomes a prerequisite to normal functioning. It includes acute intoxication, periodic or habitual drinking to excess, and the inability of the individual to go one day without drinking. All presume dependence upon the drug for one reason or another. Intoxication is defined as that state in which the person's coordination, speech, and behavior are so impaired or altered as to reduce his ability to function effectively. It may be the result of the intake of alcohol or other drugs. Episodic excessive drinking means the presence of alcoholism and intoxication as often as four times a year. Habitual excessive drinking means the presence of alcoholism and intoxication more than twelve times a year, or that the individual is obviously under the influence of alcohol more than once a week, even though not intoxicated.

ANTISOCIAL BEHAVIOR

The individual with this kind of behavior is one who gets into frequent, repeated difficulty with the law; it is sometimes called delinquent behavior. It is as if the individual were deliberately or compulsively delinquent. His actions are often irrational and represent a repetitive acting out which he is unable to inhibit or control. Therefore, we see the compulsive continuance of behavior, which rather than helping to satisfy his needs does the opposite, that is, creates further frustration. It is a self-destructive way of behaving. The child who knows perfectly well that if he steals money from his mother's purse he will not only be punished but rejected as well takes the money anyhow and leaves the purse open so that the theft will be all the more obvious.

The adolescent who knows he will be caught if he steals an automobile does so anyway and drives down Main Street exceeding the speed limit so as to make his actions all the more evident. The adult who knows when the police make their rounds robs the corner grocery just at the time when he will be sure to be caught. The criminal who has been a model prisoner breaks out the night before he is to be paroled, thus insuring that he will spend a considerably longer time incarcerated.

There are many explanations as to why the individual behaves in such a self-defeating fashion, but it is certain that if he could behave differently he would not choose this route. Some people think it is a constitutional problem; that is, the person is born with some kind of genetic weakness or inferior makeup. Others believe this behavior is due to some kind of organic disorder of the brain. Another theory is that it stems from faulty interaction with the environment, resulting from serious defects in an individual's personality structure. All of these explanations have some validity and substantiation in fact, and all of them see the problem as centering around the person's inability to learn the necessary lessons for successful living. Our discussion will focus upon what seems to interfere with the individual's adjustment as it relates to the pattern of his growth, development, and function.

In reaction to frustration, sometimes in the form of rejection, the child experiences hostility toward his parents. His unacceptable impulses, particularly aggression, find their outlet in actions rather than disturbances in feeling, distortions in thinking, or physical symptoms. He does not learn to separate himself from the environment and develop strength and integrity within himself, nor does he learn how to postpone satisfaction and still maintain peace within himself. He is unable to control or inhibit or direct his basic impulses and promote harmony with his environment. He remains as he came into the world—all needs, lacking in self and conscience. He maintains the personality characteristics of the infant—demanding, dependent, receiving—and continues to interact with the world in these terms, even though the opposite is expected of him.

The inability of a child to grow up and function as a responsible adult is expected to function may result from different kinds of faulty interactions with his environment, particularly with his parents during his formative years. He may be completely rejected so that he never learns to modify or channel the hostility he experiences because he does not have the opportunity to do so. He may be so over-indulged or over-protected that he never learns where he ends and the world begins because there are no limits set for him. He may be ignored and isolated and may never learn that he is a person of some worth and dignity who really belongs to the group. He may be so severely criticized or punished that he never learns the joys and pleasures that can result from socially acceptable interactions.

A child may have been expected to behave in such impossibly virtuous ways that he can escape the sense of complete and utter failure only by annihilating the strictness and rigidity. Whatever the reasons for his failure to incorporate limits, controls, coping methods, a sense of identity and strength, he winds up in serious trouble with himself and in conflict with his environment.

Antisocial acts may become a means of defense against (1) more disruptive reactions to stress, such as depression; (2) more devastating feelings, such as fear or loneliness; (3) more destructive experiences, such as failure or rejection. The individual may adopt a devil-may-care attitude toward life including his own, and run rough-shod over everyone in his path. His behavior may include a mixture of symptoms from all four of the categories of illness which we will discuss: antisocial personality, sexual deviations, drug addiction, and alcoholism.

Often the individual with antisocial personality is described as lacking purpose in life. He seems to have no long-range goals and lives for the moment. This is perhaps related to his need for immediate satisfaction and his low-frustration tolerance. He often makes a very good first impression, but his instability and lack of consideration for others may cause great suffering for his friends and family. He seems deficient in moral sensibility and the sense of responsibility expected of adults. Often he displays the symptoms of lying, stealing, showing off, manipulating, promiscuity, temper tantrums, or destructive outbursts. He seems to have little feeling for anyone or anything. He often uses people like objects, considering only his own pleasure and discarding them heartlessly when they are no longer useful to him. Often he is described as selfish, amoral, cruel, and impulsive. He seems unable to suffer guilt or to learn from his experience that he should or must behave differently.

The person with an antisocial personality gains little satisfaction from his way of behaving, and his ways are not only unacceptable but are also attacks upon society. The core problem of the illness is lack of control and rejection of authority, with aggression, hostility, and basic impulses acted out against society. He develops a distorted picture of himself and the world he lives in, has little self or conscience, is emotionally immature, and is unable to postpone satisfaction.

Antisocial acts may occur at any stage in the life cycle. In childhood, as with other kinds of disturbed behavior, people often tend to write these acts off as a phase the child is going through or something he will outgrow. Frequently, antisocial acts of the problem child are first dealt with in the school system. The child may exhibit such symptoms as poor scholastic achievement, aggressive behavior with other children, hyperactivity, lying, stealing, truancy, temper tantrums, or showing off. In adolescence, or even pre-adolescence, the child may get into difficulty with the law with such acts as stealing, fighting with other children, particularly those younger than himself, cruelty to neighborhood pets, and destruction of property. He may commit arson, vandalism, theft, burglary, assault, sexual offenses, murder. He may use or abuse drugs, including alcohol. In fact, a youngster's behavior may be as offensive as an adult's, thereby throwing him into a life situation in which he is repeatedly punished for behavior that he seems unable to correct.

As an adult, he may commit any of the antisocial acts mentioned so far and they almost invariably lead to some kind of legal action being taken against him. The range of behavior may vary from the immature, irresponsible husband to the alcoholic, abusive parent; from the successful Don Juan to the flagrantly deviant sexual behavior of exhibitionism; from the social drinker to the hopeless derelict on skid row; from the occasional pot smoker to the confirmed dope addict; from the ready fighter to the psychopathic killer. One winds up in divorce court or civil court, and another in criminal court, but all are asked to pay for their misdeeds.

As a child, the disturbed person is referred to as a behavior problem; as an adolescent, a juvenile delinquent; as an adult, a psychopath, offender, or criminal.

SEXUALLY DEVIANT BEHAVIOR

In our society we have strict rules and regulations governing the expression of sexual as well as aggressive impulses. Violation of these controls reflects serious personal and social problems which may severely interfere with the individual's healthy functioning. Each person is expected to incorporate the standards of behavior, including sexual behavior, for his particular social group through the process of identification and the development of self and conscience. If he obtains sexual satisfaction in ways that are different from the accepted heterosexual practice of coitus, then something is amiss in his sexual adjustment. The degree to which his methods interfere with the satisfaction of his basic needs, and the extent to which they are viewed in the general society as unacceptable, determine the seriousness of the symptoms. For example, it is not uncommon for husband and wife to punish one another, either consciously or unconsciously. However, when punishment becomes a major source of sexual gratification in such a relationship, then we say the behavior is unhealthy or deviant.

In the process of developing physically, emotionally, and socially, the individual also develops sexually. He must learn how to control and express his basic impulses involving sexual desire and aggression. He learns from interaction with his environment how to fulfill his sexual role in life. As a child, he learns how to behave as the adult he becomes through the process of identifying with significant people in his environment and incorporating their expectations of how to behave. If the significant others are faulty models, or he incorrectly perceives what they expect of him, or he experiences repeated failure in his attempts to imitate them, then he may not develop the necessary sense of identity and the appropriate sexual behavior which accompanies it. For example, if the little boy is surrounded with female figures, his identification will be faulty, and he may express himself in feminine ways. If the little girl takes her father's place as her mother's champion and protector, then she may behave in more masculine ways than her role in life calls for. If sexual expression and aggression are equated in the behavior of the adults around him, these two may be fused in the child's mind, and he will get sexual pleasure by being cruel. If he is repeatedly rejected or abandoned by his parents, he may begin a desperate search for the missing affection, turning from one stranger to another. In other words, as a result of his learning experiences in childhood, the individual may turn to sado-masochistic or promiscuous ways of behaving in an attempt to satisy his needs.

Very often, as in all kinds of sociopathic behavior, sexually deviant behavior is seen as weakness, immorality, or wrongdoing rather than illness. We have a tendency to condemn the behavior and punish the person who commits the offense without understanding the nature of it or bothering to correct the cause. The behavior represents an attack upon the mores of society, and the response is a defense against that threat to the security of the group.

The stage in the life cycle in which the individual struggles for a sense of identity, leaving behind the sexual behavior of childhood, is adolescence. He is expected to turn into the adult form of male or female after successfully negotiating this period, leaving behind him previous forms of sexual expression and pleasure, and turning to the mature adult form of heterosexual relationships. He may be successful in negotiating this period without fully developing his sense of identity, and may embark on a heterosexual course in adulthood, marry, and raise a family. However, his experiences with heterosexuality may be unsuccessful, or the stress of a particular period or circumstances in life may be sufficient to cause him to search for sexual satisfaction and identity in deviant ways.

Sexually deviant impulses may be either overt or covert. That is, the individual may be aware of such desires and acting upon them (overt), or he may be unaware of them, or aware of them but not acting upon them (covert). An individual learns how to express his sexual desires and aggression in acceptable ways, how to direct basic impulses into constructive channels. It is not unhealthy or abnormal to love people of the same sex, or to love children, or to want to be noticed, loved, or taken care of, or to feel angry, destructive, or aggressive. It is, however, considered unhealthy or abnormal to express those feelings or thoughts or desires in certain kinds of ways—pedophilia, sado-masochism, or prostitution. It is unhealthy or abnormal because it is contrary to the regulations of our society, and we are products of that society.

Further, sexually deviant behavior tends to interfere with the satisfaction of basic needs rather than promote it. People who engage in sexual acts that are contrary to what society has determined as acceptable often feel guilty and not quite respectable, despite the fact that they may derive pleasure from the experience, or feel that they are unable to control their behavior or redirect it. The person often feels inadequate, inferior, or unworthy to begin with and such behavior often makes him feel worse instead of better as a person. The use of drugs, including alcohol, is sometimes introduced to relieve the feeling of guilt, remove the severe self-criticism, and at the same time, punish the participant for his wrongdoing.

THE USE AND ABUSE OF DRUGS

This is an age of drug use and abuse. Different ages have different ways of dealing with anxiety; we take drugs. People take drugs to keep them awake and put them to sleep, pep them up and calm them down, increase and decrease their appetites, speed up and slow down their elimination, stimulate or inhibit their estrogen production; and today we even have "the pill" which can control the creation of life itself. We have become a nation of pleasure seekers, concerned with what we can buy and how we can enjoy ourselves.

It used to be that drugs were used mostly by the socially deprived in an attempt to experience some of the joy and pleasure they were denied in real life. Now drug use cuts across all social classes. It used to be that drug users were in their late teens or early twenties. Now 15- and 16-year-olds, even 10- and 12-year-olds, are experimenting with and are generally knowledgeable about drugs, including marihuana and narcotics. Youngsters see and imitate their parents, but instead of liquor they are looking for something new, different, untried—their "own thing." Furthermore, youngsters have ready access to the medicine cabinet which often contains all kinds of drugs, including amphetamines, barbiturates, and tranquilizers.

There is great concern for the increased use of drugs, particularly among the youth of the country, partly because dependence upon drugs becomes a way of life and adds to, rather than resolves, underlying emotional problems. Young people take drugs for a variety of reasons. A great many just experiment, taking them once, or a few times, to satisfy their curiosity, display rebellion or courage, or conform to the group. The majority do not need drugs, so they can take them or leave them alone much as adults use alcohol. However, for the person with deep-seated emotional difficulty, the road from marihuana (pot) to heroin (H) is all downhill.

Sometimes youngsters turn to drugs because they feel unwanted or rejected by their parents. They may try to find the acceptance they need with their peers, some of whom may be maladjusted or use drugs, and when they follow suit, they get the affection they so sorely need. Sometimes youngsters feel ignored, almost as if they did not actually exist as people, only offspring, by their parents. They may turn to drugs to attract the attention of their parents in a rather desperate plea for recognition. Sometimes youngsters have so much permissiveness or so little in the way of expectations from their parents that they become passive receivers in the world, not givers. They stand in the receiving line, taking anything that comes along for the comfort and pleasure it gives. Sometimes parents have completely unrealistic ambitions for their children regardless of their capabilities, so they are constantly disappointed in them. Youngsters, in their defeat and frustration, may turn to drugs for some kind of comfort and solace. Sometimes youngsters come from homes where they have not had the proper models to follow so that they might develop into responsible, giving adults. Instead, they remain at an infantile, expectant stage, and turn to drugs for warmth and comfort.

The increased use of drugs reflects a change in social values and a general breakdown in family relationships. Most young people feel that their parents do not understand, accept, or care about them. This is commonly referred to as the "generation gap." The youth of today have been called the "turned on" generation partly because of their inclination to take anything they can get their hands on—not only LSD, STP, DMT, and marihuana, but antihistamines, airplane glue, barbiturates, amphetamines, tranquilizers, cold remedies, heart stimulants, nasal inhalants, and aerosol ingredients. For example, amyl nitrite, a heart stimulant, was used as a pep pill by youngsters until it was taken off the pharmacy shelves. An asthma remedy, Asthmador, was brewed as a tea or imbibed with Coke in a mixture called "mud" to give the users a "trip." Contac, which contains atropine, has been used to produce hallucinations. Throat discs, which contain chloroform, have been chewed like candy to produce a "high."

Cough syrup is one of the oldest abused drugs on the market. For one thing, it has been, until recently, readily available in over-the-counter sales. It is often used by heroin addicts to "kick the habit." During World War II, elixir of terpin hydrate and codeine (ETH) was called "G.I. gin," and used for the same purpose, to get "high." It contains codeine and 40 percent alcohol. Other popularly abused cough syrups have been Robitussin and Romilar. Even when the codeine is removed and other cough-suppressing drugs are substituted, a person can get high from it if the mixture is taken in sufficient quantities and in combination with other drugs.

One of the very real dangers, of course, is that a drug which is capable of altering perception or mood may also prove fatal. Enough youngsters have suffered from the lethal effects of glue sniffing that some states have passed laws restricting its sale. Warnings have been issued against the use of cleaning fluids containing carbon tetrachloride and aerosol refrigerants like Freon. Any drug can be misused to produce reactions for which it was not intended. It is impossible to eliminate drug abuse completely, but efforts have been made to cut down on the practice. State Pharmacy Boards have taken many drugs off the pharmacy shelves and put some exempt narcotics back on prescription. The list of dangerous drugs has been increased. Hospitals and pharmacies have placed restrictions on access to drugs and instituted control measures in an effort to decrease drug abuse. More legislative control and less accessibility are recommended, along with more education and knowledge of the dangers of drug abuse. Of course, the real answer is to eliminate the emotional problems that lead to drug use, abuse, and dependence.

Amphetamines. The most commonly abused drugs in this group include Benzedrine and Dexedrine, and are called "Bennies," "pep" pills, or "up" pills. They are usually taken by mouth to give the person a feeling of well-being, confidence, boundless energy, and great good humor. They are stimulants which affect the CNS, so that misuse of them may result in permanent damage to the brain or produce toxic psychosis. On large doses the individual becomes hyperactive, agitated, tremulous, and easily distracted. Since the drug reduces appetite, he may lose weight and become thin and haggard in appearance. Amphetamines are readily available, and may be used a few times by youngsters seeking a thrill or a new experience, or by students studying for exams or preparing term papers in order to stay awake. Although they are not addictive, in the usual sense, a person may become emotionally dependent upon them, especially if he has strong feelings of inadequacy and inferiority. He may use amphetamines to defend himself against more serious emotional problems, such as depression, schizophrenia, antisocial personality, or neurosis. If he misuses them over a period of time, he may precipitate a psychotic illness rather than helping to effect a more successful adjustment.

Marihuana. Marihuana is a variety of *Cannabis sativa* (Indian hemp plant), which grows wild in many parts of the United States and Mexico. It is also known in other parts of the world as hashish and bhang. The flower of the plant is dried, rolled into brown paper, and smoked like a cigarette, called a *joint.* (Terminology changes with the years; at one time, the most popular terms were *reefer* and *stick.*) The practice is referred to as "smoking pot," and results usually in a pleasant, dreamy state of euphoria and sense of well-being. There is generally a peculiar distortion of time and space, an increase in imagination, hallucinations of a pleasant nature, and loss of discriminatory ability, so that everything seems wonderful. Under the influence of marihuana, a person's behavior is impulsive, his mood is elevated, and random ideas are quickly translated into action. He gives the appearance of being intoxicated, with a tendency to giggle or laugh inappropriately, lack of coordination, and wandering thoughts. Like the amphetamines, marihuana is not addictive in the usual sense, but the individual with underlying problems in adjustment may develop an emotional dependence upon it. Chronic use tends to release inhibitions and thereby expose the basic problem of the inadequate person. People with strong feelings of inadequacy, inferiority, and insecurity may be attracted to its use. But, again, like amphetamines, rather than helping the individual to live more successfully, it tends to interfere with his relationships with others and may get him into difficulty with the law. Contrary to public opinion, there is no firm evidence that the use of marihuana increases antisocial behavior or criminal acts. However, the possession and use of marihuana is illegal so that procurement and smoking of pot may be surrounded by illicit or illegal circumstances.

Lysergic Acid Diethylamide. LSD, or "acid," as it is commonly called, is a drug which produces symptoms resembling or mimicking those generally occuring in psychoses, such as hallucinations. For this reason, it is called a psychotomimetic or hallucinogenic drug. The user takes the drug, usually in a cube of sugar, to experience a "trip," which includes thoughts, feelings, and perceptions that are described by users as ecstatic, terrifying, or bizarrely fascinating. LSD has often been advertised as a "mind-expanding" drug, which aids the person to be more creative. However, as with other drugs, there is no evidence that a chronic user of LSD is indeed more creative or productive. The user may "feel" more creative, but creativity requires that the artist make discriminating judgments and apply himself to the work, and this the use of LSD and other drugs prevents. It is true that LSD is a "mind-altering" drug because it produces changes in the user's perceptions and thinking. Not enough is known about LSD to definitely determine whether it is addictive or not, and there is a great deal of controversy about this. However, its use is considered dangerous and is illegal. It may lead to the use of even more dangerous addictive drugs such as heroin, or it may lead to psychotic behavior. In a "bad trip" the user may experience feelings of detachment, rapid mood swings, and terrifying hallucinations. He usually winds up in the hospital, sometimes a psychiatric hospital. The drug is often used by people with severe underlying emotional problems, "social drop-outs," to give them a sense of comfort which their social interactions do not provide.

Narcotic Addiction. The most common narcotics to which people become addicted are heroin and morphine, occasionally Demerol, Dilaudid, and codeine. Drug addiction usually begins with a person being introduced to the use of the drug through an acquaintance, himself an addict, who may be trying to support his own "habit" by selling to others. A person takes the drug, usually administered I.V. by either himself or someone else, in order to obtain a sense of comfort, well-being, and relief from turmoil. Thus, he develops first an emotional dependence on the drug because it gives him the pleasant sensations which he desires. If he continues to take the drug, however, he develops also a physical dependence which completes the picture of addiction.

Narcotics are sedative drugs which affect the CNS. With continued use of narcotics, the CNS develops a physical tolerance to the sedative effects, and attempts to counteract those effects with a continual discharge of nervous energy or impulses. Thus, the addict begins to require greater amounts of the drug at more frequent intervals in order to achieve the desired relaxation and pleasure. When the drug is abruptly withdrawn, the addict's CNS continues to discharge the messages, which in the absence of the sedative drug cause excitation of the CNS and account for the various symptoms which we see in withdrawal—tremor, profuse perspiration, nausea, vomiting, stomach cramps, convulsions, and coma.

The Harrison Narcotics Act strictly regulates the use of narcotics so that an addict can only get the drugs, usually heroin, by illegal means. As his habit increases, and his physical, emotional, and social functioning begin to deteriorate, he sinks lower and lower into the underworld of drugs, deception, and danger. Often he cannot hold a steady job, so in order to support his habit he must resort to criminal acts—burglary, theft, assault, prostitution, forgery—or he becomes a "pusher" to get the necessary money to purchase the drug. He becomes, as some addicts themselves admit, truly a "dope fiend." He lives for his habit, in a world alone, and will do whatever is required in order to maintain it. It is very difficult, if not impossible, for him to rise out of the morass and "kick the habit." He needs all the help he can get, and then he may not be able to "stay clean," because of his alienation from family and friends, contact with his former associates, his rejection by society in general, his physical dependence on the drug, and the severe underlying emotional problems that got him "hooked" in the first place.

Usually, the person who becomes an addict has strong feelings of inadequacy, inferiority, insecurity, and he turns to drugs for relief from these painful feelings. He may also be unable to form successful relationships with others because of his self-centeredness. He may have a defective sense of guilt and social responsibility, and may be unable to tolerate frustration or postpone satisfaction, so he proceeds from one impulse to another without consideration for the long-range results of his actions.

In childhood, the narcotic addict has usually had traumatic relationships with both parents. Since he did not have the love and acceptance he needed, he was unable to develop the necessary sense of identity and belonging. Thus, his addiction becomes an expression of rebellion, hostility, and terrible self-punishment which often leads to suicide. Underneath it all, he often craves the mothering, the care that he has been denied in real life and that he tries desperately and unsuccessfully to find in narcotic oblivion.

Barbiturate Addiction. A person who takes as much as 800 mg. of barbiturates per day for six weeks or more develops marked withdrawal symptoms upon stopping. Often the individual begins to take the barbiturate, commonly Seconal or Amytal Sodium, for some specific physical symptom, and then, gradually, he develops an emotional and physical dependence upon the drug. "Down pills" or "goof balls," as they are popularly called, are often used in conjunction with other drugs—amphetamines, marihuana, LSD, narcotics, and alcohol. Sometimes the individual uses one drug to get "high" and another drug to get "low" or "come down" or return from a "bad trip."

Barbiturates are CNS sedatives, and are taken by the individual usually to relieve anxiety, tension, pain, sleeplessness, and irritability. Usually the addict has severe emotional problems underlying the misuse of the drug and is in need of treatment. There is a tendency to increase the dosage, due to the development of tolerance; to use the drug for other than the purpose for which it was originally prescribed; and to generally disregard the medical instructions regarding its use.

The individual who becomes addicted to barbiturates often winds up in a general hospital from an overdose, taken either deliberately in a suicidal attempt or accidentally in his mental confusion or semi-conscious state. He may end up in a psychiatric hospital with acute intoxication or a toxic psychosis. The symptoms of addiction are those of acute intoxication—blurred speech, ataxia, impairment of mental function with confusion, poor judgment, loss of emotional control, vomiting, and stupor.

Cocaine Addiction. Cocaine is becoming an increasingly popular illicit drug. It is estimated that approximately 10 million Americans now use "coke" with some regularity, and another 5 million have experimented with it. The actual number of users is probably twice that. Although it is an expensive drug (five times the price of gold per ounce), it is used by all classes of people, rich or poor, high and low on the social ladder, young and old. The cocaine "high" is what users find pleasurable; it is described as an intense kind of euphoria, a rush of well-being and confidence, that leaves the person yearning for more. It is commonly sniffed but can be taken by smoking or I.V. The "high" is often followed by a letdown. The use of cocaine can lead to depression, weight loss, paranoia, hallucinations, physical collapse, and destruction of the nasal membrane.

ALCOHOLISM

One of the foremost health problems in the United States is that of alcoholism. The manufacture, sale, and consumption of alcoholic beverages is a matter of social concern. Nationwide, most adults (about 75 per cent) drink. In fact, drinking has become such an established social practice that the man or woman who does not drink at all is looked upon with some mistrust. We spend more money on alcohol in this country than we do on education, and it has become big business. The hidden costs to industry and social agencies in lost man hours and required services related to the consumption of alcohol cannot even be accurately estimated. For example, in 1965 two million arrests, one out of every three, were for the offense of public drunkenness, thus putting a great burden on police, courts, public institutions, and private industry.

When we talk about alcoholism, we are generally referring to the uncontrolled, compulsive, self-destructive drinking pattern of some alcoholics. However, alcoholism is defined as the consumption of sufficient amounts of alcohol to interfere with the individual's physical, emotional, and social functioning; or dependence upon alcohol to the extent that the individual cannot function without it; or inability on the part of the individual to control his alcoholic intake. Probably more than one-third of the adult population of the United States fits one of the above criteria.

Alcoholism is no longer associated only with the derelict on skid row, but has become a disease or symptom of an affluent society. It cuts across all socio-economic, cultural, and intellectual levels of our society. It includes professional people, successful businessmen, white-collar workers and laborers as well as the unemployed, the socially and culturally deprived, and the welfare recipient. It includes men who become intoxicated in public, and women who drink alone at home; it includes the respected and the rejected.

For years various efforts have been made to recognize alcoholism as a disease rather than as a question of morality or a criminal offense. Only recently have the courts begun to rule that alcoholism is an illness and its symptoms are therefore not punishable as criminal acts. However, criminal offenses associated with the use of alcohol are punishable criminal acts. For example, a person cannot be arrested for drunkenness alone in some states, but when he is driving a car he may be.

The social stigma attached to alcoholism has led to many misconceptions which people use to deny or defend their drinking habits. Some people who drink to excess say they are not alcoholic because they can stop whenever they want to, and yet they keep right on drinking. Others believe they are not alcoholic because they do not drink alone, or they do not drink before noon, or they drink only beer. Others maintain they are not alcoholic because they drink to excess only periodically or on weekends. However, anyone who drinks sufficient alcohol to cause significant physical, emotional, and social malfunctioning has a problem with alcohol and needs to take appropriate action to resolve it.

It is difficult to determine definitely where socially acceptable drinking leaves off and alcoholism begins, or why one person who drinks becomes addicted and another one does not. According to the National Institute of Mental Health, attempts to identify physiological, nutritional, metabolic, or genetic defects which could explain excessive drinking have not succeeded. However, it is generally accepted that there are physical, emotional, and social factors which contribute to the development of alcoholism. It is probably better to recognize drinking as a psychological problem for which an individual may seek treatment than to try to identify alcoholism as a specific disease entity, because there are so many varying symptoms and underlying causes.

People drink for many different reasons, turning to alcohol to relieve the stress from underlying emotional problems. The excessive use of alcohol is associated with many different kinds of behavior from healthy to psychotic, so it is probably more accurate to call alcoholism an illness symptomatic of underlying emotional difficulties rather than a disease in itself to which we can assign specific causes and resulting behavior. In any case, it is an attempt on the part of the individual to disguise, distort, or alleviate the anxiety that he experiences in reaction to the stress in his life.

The individual who comes to rely too heavily upon alcohol is generally a dependent person with marked hostility, self-centeredness, and low-frustration tolerance. Usually, his dependency is combined with high expectations of himself which he cannot always fulfill. As a result, he sets up a pattern of repeated failure which adds to the ordinary stress of living and requires increasing reliance upon the effects of the drug. With the help of alcohol, he tries to overcome his strict inhibitions, intense feelings of inadequacy, or severe self-criticism. He may escape from his conflicts in a regressive fashion, becoming carefree, passive, or childlike with the help of alcohol. The use of alcohol may give him a false sense of confidence, courage, or accomplishment. It may dull his self-depreciation and sense of failure. It may allow the expression of feelings of ambivalence, feelings which he ordinarily keeps bottled up inside himself because of his strong need for approval. Since alcohol is a depressant, not a stimulant, it tends to decrease his power of discrimination, impair his judgment, and lower his critical ability. Although he may experience some temporary relief, the usual picture is that of a vicious circle. The individual feels guilty because of his misuse of alcohol, his actions under the influence of it, and his weakness in needing it in the first place. As a result, he feels more anxious, and becomes more dependent upon alcohol for relief. Frequently, it interferes further with his effective functioning and makes things worse for him instead of better.

The excessive use of alcohol may be a defense against or a symptom of more serious illness. The depressed patient may drink to ward off his feelings of despondency and suicide. The schizophrenic patient may drink to counteract his feelings of loneliness and isolation. The neurotic patient may drink to overcome his feelings of overwhelming anxiety, panic, or fear. The psychosomatic patient may drink to deaden the pain and dread of his illness. The sociopathic patient may drink to alleviate his feelings of inadequacy, inferiority, and insecurity. In most cases, the purpose of the excessive alcoholic intake is to somehow ease the misery and suffering that he experiences. The trouble is, as with all sick or maladjusted behavior, it doesn't work. The alcoholic road leads to increased misery, suffering, and self-destruction.

Because of the sedating effect upon the CNS, chronic excessive use of alcohol may result in permanent brain damage. It acts first on the cerebral cortex to impair judgment and intellectual alertness. Because it also relieves the individual's inhibitions, he tends to think of himself as more capable than he really is, and this adds to the dangerous possibility of serious error in whatever he does. As the level of alcohol in the blood increases, it affects the motor areas of the cortex with a resulting difficulty in coordination and locomotion. Very high blood levels of alcohol may cause malfunction of vasomotor, cardiac, and respiratory centers in the brain. Large doses of alcohol over an extended period of time may lead to acute alcohol intoxication, delirium tremens, Korsakoff's syndrome, alcoholic psychosis, serious physical disease, or fatal coma.

Acute alcohol intoxication means the depression of CNS function, characterized by delirium, coarse tremors, and frightening visual hallucinations. Korsakoff's syndrome is a variety of chronic brain syndrome associated with long-standing, excessive use of alcohol characterized by memory impairment, disorientation, peripheral neuropathy, and confabulation. Alcoholic psychosis includes a paranoid state characterized by excessive jealousy, and hallucinosis characterized by accusatory or threatening auditory hallucinations in a state of relatively clear consciousness.

Frequently, the physical complications of alcoholism are associated with nutritional deficiencies accompanying chronic, excessive drinking. The most common physical conditions due directly to the chronic excessive use of alcohol are disturbances of the gastrointestional tract. These gastric disturbances include nausea, discomfort, vomiting, distention, diarrhea, and hemorrhage. Another common physical condition associated with prolonged use of alcohol is liver dysfunction, particularly cirrhosis, because the metabolism of alcohol takes place largely in the liver. Other medical complications such as pancreatitis, pneumonia, diabetes, cardiovascular disease, and injuries from accidents are common. The neurological syndromes associated with alcoholism, including polyneuritis and Korsakoff's syndrome, are largely due to the lack of vitamin intake, particularly vitamin B deficiencies.

There is some question as to whether the individual becomes physically addicted to alcohol in the same way as he does to narcotics. However, there is no doubt that some people become physically dependent on alcohol and suffer symptoms of withdrawal when they are denied its use. It may be more like the habit of smoking, which is extremely difficult to give up even though we know it is physically harmful. But whether it is addiction or habituation, excessive drinking carried on for a long time may result in alcoholism.

As the illness progresses, the alcoholic finds that the occasional social drink or party is not enough. He may take a drink the next morning to recover from the after-effects of the night before or in order to face the day. This may turn into a daily "eye-opener." At first, the alcoholic may find one drink or a morning beer sufficient, but gradually, more and more alcohol is needed to maintain the sedative effect. He may carry a quantity of alcohol with him, or hide it in convenient places, or arrange to have a "quick one" frequently during the day.

As the individual's need for alcohol increases, his ability to function decreases. He begins to lose friends and may lose his job because of lack of emotional control or ability to think clearly. He may become evasive, irresponsible and unreliable. He may lie profusely, deny his drinking although it is obvious, and blame others for his difficulties. As he loses his ability to hold a job, he becomes dependent upon his family or relatives. He may lose interest in people and activities, become increasingly self-centered, lose his sense of decency and integrity, and live only for the drink that is the focus of his life. His progressive deterioration often causes great suffering not only for him, but for his family, relatives, and friends. He often winds up sick and alone, not caring about anyone and with nobody caring about him. Frequently, such a person develops a physical illness which brings him into the emergency ward of the general hospital for treatment. Occasionally, he develops the symptoms of alcoholic psychosis, D.T.'s, or hallucinosis, and he is admitted to the psychiatric hospital for treatment.

EXAMPLES OF SOCIOPATHIC BEHAVIOR

Now let us look at some actual case histories of patients with sociopathic behavior which will demonstrate the types, symptoms, process of development, and progression of the illnesses as we have discussed them.

Case Example No. 1 (Antisocial Behavior)

Patient is a 25-year-old, single man. After spending much of his adolescence in mental hospitals, he has been on terminal leave for the past 14 months and did well until 2 months prior to admission. He impulsively quit his job, began to neglect the care of his diabetes, and finally broke into a school, allegedly to perpetrate vandalism, arson, and theft. He was apprehended and returned to the psychiatric hospital.

On admission, patient was described as tense, apprehensive, but socially appropriate. He had difficulty concentrating and told about his recent experiences in a somewhat disoriented but factual manner, justifying his behavior with bizarre logic. His story was full of inconsistencies in motive and emotional tone, which, when pointed out to him, became increasingly divergent. For example, he told one event twice as if it were two separate events with completely separate particulars and associated feelings. In many areas he was unable to discuss his thoughts, and this reluctance seemed to stem from a genuine fear of reflection in these areas rather than a concern of self-incrimination or of indiscreet frankness. Physically, he complained of vague numbness of the right hand and both feet, with decreased cutaneous sensation to pain, touch, cold, and heat. He had a mild hypertension of 140/95. He had an avid appetite, felt continually thirsty, and drank 20 cups of water a day. Urinalysis showed 4 plus sugar. Otherwise, physical and laboratory exams were negative.

Patient is an only child of a difficult marriage. His mother, who contracted tuberculosis in adolescence, spent the four years prior to the patient's birth in a sanitarium. She was able to be released briefly for the patient's birth, but before he was six months old, she had to return to the sanitarium where she spent six more bedridden years. The patient's father, an unskilled laborer, is described as unstable, prone to psychotic episodes, with a history of overuse of alcohol. With mother's return to the sanitarium, patient was placed in the home of a friend of father's. In his early years, patient had four sets of foster parents.

Patient is described as a shy, retiring youngster who was overly cooperative and carried a constant concern about being unwanted. When the patient was 10 years old, his mother was released from the sanitarium and was able to resume her marriage. For the next four years, the patient lived with his parents. Records show that both parents drank to excess at this time, and the patient was caught between alternating harsh discipline and no supervision at all. Frequent threats of violence were exchanged between him and his father during this time.

By the time the patient was 12, he was described as stubborn and sulky, and came to the notice of the authorities as a runaway. By the age of 13, he was a chronic runaway with multiple brief detentions in various juvenile facilities. His formal schooling stopped at the eighth grade at age 14. Acts of truancy and delinquency made it necessary for him to be housed, at age 14, in a juvenile detention home. He was transferred from there to a juvenile correction and treatment center because of flagrantly rebellious behavior. Here, also, his inability to respond to human warmth was outstanding, and his antisocial acts continued.

Patient was committed, at age 14, to the psychiatric hospital as a psychopathic delinquent. However, he was returned to the juvenile facilities shortly after admission because of lack of psychotic symptoms and lack of treatment facilities for youthful offenders. In the juvenile detention home, his behavior continued and in fact, got worse; and three months later, he was again sent to the psychiatric hospital where he spent the remaining four years of his adolescence.

At the psychiatric hospital, he was treated with psychoactive drugs without significant response. At approximately yearly intervals he ran away from the hospital. He would usually hop a freight train, travel some distance away, commit some serious offense, and be returned to the hospital. For example, on one of these escapades, at age 15, he set fire to a motel.

A sixth escape from the hospital was successful, and four months later he enlisted in the army. He finished basic training without difficulty and was completing a radio repair school when symptoms of diabetes began. Since the military service was aware of his past psychiatric diagnosis, he was medically discharged as unsuited for military service with the diagnosis of schizophrenic reaction, chronic undifferentiated type.

At age 19 now, he returned to his home state, held down several unskilled jobs, which were shortlived because of his diabetic symptoms and his personality difficulties. A year later, he was apprehended for burglary and held in jail for several months. He was then sent to the psychiatric hospital where he spent four more years. Here again, he continued to run away periodically and committed such serious crimes as setting fire to a restaurant, attempting to derail a train, and armed theft of an automobile. He was transferred to the maximum security ward of a psychiatric hospital, where he spent 18 months in a prisonlike setting.

He was now 21, and for the first time he showed a sustained effort to help himself. After a self-study program, he passed a GED test. As part of the plan to help him work toward self-sufficiency, he was placed on terminal leave in order to qualify for a grant to attend a business college. His vocational counselor terminated his business course after eight months of study because of his waning interest, and helped him find a job. He worked alone with acceptable efficiency for four months until he impulsively terminated, stating he wanted to go to college. Out of work, he became increasingly restless, began to bicycle over the countryside, neglected his diabetes, and slipped back into antisocial behavior. He allegedly entered a school warehouse, took several salable objects, and started a fire. He was apprehended and after psychiatric consultation, returned to the psychiatric hospital.

Diagnosis: Schizophrenia, undifferentiated type with antisocial behavior.

Case Example No. 2 (Antisocial Behavior)

Patient is a 19-year-old, single man, transferred from another psychiatric hospital because he has presented an exceedingly severe management problem there. He has left the hospital on numerous unauthorized leaves, during which he committed burglary and set fires, among other things, in the local neighborhood. Despite attempts to improve the situation, the patient's behavior has remained unchanged. It was felt that a move would probably be beneficial to the patient in the sense that a new place would enable him to start fresh.

His first admission to a psychiatric hospital was five and a half years ago when he was admitted for a 90-day observation ordered by the juvenile court. A diagnosis of schizophrenia, childhood type was made. Subsequently, he was committed upon regular court order at the age of 13 to a psychiatric hospital with facilities for child care. He remained there for the next five years until he was transferred to the second psychiatric hospital.

On admission, patient was described as alert but relatively unspontaneous. His affect was flattened and he was somewhat sullen, but smiled appropriately with a somewhat childish, happy grin. He was mildly anxious and restless, and had some difficulty in enunciating words. His orientation was correct and his memory intact. He acknowledged feelings of restlessness at times and transient thoughts of stealing. He felt that the staff at the other psychiatric hospital did not like him and made fun of him. The physical and lab exams were negative except for the EEG which showed marked generalized disturbance of brain function suggestive of subcortical impairment. Epileptiform activity was present over the left mid- and posterior temporal regions.

Patient was adopted during the first week of life. He was the illegitimate child of a 17-year-old girl, father unknown. The mother gave the baby away for adoption immediately following delivery which happened in the eighth month of pregnancy. The infant patient was kept in an incubator for one month following delivery. Patient's adoptive father is 60 years of age, a carpenter. He describes himself as even-tempered, gets neither very angry nor very happy. This is his first marriage, and he and his wife have one son, six years older than the patient. Father has taken patient to recreational activities such as swimming, roller skating, picnicking. He has tried to whip the patient by hand or with a stick half a dozen times, but gave it up when he realized it did no good. Patient's adoptive mother is 55, works in a restaurant. She stated she is generally cheerful, but has a nervous disposition and is easily agitated or aroused to anger. She spoke slowly with a rather whining voice. She has been married twice before her present marriage. She has not tried to spank the patient for wrongdoings for three or four years. She said she began working because she could not handle the patient.

The only child of the patient's adoptive parents is 24, married, and has one child. He is of very calm disposition, easy-going, very friendly, quiet about his personal affairs. He and the patient seemed fond of each other, but it has long been impressed upon this foster brother that the patient is "different" and requires special handling.

Patient went to fifth grade in school, then he was expelled when he pushed another boy through a first-floor window. He went to a boarding school for a short while, but stopped going because he did not do his work. He stated that he hated all the teachers because they made him "toe the mark." He had temper tantrums at school and threw things, which upset the other students. The other children teased him at school, and although he liked to tease others, he could not bear to be teased. They said he was "crazy," "tetched in the head," and "had been dropped on his head." When he was younger, he tried to play with others, but he could not understand the games and usually got angry and started a rock fight.

Patient has had trouble in school since he started. He spent two years in the first grade. He has stolen cigarettes, candy, and money, not only from his parents but from others. He was picked up several times by the police for breaking into homes and stealing things. The police returned him to his home each time. At home he went into many temper tantrums, and repeatedly threatened to kill his adoptive parents. He lied when he was accused of something but also for the pleasure of it. He stole beer and drank it, stole cigarettes and smoked them. He was described as lacking ambition, natural curiosity, interest in anything scholastic, and affection toward anyone. He was still wetting the bed at 13 and biting his nails.

He stated that he had frightening dreams, but cannot say what was frightening about them. His father finally went to the juvenile authorities for help; the court recommended psychiatric evaluation, and he was sent to the psychiatric hospital for a 90-day observation period. At the end of that time, he was returned to juvenile court with the diagnosis of schizophrenia and the recommendation that he have treatment, so he was committed to a psychiatric hospital with facilities for child care.

During his five years at the first psychiatric hospital, further evaluation was done. Psychological tests pointed to marked disturbance of intellectual functioning with many psychotic symptoms. He showed distorted thinking, inappropriate laughter, bizarre gesturing, extreme lability of mood, obsessive-compulsive behavior, I.Q. of 58, and grossly abnormal EEG.

His hospital stay was characterized by little, if any, progress and innumerable escapes. On the children's ward, he was hyperactive, impulsive, uncontrollable. He was frequently involved in sexual activities with other children whom he aggressively sought out. He could not keep still, paced about, asked numerous questions about why he could not do things. When he went out with his parents, he ran away from them and stole things. He went on unauthorized leave and committed a series of burglaries, ransacking homes and business establishments, setting fires, and leaving behind him damage amounting to several thousand dollars. He was quiet and cooperative on the ward.

Diagnosis: Schizophrenia, with antisocial behavior.

Case Example No. 3 (Drug Addiction)

Patient is a 55-year-old woman committed to the psychiatric hospital with a long history of addiction to Amytal Sodium. Over the past two years she has suffered despondency and depression, with overdoses of barbiturates and suicidal ruminations. She was pleasant and cooperative, but somewhat angry over being committed to the hospital. She stated she did not want treatment, but appropriately evaluated the reasons for the court commitment.

On admission, patient was described as a small, undernourished woman with multiple bruises over her legs, ankles, and feet. She seemed to be of average intelligence and was oriented as to place and person but not as to time. Her speech was slurred, eyes droopy, and her facial expression was fatigued and depressed. Her gait was unsteady, and generally she gave the impression of being under the influence of drugs; she made no attempt to cover up the addiction to Amytal Sodium. She denied any emotional problems, or any feelings of depression or anxiety. Multiple physical complaints were present, mostly related to her gastrointestinal system, for which she felt she needed Amytal Sodium. She was strongly opposed to any plan of withdrawal from the drug because she did not believe that she could get along without it. She was unable to accept the possibility that underlying her physiological symptoms was chronic suppression of her emotions, resentments, and hostilities, and she continued to demand medical attention for her physical complaints. Patient's affect was appropriate to her depressed mood and ideation. There was mild impairment of recent and remote memory with some difficulty in concentration.

Patient's father was a successful businessman and was considered brilliant in his field. Mother was described as a nervous person who had several nervous breakdowns. Father died six months ago, mother five years ago. When mother got sick, she was usually sent off somewhere and maternal grandmother came and took care of the children. Father was often unfaithful, and one time mother left home over this, but returned at patient's request. Patient has three older brothers, one younger, who are said to be successful, well-educated, stable men.

Patient graduated from high school at 15. At age 19, she received training as a dental nurse and worked in a dental office until her marriage. Her marriage lasted approximately five years. They lived with the husband's rich parents, and he either played golf or was involved in some other kind of entertainment. Patient was so unhappy that she left her husband and returned home. Subsequently, she got a divorce and returned to work as a dental assistant.

When patient was 15, her parents took her to a doctor for treatment of "nervous stomach." It was during this time that her parents' marriage underwent its most severe crisis. The doctor prescribed Amytal Sodium, which the patient was to take a half hour before meals. Parents kept the patient provided with this medication as long as she was at home. Later she always found physicians who renewed her prescription for it even though she has been advised many times to enter the hospital and be withdrawn from it.

At age 41, she was found to have far-advanced, bilateral pulmonary tuberculosis with a large cavity in the right lung, and she was hospitalized in a sanitarium. She was treated with bedrest and medication, and finally a right upper lobectomy with thoracoplasty was performed. Two years later she was discharged with the recommendation that she continue on medication for an indefinite period of time. She has remained under the supervision of the Public Health Department and the family physician since then.

Over the years she has increased her intake of Amytal Sodium gradually, taking it not only prior to meals, but for any minor upsets and frustrations as well. She would regularly take 400 mg. before meals, 400 mg. at bedtime, and 400 mg. whenever she awoke in the night. Her friend and landlord stated that she took additional capsules whenever she did not get her wishes fulfilled as she could not take a "no." The landlord is an old friend of the family, and he stated that she has always thrown temper tantrums whenever her wishes were not fulfilled immediately.

As long as the patient has lived in the house of the landlord, she has been fatigued and somnolent. She was usually too sleepy to eat her meals, and often fell over while eating. As a result, she has had a significant weight loss in the past two years. The landlord would be unable to get her to go to bed and would cover her up wherever she was sitting or lying. Her lack of alertness, her lackadaisical attitude, and her impulsivity when angry made her a suicidal risk in his eyes, and he did not want to be responsible any longer for her welfare. On several occasions he asked her to move out of his house, and she has done so, but he has always taken her back again when she returned.

Since her father's death six months ago, she has become increasingly depressed. She has been seen regularly by the public health nurse and a case-worker from the Department of Public Assistance; they became concerned about her and felt she needed treatment. Arrangements were made for her to be seen in a community mental health clinic. Her gait, speech, and general behavior were those of a person under the influence of drugs. The depression became evident when she said that she saw herself as a worn-out woman dependent on drugs with a tremendous fear of withdrawal. Psychiatric treatment was thought essential and commitment procedure was initiated.

Diagnosis: Drug addiction with chronic psychophysiological gastrointestinal reaction and depression.

Case Example No. 4 (Alcoholism)

Patient is a 25-year-old married man with two small children who came to the psychiatric hospital for the first time as a voluntary admission. He is reported to be an habitual heavy drinker. Recently, he stayed off work, drank excessively to the point of blacking out and falling over in his own vomitus. He has been hospitalized several times in general hospitals and his private physician suggested he come to the psychiatric hospital.

On admission, patient was extremely agitated and nervous. However, he was well-oriented, and admitted to having had hallucinations earlier in the day. Mental exam was normal except for auditory hallucinations. The hallucinations started while he was drinking, and consisted of voices coming from the lawnmower, his car, the devil, and God. He also stated he hears his wife's voice saying, "Don't leave me." He stated he has heard voices before when he was drinking heavily. He reportedly has duodenal ulcers with episodes of profuse bleeding in the past year. Gross tremor of the hands was evident. Otherwise, the physical and laboratory exams were negative.

Patient is an only child. Father was disabled at the time of his birth, and later died of tuberculosis when the patient was four years old. Patient went to live with maternal grandmother and aunt, a living pattern which persisted off and on until he joined the service at age 18. Patient does not remember his father. He described his mother as being rather irresponsible toward him, a gambler who now tries to buy his love with money. His mother remarried shortly after his father's death, and she took the patient with her to start school. His twelve years of schooling were divided between his mother's place of residence and his grandmother's. He was frequently sent to his grandmother's home when he interfered with his mother's social plans or pleasure, or when he was not doing well in school, or got into other difficulties. Apparently, in school he achieved good grades until adolescence, at which time his grades fluctuated from poor to good. Patient remembers his stepfather as having spanked him often, and recalled many fights between the parents. He described his aunt and grandmother as stern disciplinarians. However, other family members describe his relationship with them as similar to that with his mother, one in which he could manipulate them with threats.

He met his wife while staying with his grandmother, and dated her for several years. After he was in the service, he learned that she was pregnant and returned to marry her. At age 22, he was honorably discharged and he got a job working in a factory belonging to the aunt who had helped raise him. His wife described the marriage as satisfactory until the patient began drinking heavily. The patient thought the marriage was poor from the start. He stated that his wife is a poor housekeeper, he felt no companionship with her, the children irritate him, and he drinks to feel human; otherwise, he is depressed.

Though the patient drank frequently and had a bad temper, this has all worsened in the last two years. He drank more (up to a gallon of wine a day), began to stay out at night, spent the family money on liquor, and missed work for up to a week at a time because of drinking. He had frequent temper tantrums, and became physically abusive to his wife and children. He has had visual hallucinations after some drinking spells, and has been hospitalized several times in the general hospital when his ulcer began bleeding. He has alienated his wife's parents and his maternal aunt, his job is in jeopardy, and the family's financial resources are depleted.

Diagnosis: Alcoholic psychosis with hallucinations and depression.

CARE AND TREATMENT

The care and treatment of patients with sociopathic behavior, including antisocial acts, sexual deviations, drug addiction, and alcoholism, is one of the most controversial and difficult social problems of our time. There seems to be ample evidence that punishment is not the answer; yet we are generally reluctant to accept this kind of behavior as symptomatic of an illness which must be treated if it is to be corrected. Furthermore, treatment efforts have been widely varied and not too successful, so that there are no established patterns or guidelines to follow. It is difficult enough to change one's attitudes, or mores, or standards of behavior, when there is good indication that it will be advantageous. It is almost impossible to do so when there is not clear evidence that we will profit from doing so. Even psychiatrists and other specialists in the field disagree as to the treatment, or even the treatability, of such behavior.

Antisocial Behavior

An essential part of the treatment for such behavior is the institution of the necessary control or restraint which the patient himself seems to lack. This control is often necessary for the protection and safety of the patient as well as the community. Such control frequently takes the form of incarceration, locking the offender up, and this may be the first step in interrupting the antisocial behavior. It should, however, be kept in mind that it is only a first step. It does not provide an opportunity for correction of the behavior; it only stops it for as long as the patient is locked up. It is not unusual to hear people say, "He should be locked up and the key thrown away," when the patient's behavior has been particularly threatening or offensive. Obviously, that is not a therapeutic solution to the problem, if it is a solution at all.

A second way of providing control or restraint is through the use of somatic treatment. Frequently, tranquilizers are used for impulse control during the day, and sedation at night. Sometimes Amytal Sodium is given I.V. or I.M. to interrupt destructive behavior in a hurry, but the tranquilizing drugs I.M. have been most helpful in treating the psychiatric emergency. An EEG should be done, and if there is evidence of an epileptiform tracing, often an anticonvulsant drug, such as Dilantin, is given. If there is evidence of a slowing down of brain function, a CNS stimulant such as Dexedrine may be given. Sometimes ECT is used to discharge the pent up physical and psychic energy which the patient seems to accumulate.

Probably one of the most effective means of providing restraint or control is by providing productive energy outlets. The patient needs to get rid of his aggressive, hostile impulses, and, like a child, if he is not provided with constructive channels, he will find his own which may very well be destructive. Physical exercise is essential to the release of feelings and tension within the patient. R.T., O.T., and industrial therapy are all of great importance in the structuring of the environment and channeling of the patient's energy. Work, particularly, not only provides for the discharge of unacceptable feelings in constructive ways, it also offers a correctional experience for the patient by helping him to satisfy his needs more effectively.

Another way of providing restraint or control as well as corrective experiences is through relationships with the staff and other patients. Psychotherapy is often provided in the form of group therapy. One of the problems of the patient is that he feels he is different from others, and therefore, not subject to the rules and regulations governing other people. In group therapy he may learn that he is not so different from other people as he thinks. He also has the opportunity to express his ideas and feelings freely, and he experiences the feedback which may help him to correct the distortions he has of himself and the world he lives in. He learns to face and deal more honestly and responsibly with his own behavior. He begins to learn that he is not the world, but a person in it, and through his therapeutic relationships with others, he begins to develop some sense of identity and selfhood. He begins to learn how to behave so that his needs are met more effectively. He begins to grow up, and assume more responsibility for himself and his behavior.

Drug Addiction

Withdrawal. The first essential step in the treatment of the patient with drug addiction is to get him off the drug as rapidly and safely as possible. Drug withdrawal can be accomplished in a number of ways and is dependent upon the addicting drug, and the capacity of the patient to endure withdrawal symptoms. *Abrupt withdrawal* of the drug is sometimes called "cold turkey," and refers to taking the patient off the drug abruptly without using a substitute or otherwise treating the withdrawal symptoms. It is often what happens in jails or prisons when the patient is incarcerated. It can be physically and psychologically traumatic, even inhumane, and may result in convulsions, coma, and death. Since most addicts are extremely apprehensive about withdrawal and are afraid they will not be able to withstand the extreme suffering involved, abrupt withdrawal may make them all the more apprehensive. On the other hand, it has been used by addicts themselves and sometimes quite successfully.

Another method is *prolonged withdrawal,* which is a system of gradual reduction of dosage of the drug. It reduces the physical reaction to withdrawal, but often increases the anxiety over an intolerably long period of time. Probably the most commonly used method is rapid withdrawal, using a substitute drug or simply reducing the addicting drug dosage, usually over a period of ten days. For narcotic addiction, specifically heroin or morphine, a synthetic drug similar to opium, Methadone, has been used successfully. The patient does become dependent upon Methadone, but it can be withdrawn abruptly without the patient suffering severely. In barbiturate addiction, tranquilizers are often used as substitute drugs because of their nonaddicting, calming action, and their relief of anxiety and physical tension. In the treatment of intoxication from the overuse of stimulants, such as the amphetamines, sedatives and tranquilizers are the agents of choice. For treating psychotic reactions to the use of the hallucinogenic drugs such as LSD, tranquilizers are used in much the same fashion as in the treatment of the functional psychoses, schizophrenia, and depression. Sometimes an anticonvulsant drug such as Dilantin is added to the medications in order to reduce the possibility of convulsions as a withdrawal symptom.

Convalescence. The second essential step in the treatment of the patient addicted to drugs is a prolonged period of convalescence. Drug addiction causes a profound physical, emotional, and social deterioration which requires intensive and prolonged treatment. Medical treatment is usually required for the effects of malnutrition and physical neglect which accompany addiction. The patient must rebuild his badly shattered self-esteem, personal integrity, and self-confidence. This is a long, slow process, usually accomplished through relationship therapy in the form of individual or group counseling sessions. Often group therapy is more effective because the patient feels less isolated, different, misunderstood when he is with others who have had similar experiences and problems. Resocialization or readjustment consists of using all possible avenues to include the patient in social activities and help him find expression and satisfaction through productive, acceptable social outlets. Often he has become a "social dropout," so that he may have to learn social skills he never possessed before, or relearn those he has long neglected in favor of his "habit." Again, industrial therapy is an important aspect of his treatment, and may include job training or upgrading classes in a specific occupation.

Re-entering the Community. The third essential step in the treatment of the patient addicted to drugs is his re-entry into the community. California, with more than 10,000 addicts under correctional control, has a rehabilitation-oriented program at the California Rehabilitation Center at Corona. The program includes intensive and compulsory group therapy sessions five days a week. After sufficient improvement, which includes making plans for living in the community, patients move on to outpatient status which takes approximately a year. They may move into a halfway house until permanent living and working arrangements are made. They are assigned a parole officer, who acts as counselor and assists the patient in finding a job, a place to live, and in acquiring whatever training is necessary. Patients remain under supervision and treatment in the rehabilitation program as long as seven to ten years. However, if the individual remains drug-free, "clean," for a three-year period in the community, he may be discharged earlier.

Other organizations have offered rehabilitation services to ex-addicts, among them Synanon. Synanon is a group of halfway houses operated almost exclusively by ex-addicts. Because of their use of unorthodox and sometimes controversial methods, as well as their nonprofessional help, they have run into some problems in being accepted and supported by the community. However they have undoubtedly helped many ex-addicts to successfully negotiate the road back to community living. The student is referred to *The Tunnel Back: Synanon* by Lewis Yablonsky for further details about the program.

New York City's program has established therapeutic communities in the neighborhoods where drug addiction is widespread, including Community Orientation Centers, intensive treatment units, and halfway houses to aid in the rehabilitation process. The New York program trains and employs ex-addicts as "addiction specialists," as well as utilizing professionally trained psychiatrists and social workers. Both programs include group therapy, which employs attack or encounter or confrontation methods; these are sometimes called "gut-therapy" or "haircut" sessions. They are designed to strip away defenses, attitudes, and behavior that prevent the patient from honestly looking at and resolving the problems that led to his addiction. Links between the New York addict-rehabilitation program and the "real world" consist of various community organizations. One, known as Rehabilitation of Addicts by Relatives and Employers (RARE), is made up primarily of families of addicts under treatment. Another, called Addiction Workers Alerted to Rehabilitation and Education (AWARE), is composed of community leaders, businessmen, relatives, and anyone interested or concerned with the addict and his problems.

The Treatment Program. Drug addiction tends to be chronic, with a tendency toward remission and relapse. In this respect it can be compared with medical illness such as cancer, in which the patient is considered cured if there is no recurrence of the symptoms in five years. The most successful treatment, of course, includes prevention of drug addiction. Prevention might be accomplished by: (1) eliminating addicting drugs altogether, which seems unrealistic; (2) decreasing their availability by stricter law enforcement, which seems impossible; (3) reducing the desire for drugs, which seems the most promising solution. This would include the establishment of education and information programs aimed particularly at youth in school, and a long-range attack on emotional, social, and economic conditions which encourage the substitution of drug use for healthy functioning.

Treatment itself is often conducted in a closed institution equipped to handle the special problems that face the drug addict, because it is well known that neither the psychiatric nor the general hospital is adequate to the task. The treatment should comprise a great deal more than the detoxification process or the withdrawal of the drug. It should consist of a prolonged period of intensive medical and psychiatric treatment, convalescence, and rehabilitation. The rehabilitation process should begin even before admission, and continue for an extended period of time after discharge. Community assistance in the re-entry phase is crucial to the success of treatment because unless the patient can find his way forward in the community, he will find his way back to the drug.

There are a number of drug treatment programs across the country administered by federal, state, and local governments. The best of these programs include comprehensive medical treatment, psychiatric assistance, and occupational rehabilitative facilities.

Alcoholism

There are a number of degrees and kinds of alcoholism. Some alcoholics stop drinking without any medical aid because of changes in their life situations or their attitudes toward life. Some stop with assistance such as psychotherapy, somatic therapy, or social and vocational rehabilitation programs. Probably more than half continue to drink throughout their lives, with the occasional treatment of medical problems related to their alcoholism. A few develop serious physical illnesses which require treatment and from which they may recover, become disabled, or die. Generally, however, when we use the term alcoholism, we are referring to the excessive, compulsive, uncontrolled, and self-destructive intake of alcohol. It is that person whose dependence upon alcohol has resulted in his physical, emotional, and social deterioration that we refer to as the alcoholic. The care and treatment of such a person is similar to that of a drug addict described above, but there are some pertinent points to be mentioned.

Detoxification. The first step of the treatment is the detoxification or "drying out" process. The patient is usually admitted to a hospital where he can be cared for medically, and where he cannot get any alcohol to drink. This part of the treatment consists of intensive care to combat the acute toxic state and to return the patient to self-care as rapidly as possible. It takes anywhere from twenty-four hours to several days. It consists of correcting his fluid balance by giving I.V. glucose and saline. Nutritional deficiencies are corrected with I.M. or I.V. vitamins, particularly vitamin B complex. It may be necessary to give the patient supplemental or reenforced liquid feedings until he can tolerate a regular diet. Tranquilizing therapy has been remarkably effective in shortening the acute toxic state and rendering the patient capable of responding to further treatment. He is usually given tranquilizers during the day, such as Librium or Thorazine, and sedatives at night, such as chloral hydrate. He should be carefully examined and treated for any medical complication such as diabetes, polyneuritis, or upper respiratory infection.

Psychotherapy. The second step in the treatment program is the resolution of underlying emotional problems through individual or group psychotherapy. It is essential for the alcoholic to admit his problem with drinking and accept the fact that he must abstain from alcohol completely. He cannot remain a moderate or social drinker because that first drink is enough to make him slip back into his particular pattern of alcoholic excess. He must be persuaded that life without alcohol is not only possible, but better than life with it. He needs assistance in handling the anxiety and tension that he has previously allayed with alcohol, and this can sometimes be achieved in the prolonged use of tranquilizers. The counseling sessions may deal with the underlying feelings of inadequacy, inferiority, and insecurity that led him to drink in the first place. They may deal with the underlying symptoms of depression, schizophrenia, neurosis, or a psychosomatic or sociopathic condition. They are directed toward helping the patient realize the need for changing his behavior so that he will be more successful in his relationships with others.

Rehabilitation. The third step is that long process of rehabilitation, or readjustment to life without alcohol. He may receive psychiatric care on an outpatient basis, continuing regular counseling sessions and tranquilizers for a prolonged period of time. Often family therapy is instituted while the patient is in the hospital and continued after hospitalization to provide support and assistance to the people directly concerned with the patient's drinking problem, and to correct faulty patterns of family interaction that may be a factor in the patient's drinking.

Sometimes disulfiram or Antabuse therapy is useful in establishing long-range control of alcoholism. Antabuse is an alcohol-sensitizing drug, so that if the patient drinks while he is on the drug, he suffers severe discomfort in the form of nausea, vomiting, and cardiovascular symptoms. If he associates drinking with the severe discomfort, it serves as an additional deterrent.

The patient may be referred to social and vocational rehabilitation programs available to him in the community. Often he needs help in developing more successful ways of interacting with people and more acceptable social outlets that will replace the necessity for alcohol and change his major source of satisfaction from alcohol to people. Vocational counseling, job training, and placement may be required for some patients who have become dependent socially and economically and who need help establishing themselves as productive members of society.

Alcoholics Anonymous has helped thousands of alcoholics lead successful lives without the use of alcohol. It is composed of reformed alcoholics who band together to help themselves and their fellow members abstain from alcohol. Although they do not rely upon psychiatric professionals, they use many of the principles of group therapy. Membership requires that the alcoholic admit his drinking problem, resolve to abstain from alcohol, and help others to do so. If a member of AA is tempted to drink, he may call other members who will come immediately to his aid and give him whatever assistance is required.

Often only the first step of the care and treatment program is completed—the detoxification process. Very often the patient returns to the hospital again and again, sometimes in increasingly serious toxic states. Without some resolution of the underlying emotional problems and assistance in the long process of readjustment to life without alcohol, it is very likely that the patient will again resort to the use of alcohol in a vain attempt to ease the constant, intolerable pain in his life by numbing his sensitivity.

Case Example No. 1 (See p. 269)

Following his admission to the hospital, the patient was treated with 75 units of NPH insulin and covered for additional sugar with regular insulin. The staff decided to risk the further lack of control of his diabetes by insisting that the patient take care of his own diabetes. After several days in which his diabetes went uncontrolled, including one day on a medical ward, he brought his diabetes under his own control. By the sixth hospital day, his urine was completely free from sugar. As the weeks passed, the patient's insulin requirements decreased from 75 units of NPH to 40. The patient ate a regular diet and used good judgment in regulating the amount of insulin he needed.

For the first week, the patient was on Serax 15 mg. t.i.d., Navane 10 mg. t.i.d., Cogentin 2 mg. q.d. He began to work very hard keeping the ward clean. When the staff did not praise him for his effort, he suddenly quit, and for a couple of weeks did little constructive work beyond self-centered tasks for his own amusement and diversion. He was seen for a month in weekly individual psychotherapy. It was soon evident that the patient could not utilize the sessions sufficiently to effect any major change. During these therapy hours he was quite constricted in what he could discuss, fearful of introspection, and repeatedly attempted to maneuver the therapist into a direction-giving role. Treatment at a more action-oriented level with a social worker brought the patient to the point of doing some realistic social planning. Despite the fact that he was apprehensive over having to face legal charges, he began laying plans that included eventual residence in the community, seeking employment, and initiating part-time study.

After about three months of hospitalization, it was apparent that the patient had reached the maximum point that inpatient treatment could achieve, and that the next step was either a well-supervised community placement or a return to court jurisdiction to face his pending charges. It was felt that the patient could handle a court appearance, so he was discharged and transferred to jail.

Case Example No. 2 (See p. 271)

Patient was put on medication: Haldol 10 mg. t.i.d., Cogentin 2 mg. q.d., and he showed a remarkably positive response to treatment the first few weeks of hospitalization. He became markedly less resistive, appeared happier and more relaxed and participated in ward activities, O.T., and R.T. He got along with fellow patients, socializing, playing cards, and making conversation. His dress was appropriate and he took great pride in his appearance. He seemed eager to please the ward staff, and was generally happy and comfortable.

It was felt that if his improvement continued, plans should be made for his discharge, including some kind of suitable employment. His parents were seen in family therapy to help them understand and support the patient.

A home visit a month after admission did not go well, and his behavior in the hospital began to deteriorate. There follows a long list of escapes from the hospital, acompanied by acts of burglary, arson, and theft. He was included in every available type of program the hospital had to offer, all without great benefit to him. For periods of time it was necessary to keep him locked in his room or in restraints, in order to control his impulsive antisocial behavior. Whenever he was released for freer movement about the ward, there were further episodes of escape with antisocial acts.

After about six months, he has begun to show some improvement. His current medications are Haldol 10 mg. t.i.d., Haldol 30 mg. h.s., Cogentin 2 mg. q.d. He gets along well with staff, but is quite selective about patients he associates with; usually they are the younger, better-oriented patients. He has become increasingly self-reliant and trustworthy. If he continues to improve, an attempt will be made to find him a well-supervised community placement and he will be referred to the mental health clinic.

Case Example No. 3 (See p. 273)

Because of the patient's history of having been in chronic and semicomatose states, she was placed on a withdrawal program. This consisted of a reduced dose of Amytal Sodium before meals and h.s., repeated upon awakening, and Dilantin to prevent seizures. In addition, she received Navane 10 mg. t.i.d., Kemadrin 5 mg. b.i.d. She was placed on between-meal nutriment to promote weight gain. She went through withdrawal without any particular difficulty.

Prognosis is considered poor in regard to future relapses because of patient's low-frustration tolerance, her almost lifelong drug habituation, and her gastrointestinal symptoms when under stress. It is planned to keep her in the hospital until she has gained weight and received more specific treatment for her depression. She was put on Ludiomil 50 mg. t.i.d., Sinequan 100 mg. h.s.

After about six months, she was discharged from the hospital and referred to the mental health clinic for further counseling and medication supervision.

Case Example No. 4 (See p. 275)

On admission the patient was given Dilantin 100 mg. t.i.d., Trilafon 8 mg. t.i.d., Elavil 150 mg. h.s., chloral hydrate 500 mg. p.r.n. for sleep. The patient had trouble relaxing at first, and at times he was hostile and withdrawn. He reported hearing voices and was somewhat anxious and agitated at times. At other times he was pleasant and cooperative. He was put on self-medications and assigned a counselor and an activity group.

He was consistently angry, demanding, and rude toward the nursing staff. He found a few patients he could socialize with, and constantly criticized the hospital program. In counseling sessions, he alternated between being verbally seductive when he wanted something from the counselor, and verbally hostile when he was not getting his own way or was criticized for his behavior.

Marriage counseling was instituted at the request of the patient and his wife. It became evident that the wife was too frightened of the patient to discuss any problem unless protected by a third party. It was equally evident that the wife was unable to stand up to her husband when he was verbally seductive with her—she would "melt" under the persuasion and never make her point. The patient made promises that all would be well at home if she would only clean the house. She cleaned, but nothing changed when he was at home on visit. He drank while he was at home and hid the bottles from his wife.

He was discharged from the hospital and referred to the outpatient department for weekly counseling sessions; however, the patient resumed drinking and refused to come in for the counseling sessions. His wife requested to be allowed to come in alone for the sessions and did so.

The patient was readmitted to the hospital twice following his discharge. Five months following discharge, he was readmitted suffering from auditory hallucinations and suicidal ruminations. Two months later, he was admitted again, following a suicidal attempt with an overdose of barbiturates and phenothiazines. He was taken to the general hospital for emergency care each time and then to the psychiatric hospital for treatment. This time the patient seems sincere in his cry for help, and it is hoped he can be more cooperative with treatment plans now than in the past.

NURSING CARE AND TREATMENT

The nurse may not be involved directly in the care and treatment of the patient with sociopathic behavior because he is often treated in a facility where nursing is not a traditional part of the treatment program, such as correctional institution, detention home, special school, or treatment facility. However, as nurses become more involved in comprehensive mental health care they may find themselves having to deal with this kind of illness in various health programs in schools, public health departments, social agencies, social and vocational rehabilitation programs, and general hospitals. The nursing care and treatment follows the general guidelines set down in the preceding section, so we will discuss only some of the more pertinent points and problems pertaining to nursing.

Establishing a therapeutic relationship and creating a therapeutic environment for the patient are two primary areas of responsibility for the nurse. How therapeutic the relationship and environment are depend to a great extent upon the attitude of the nursing staff toward the patient, his illness, and his response to them. Let us deal first with the negative attitudes nurses frequently have toward this kind of behavior that interfere with their effectiveness in helping the patient. Indeed, the patient often has three strikes against him before he ever steps up to bat.

An attitude is defined as an enduring, learned predisposition to behave in a consistent way toward a given class of objects, situations, or people. Attitudes are conscious or unconscious stands that people take in response to the knowledge and experience they have gained from life. If a person approaches a problem or situation or another person with a negative predisposition, he tends to react negatively regardless of the merits of the existing circumstances. He tends to react in accord with his already drawn conclusions rather than drawing more accurate or realistic conclusions from the experience itself. The more fixed and negative his predisposition, the less likely he is to be intelligent, appropriate, or helpful in his interactions.

Negative attitudes of nurses toward sociopathic behavior are based upon three interrelated and common misconceptions about the illness: namely, *the patient is not sick, the patient is just bad,* and therefore, *the patient should be punished.* Indeed, on the surface, the patient's behavior seems to indicate that he is not desirous, or in need, or deserving, or appreciative of the nurses' help. The notion that the patient is not sick is generally supported by certain facts: he is not out of contact, he is not hallucinating or delusional, he is not psychotic. In other words, he talks all right, he takes good care of himself, and he appears in general to be healthy. The implication is that he could control his behavior if he really wanted to. As a result, he very often is expected to behave as if he were well, as if he were not sociopathic, as if he were not sick. It is illogical and nontherapeutic to expect him to be able to do the very thing that he cannot—correct the core problem of his illness and control and constructively channel the expression of his basic impulses and negative feelings. When he is expected to behave as if he were well, he is doomed to certain failure. The nursing staff's reaction to his failure to behave as expected is often one of disappointment, rejection and punishment.

The patient must be accepted just as he is if he is to be helped at all. That does not mean that his destructive behavior must be ignored or condoned, or even allowed. It means simply that he is not to be prejudged and discarded as a potentially productive member of society. Any successful relationship begins where the participants are, not where they were last year or where they hope to be ten years from now. Learning, progress, and change take place when a person is accepted, not when he is rejected. The nurse must be realistic in her expectations of what the patient is capable of accomplishing; otherwise, she encourages the patient's repeated experience of failure and frustration. Because he talks intelligently and presents himself well does not mean that he is capable of holding down a demanding, stressful job. Often a patient is placed in a job situation that requires more than he is capable of giving, and we tend to blame him rather than ourselves for his failure. Furthermore, the nurse's expectations of him must be made as clear and explicit as possible, so as to decrease the necessity of testing behavior on the part of a patient. He should also understand the alternative courses of action that may be taken and what their anticipated outcome may be, so that he can choose more appropriate ways of behaving based upon cause and effect and assume increasing responsibility for his own behavior. He cannot really help what he does, and if he could, he would certainly not need the nurse's help.

The second part of the threefold misconception, *that the patient is just bad,* is based upon the symptoms of his illness. Often, because his behavior represents an attack upon society and the nurse is a product of that society, she feels personally attacked and defends herself accordingly. She tends to hold him accountable, not only for the way he behaves, but for the way he makes her and others feel. The behavior itself may evoke such strong feelings of fear or revulsion or anger that it is extremely difficult not to retaliate. His self-centeredness, his lack of concern for the welfare of others, and his cruelty are often contrary to the best interests of his fellow patients, whom the nurse feels called upon to protect. He is often at the bottom, or close to the source, of problems on the ward, like the eye of the storm, and this provokes further resentment on the part of the nurse.

The nurse's relationship with him must help to provide him with the essential material for successful living which he does not have. The nurse does for him what he cannot do for himself. She must provide the necessary restraint and control until he is able to do it for himself. She must help him learn how to postpone satisfaction and tolerate frustration. Like the child he resembles in personality structure, he must experience satisfaction and security before he can master the stress of his environment. He needs to learn safe outlets for his pent-up feelings. He needs to learn self-respect, esteem, and confidence from successful interactions with those around him. He needs to know himself as a person of importance, worth, and dignity in relationship to the world he lives in. He needs to learn how to live in peace and harmony. He can only learn these things in interaction with people who are calm and matter-of-fact, stable and mature, honest and accepting. Only from the "treatment models" around him can he learn to correct the distortions he has of himself and others.

The third part of the misconception—*the patient should be punished*—stems from the kind of behavior he exhibits and the feelings he evokes in others. He has to learn how to control his impulses, postpone his gratification, and find acceptable social outlets for his feelings. He does not learn how to do this by being told what to do or being punished when he does not do it. He must learn through his experiences with others that if he behaves in certain ways certain results will accrue, and other ways of behavior will bring other results. He must be confronted with his behavior, not to put him down or make him feel bad or "teach him a lesson," but to help him alter it so that he can be more successful in the future. His environment must provide him with a sense of identity, belonging, success, and responsibility. Therefore, it must be full of opportunities for him to learn and full of support for him in case of failure. He must learn who he is, what is expected of him, and how to achieve that. Only after his self-concern has been satisfied can he afford to be concerned about others. He must learn what his limits are and how to relate with others in order to experience some degree of comfort, success, and health. It is unfair to expect him to magically become the mature adult—independent, cooperative, giving—when he has not yet negotiated a successful childhood. We must help him start at the beginning, rework the fibers, and come out with a whole cloth. It is a long hard road to health for him, so the sooner he gets help, the better, and the better it is for society.

Sociopathic behavior refers to a severe disruption in the person's interaction with society. It reflects a basic disturbance in his ability to live in peace and harmony with his world. The disorders can be grouped into personality disorders, sexual deviations, drug addiction, and alcoholism. All of these include antisocial acts, behaving in ways which are usually in conflict with the law.

The symptoms of the disorders are difficult to regard or to accept as indications of illness because by their very nature they represent attacks upon society of which all people are a part. The tendency is to react or interact as if we had been personally attacked, as indeed we often are, and retaliate by counterattacking, punishing, or rejecting the patient for his sick behavior.

Care and treatment of patients with sociopathic behavior is one of the most controversial and difficult social problems of our time. People disagree as to treatment, or even the treatability, of such behavior. It is generally agreed that the core problem lies in the individual's lack of impulse control, rejection of authority, and the direct expression of hostile, aggressive, and sexual urges in ways that are contrary to society's rules and regulations. Current emphasis is placed upon prevention, treatment, and rehabilitation rather than upon punishment. A wide variety of physical, emotional, and social approaches may be used that are appropriate to the form of the illness and the requirements of the particular patient being treated.

If the nurse is to be helpful, it is essential for her to see and resolve the negative attitudes based upon the threefold misconception—that the patient is not really sick, that he is just bad, and that he should be punished—since these attitudes interfere with therapeutic relationships.

REFERENCES

Bakdash, Diane P.: "Becoming an assertive nurse," *American Journal of Nursing, 78* (October, 1978) pp. 1710–1712.

Dostoyevsky, Fyodor: *Crime and Punishment,* Pendulum Press, West Haven, Connecticut, 1979.

DuPont, Robert, et al.: *Handbook on Drug Abuse,* Metrotrec Research Associates, National Institute of Drug Abuse, Washington, D.C., 1979.

Fortin, Mary Lynch: "A community nursing experience in alcoholism," *American Journal of Nursing, 80* (January, 1980) pp. 113–114.

Futz, John M., Jr., et al.: "When a narcotic addict is hospitalized," *American Journal of Nursing, 80* (March, 1980) pp. 478–481.

Kaplan, Helen Singer: *Disorders of Sexual Desire,* Simon & Schuster, New York, 1979.

Kurose, Kasi, et al.: "A standard care plan for alcoholism," *American Journal of Nursing, 81* (May, 1981) pp. 1001–1006.

Menninger, Karl: *The Crime of Punishment,* Penguin Books, New York, 1977.

Miller, Eugene, ed.: *Corrections in the Community,* Reston Publishing, Reston, Virginia, 1977.

Poley, Wayne: *Alcoholism: A Treatment Manual,* John Wiley & Sons, New York, 1979.

Roth, Lillian: *I'll Cry Tomorrow,* Frederick Fell Publishers, New York, 1977.

Steckel, Susan Boehm: "Contracting with patient-selected reinforcers," *American Journal of Nursing, 80* (September, 1980) pp. 1596–1599.

Valle, Stephen K.: *Alcoholism Counseling,* Charles C Thomas, Springfield, Illinois, 1979.

Westermeyer, Joseph: *Primer on Chemical Dependency,* Williams & Wilkins, Baltimore, Maryland, 1976.

Yablonsky, Lewis: *The Tunnel Back: Synanon,* Macmillan, New York, 1965.

Chapter 15

Neurotic Reactions to Stress

It is common for people to express and react to their emotions through bodily functions. For example, sad feelings stimulate the tear glands to produce tears, happy feelings stimulate the muscles of the throat and larynx to produce laughter. Often the physical reaction to emotion is involuntary and uncontrollable, sometimes embarrassing and inappropriate. For example, one suddenly thinks of how much he misses a person from whom he has been separated, and it is like a physical blow. His eyes may fill with tears and even run down his face, no matter how inopportune or how unwanted the reaction may be at the time, and no matter how valiantly he tries to control or shut off the reaction. Who has not experienced, and even succumbed to, the wild uncontrollable desire to laugh in a serious situation, such as in church, class, or meetings where sober, contemplative behavior is expected?

Often the expression of, and reaction to, emotion is internal, invisible, and not even perceived by the individual himself. For example, a person may find himself unable to move after the completion of an intensely emotional speech with which he has identified and to which he has listened attentively. He may go home exhausted following a day of frustration and disappointment, without realizing that his physical condition is a reaction to the emotional stress of the day. He may experience increasing physical fatigue which he blames on getting old, not realizing that it is related instead to the emotional satisfaction which his daily activities fail to offer him.

Under stress, when an individual is tired or run down, unhappy or morose, defeated or discouraged, he is more susceptible to the enemies of health that inhabit his environment all of the time. He is a more ready host for infection, injury, or malfunction. When he is in the opposite emotional state—secure, safe, satisfied—he is physically stronger, more adept in handling stress, and more resistant to the enemies of health.

EMOTIONS AND BODY FUNCTION

In certain situations in life when an individual's comfort or security is threatened, he is likely to have physical, as well as emotional and behavioral symptoms. Most of us have experienced a variety of physical symptoms associated with emotional disturbances in our lives. For example, for most people public speaking is a particularly frightening experience, because it places the individual in a position of vulnerability. He stands in front of the audience, exposed, alone and unarmed, an easy target for any critical assault. The knowledge that he is not likely to be attacked does not lessen the individual's reaction to that very possibility. He may suffer all kinds of physical symptoms, many of which can seriously interfere with his effective functioning. He may tremble all over, as with some nervous disorder. He may blush or blanch or break out in blotches, as with some circulatory dysfunction. He may feel the urge to vomit or urinate or defecate, as with some disorder of the digestive or urinary systems. He may find it difficult to breathe or get enough oxygen into his lungs, as with respiratory distress. He may find it impossible to stand, as with some deficiency of the muscular-skeletal systems. Any of his body systems, organs or functions may be affected by the stress of the moment and refuse to respond to his logical direction.

Let me give you a personal example. I was asked to prepare and read a paper at a professional meeting of some importance. In fact, I was the only nurse to present a paper at this particular meeting of psychiatrists from throughout the Northwest, so it was quite an honor. The paper contained my ideas about nursing education, particularly as it related to psychiatric nursing. I wrote it myself, recorded it several times, and knew it almost by heart. I knew when I got up to read it that I was somewhat anxious, but I was completely unprepared for the catastrophe which befell me. I had not read more than one sentence when I found myself suddenly and completely without saliva. It was as if my salivary glands had been effectively removed or tied off. If you have ever tried to talk without the benefit of saliva, you can appreciate my predicament. My lips stuck to my teeth, and my tongue stuck to the roof of my mouth. It was literally impossible to utter an intelligible word. Fortunately, the chairman of the section saw my terrible trouble and poured me a glass of water. (I could not have poured it myself because I would have spilled it all over the table.) That kind act saved the situation, and I was able to master the ordeal. Taking a sip of water, I could read a few sentences at a time until my mouth became dry again, and by repeating this process periodically I was able to finish the 20-minute paper. Now, I had no reason to be afraid of that audience; I had the paper in front of me and all I had to do was read what I had written—a very simple task. I certainly wanted to read it well, and I thought it contained some pretty good ideas. But all of this did nothing to affect the choice, control, logic or appropriateness of my physical reaction to the stress of this situation. Despite the fact that the lack of saliva only added to my stress, I was unable to change it.

Similar or different symptoms may appear in the expression of, or in reaction to, any strong emotion. Fear, anger, hate, sexual desire, love, joy are all experienced physically as well as emotionally. We say we feel "good" or we feel "bad," meaning physically as well as emotionally. They are interrelated, interdependent, interwoven to such an extent within the individual as to be inseparable. When a person gets angry, he does not decide to increase his blood pressure, it happens automatically without his doing anything about it. Even though he knows rationally that there is nothing to be afraid of, he cannot decrease his trembling because it is not based upon logic, it is based upon emotions. Although he may not wish to react as he does because it is wrong or inappropriate or embarrassing or otherwise to his disadvantage, he may not be able to change it.

The close association between our physical and emotional selves can be seen by examining our verbal communications. We express some of our strongest feelings and describe some of our strongest emotional reactions by referring to various parts of our anatomy or our bodily functions. We express impatient, painful, or stressful waiting as "sweating it out." When we are unhappy with the results we get, we say we are "fed up" or we can't "swallow" or "stomach" any more. If someone particularly bothers us, we say he gives us a "pain" which we locate "in the neck" or we say he gets on our "nerves." When we want to get rid of some burden, like guilt, we say we want to "get if off our chests" or "make a clean breast of it." If we are happy, we say "my heart jumps for joy" or "I'm heady with success." If we don't want to do something, we say we "get our backs up" or "set our feet." When we are frightened, we say "my heart stood still" or there is a "lump in my throat." If we want to be frank and honest with one another, we say, "Let's have a heart-to-heart talk" or "Let's face the issues." If we think the other fellow is a nice guy, we say he is "stout-hearted" or "has a heart of gold" or "has a heart as big as all outdoors." If he is unsympathetic, we say, "he has a heart of stone" or "ice water in his veins." People make money "hand over fist," are "up to their ears" in work, and "try to keep their heads above water," or fail and "fall flat on their faces." There are many, many more common verbalizations demonstrating the fact that our body organs, functions, and symptoms play an extremely important part in our everyday lives, and are closely associated with our emotions. Perhaps the student can think of some of his own favorite expressions.

Nobody can dispute the reality of the physical symptom or reaction, regardless of its emotional cause or nature. The pain, shortness of breath, vomiting, or lack of saliva are just as real as if they were caused by an infection, a tumor, or an injury. They are not "imaginary" or "all in the head" or "put on." Yet we often have difficulty accepting the legitimacy of emotionally caused or related physical symptoms, especially if that particular reaction to stress is someone else's major pattern of behavior or life style, not ours.

It is more acceptable to have an actual, demonstrable, organic lesion that brings about the physical reaction, as in diabetes or tuberculosis. It is more acceptable to have an emotional reaction if there is a visible threat to the individual's life or appearance or competence, as in cancer, or disfigurement, or dismemberment. Somehow, we seem to place more credence in the physical, organic, visible causes of body dysfunction, even though we all have experienced the powerful effect of emotions upon our physical health and functioning. With such social attitudes toward emotional aspects of illness, it is often difficult for us to accept, understand, and treat people who have developed physiological reactions to stress as a way of life.

Instead of turning their actions out upon society in the form of antisocial acts, as sociopathic patients do, these patients take their frustrations out upon themselves in the form of physical symptoms. Where such a patient fits in the continuum of normal to abnormal behavior, effective to ineffective adjustment, health to illness, depends upon the form of his physical symptoms, the degree to which they are acceptable to him and society, and the extent to which they satisfy or further interfere with the satisfaction of his needs.

We will discuss three major categories of illness which include physical and emotional symptoms based upon ways of reacting to stress: neuroses, psychosomatic disorders, and life-threatening physical illness.

DEFINITION OF TYPES

Neurosis, or psychoneurosis, may be defined as an unsuccessful attempt to restore equilibrium, alleviate anxiety, effect adjustment, or reach the behavioral goal of the satisfaction of basic needs in socially acceptable ways. It is, therefore, classified as a functional mental disorder, characterized by anxiety resulting from internal or external conflict, which may be felt by the patient and expressed directly (anxiety disorders) or unconsciously controlled by the patient and expressed in the form of symptoms (somatoform, dissociative, or dysthymic disorders). (See Appendix B.) The symptoms are generally ineffective substitute ways of satisfying needs. That is, the symptoms are meant to obtain satisfaction for the patient, while, in fact, they tend to interfere further with his satisfaction. The symptoms themselves are often symbolic or representative of the underlying emotional conflict. They constitute what is often referred to as "the neurotic conflict"—that is, the patient obtains some satisfaction, but even though it is not sufficient, he is reluctant or unable to give up the symptoms for something he is not sure of. It's like the old saying, a bird in the hand is worth two in the bush. Furthermore, the symptoms often represent a secondary gain for the patient—they may get him out of the situation which caused the stress in the first place.

Neurotic illness includes a wide range and variety of unsuccessful attempts to cope with life—from those that interfere very little with the person's total functioning, to those that seriously incapacitate him. Therefore, it is sometimes difficult to distinguish the former from healthy behavior and the latter from psychotic disorders. First of all, in neurosis there is generally less disturbance in the patient's thinking, feeling, and doing than there is in psychosis, less disruption in his relationships with people and his environment, and less disorganization in his personality and methods of coping with life. Here are some of the specific differences between psychosis and neurosis.

In *psychotic* disorders, the patient generally:	Whereas in *neurotic* disorders, the patient generally:
1. Denies reality	Is reality-oriented
2. Behaves in inappropriate, bizarre, or otherwise socially unacceptable ways	Continues to behave in socially acceptable ways
3. Creates a new environment	Interacts with the real environment
4. Suffers from delusions and hallucinations	Does not have delusions or hallucinations
5. Has little or no insight	Knows something is the matter with him, but doesn't know what, and doesn't know how to correct it
6. Relies upon infantile coping methods	Relies upon substitutive, symbolic coping methods

Secondly, neurosis represents a failure on the part of the person to behave in ways that help him solve his problems in life. Rather, he behaves in unhealthy ways that contribute to his difficulties. Those unhealthy ways constitute the types of neurotic illness: generalized anxiety disorder, obsessive-compulsive disorder, phobic disorders, conversion disorder, dissociative disorder, and dysthymic disorder (neurotic depression).

PROCESS OF DEVELOPMENT

In the development of neurosis, the individual usually possesses an inadequate personality characterized by faulty ways of perceiving himself and solving his problems. As a result, there is generally a lifelong pattern of maladjustment, unsuccessful relationships with others, and a high degree of insecurity and anxiety, often accompanied by physical complaints. However, an individual with healthy behavior may become neurotic if his life experiences are such as to provide sufficiently prolonged, intense, and widespread stress at a time in his life when he is least capable of handling it—that is, he faces a crisis in his life that he is unable to resolve by himself. His healthy defenses may break down and he resorts to earlier, more infantile, and less effective coping methods or ways of behaving. For example, a young husband and father who loses his leg in a serious accident may react to the stress with neurotic behavior which keeps him a semi-invalid, prevents him from returning to work, makes him dependent upon his wife, and thus interferes with his recovery.

All of us are no more a little bit neurotic than we are all a little bit sociopathic or a little bit psychotic. Each kind of sick behavior indicates a failure on the part of the individual to live successfully with a sufficient degree of peace and harmony. It is true that each of us in health contains some of the necessary ingredients for illness. However, a person is not considered sick unless his behavior fails in its essential purpose of satisfying basic needs in socially acceptable ways.

Each person who develops a neurotic illness, like every other person, is a unique individual, with different life experiences and his own particular life style. However, whatever the causes and the individual differences may be, the development and progress of neuroses seem to follow a general pattern. The individual is unable to accept himself as he is because of the unsuccessful interactions he has had with significant other people in his environment. (Remember we get our acceptance of ourselves from being accepted by others, particularly parents, as we are growing up.) He does not have the degree of self-sufficiency, adequacy, and independence which he so sorely desires. This may result from parent-child relationships in which the child is never allowed to grow up. His parents may treat him as an extension of their own thoughts, desires, ambitions. He then becomes both a source of satisfaction and a disappointment to them because he can never be what he is not. It may result from the opposite kind of parent-child relationship where he is rejected and not given the necessary parental love and support. Or it may result from faulty parent-child relationships in between those two extremes.

At any rate, the interactions that he has with other people cause him to feel inadequate, inferior, and unworthy. The goals that he sets for himself, a reflection of the goals set for him by his parents, are too high or unrealistic or impossible for him to achieve. He, therefore, embarks upon a vicious circle of frustration and disappointment. He expects impossible achievements of himself, and he is certain to suffer repeated failure and frustration from which he must protect himself. He may not have the necessary intellectual capacity to become the scholar his parents wanted him to be. He may not be the paragon of virtue that his strict parents expected. He may not even be the right sex to achieve the desired parental approval.

No matter what he does, it is never quite right, it never gains for him all the satisfaction he needs. As a result of such repeated failure and frustration, he develops a deep-seated, underlying feeling of hostility toward himself and others. He must find some way of coping with such feelings which threaten to further interfere with his satisfactions. He begins to rely more and more upon the coping method of repression. While repression tends to get rid of the displeasing, unacceptable, intolerable aspects of himself and his life situation, it also tends to interfere further with his satisfaction. It represents essentially a denial of gratification; and the more one uses repression, the less apt he is to achieve satisfaction. Also, the more he uses repression, the greater the energy and vigilance required to keep the material repressed.

Repression works like a pressure cooker. When a pressure cooker accumulates too much steam (or pressure), it is released through the escape valve. If the escape valve does not work, and the pressure builds up inside of the cooker, it will eventually blow the lid off and even blow the food out of the pot. With repression, a person keeps getting rid of those things about himself and life that he does not like by shoving them down into his unconscious. The more things that are intolerable to him, the more he must get rid of. The more he shoves out of his awareness, the less chance he has of satisfaction and the greater the pressure within himself. The first line of defense, repression, is bound to give way under continual misuse. So, when repression can no longer contain the anxiety, we see the recourse to auxiliary defenses and the development of symptoms of neurotic illness. These symptoms may be barely noticeable or overwhelming. They may not incapacitate him, but they may be sufficiently distressing that he seeks relief. They always represent a less-than-healthy way of reacting to stress.

SYMPTOMS

Anxiety States. In anxiety states, the presenting symptom is that of diffuse, inappropriate, free-floating anxiety. The patient is anxious about everything and anything and nothing. Free-floating anxiety means anxiety that is not related to or precipitated by external circumstances. The level of anxiety may vary from vague discomfort to panic, and it may be either an acute or a chronic state. Repression is only partly successful; it may push the content of the unacceptable thought, feeling, or impulse out of awareness, but its emotional charge is still felt. As many such emotional charges accumulate, due to the overuse of repression, they spill out of the unconscious and are felt by the individual.

Anxiety states are sometimes seen as the first stage in the development of all neurotic illness. Associated with anxiety neurosis, as well as with other neurotic illnesses, are the conditions of diffuse anxiety, neurasthenia, and hypochondriasis.

In Chapter 5, we defined anxiety as an unpleasant subjective experience in response to a perceived physical or psychological threat, and we stated that it was a result of conflict, ambivalence, stress, trauma, and frustration. Its purpose is to warn the individual of impending danger so that he may take appropriate action to defend himself. It is composed of an emotional response, described as fear, a physical response, described as tension, and a social or behavioral response, described as fight, flight, or paradoxical behavior. Anxiety stimulates the autonomic nervous system, which in turn prepares the individual for defensive action. However, when such action is not taken, as in neurosis, the anxiety builds up and becomes overwhelming and diffuse.

All of us, then, experience anxiety in reaction to stress situations. Any of us may have an acute anxiety attack in reaction to some overwhelming life situation. However, in anxiety states, the patient has not one attack in response to external threat, but frequent attacks (or chronic anxiety) not necessarily related to the external world at all.

The patient may be terrified and feel that some great catastrophe is about to befall him. His heart may pound; he may have pains in his chest, head, neck, stomach; he may find it difficult to breathe; he may feel sure he is going to die. Often he calls his physician or winds up in the emergency room of the general hospital. His family may react to the anxiety attack, especially the first one, with similar alarm. They may believe, along with the patient, that his symptoms are due to some grave physical disorder such as a heart attack. As the patient has repeated attacks, however, with no physical evidence to cause the condition, family, friends, sometimes physician may no longer be alarmed by his condition, although he continues to suffer the same distress with each attack.

Anxiety states may occur at any time in life from childhood to old age. They may be related to traumatic, unsuccessful experiences in childhood or adult life or a combination of the two. In other words, they may be a result of faulty methods of adjustment or overwhelming stress in the life situation. In any case, it comes about through the failure of the person's interactions with significant other people in his environment.

Often the physical and emotional distress is intolerable, and the patient goes on to develop other kinds of neurotic behavior to protect himself. He uses other coping methods to bolster the overloaded repression, which rather than helping him effect a better adjustment, cause him greater and greater distress. This results in other, and usually increasingly unhealthy ways of behaving.

Phobic Disorders. In an attempt to relieve his distress, he may displace his anxiety upon objects or situations and develop a phobia. A phobia is an abnormal, unreasonable fear of an object or situation, based upon underlying emotional conflict. The neurotic patient may have one phobia or many, but the tendency is for his unreasonable fears to multiply until he is often unable to leave the safety of his own home or room. Presumably, his distress should decrease if he has something specific to which he can attach his overwhelming anxiety; but like all sick ways of behaving, his phobias interfere further with his success as a person.

Phobias may include those common fears that most people share such as fear of illness, injury, death, danger, darkness, but they are exaggerated in neurosis. They may focus on specific objects such as fear of automobiles, airplanes, snakes, bugs, dirt, germs, storms, thunder, lightning, wind, animals, cats, dogs, mice, rats. They may include circumstances, situations, or places which may or may not ordinarily inspire fear such as fear of suffocation, impregnation, crowds, enclosure in small places, open spaces, heights, such as tall buildings, bridges, cliffs.

There is a specific term for each phobia, which names the object of the fear in the prefix followed by the root word, -phobia. The most common of such terms are *claustrophobia,* which means fear of being shut or locked in some small place; *agoraphobia,* which means fear of open spaces requiring the individual to stay indoors, usually at home; and *acrophobia,* which means fear of heights or high places. *Photophobia* literally means fear of light; however, it has come to mean sensitivity to light. It is usually associated with some organic disease, such as acute infections, which result in pain and tearing when the patient is exposed to light. *Hydrophobia* literally means fear of water; however, it is generally used to designate the disease of rabies. In the disease the patient has an intense thirst, but his attempts to drink are thwarted by choking and dyspnea.

The object of the phobia is generally symbolic of an underlying emotional disturbance. Phobias can be understood only by reconstructing the original source of an individual's fear reaction. The content of the phobia is the covering (the façade, as Freud called it) for repressed feelings or desires that are unacceptable to the person. For example, fear of high places may be based upon the unconscious fear of failure, falling from favor, or loss of approval from significant persons or circumstances in one's life. Fear of open spaces may be based upon the unconscious fear of leaving the safety and security of the home situation which generally includes the protective, comforting mother. Fear of enclosure in small places may be based upon the unconscious fear of personal closeness, being hurt, or caught up in undesirable relationships.

If the patient is faced with the object of the phobia, he is overwhelmed by acute anxiety or panic. As a result, he may become aggressive, immobilized, or physically ill. The patient may realize that his fear is unjustified and even unreasonable or he may be embarrassed by it, but he cannot logically dismiss it because of the underlying, emotional conflict from which he is trying to protect himself. He does not feel this way because he wants to, or because he thinks it is to his advantage: he cannot help it, and if he could, he certainly would. It is more comfortable for him to be afraid of high places than to face the fear of failure based upon his feelings of inadequacy. If he has a single phobia, or certain phobias, he may still manage to live a fairly successful life by avoiding that object or situation. For example, he may have such a fear of automobiles that he is unable to drive, but that need not disrupt his whole life. However, if he has many phobias or certain phobias, he may not be able to plan his life around them and still remain successful or acceptable in his behavior. For example, if he cannot leave his home, this may seriously interfere with his relationships with other people, his ability to care for himself, and the acceptability of his behavior.

Obsessive-Compulsive Disorder. Again, in an attempt to relieve intolerable anxiety, the neurotic patient may develop obsessions or compulsions, or a combination of both in the illness of obsessive-compulsive disorder. An obsession is an overpowering, repetitive, unwanted idea, which is a way of relieving the anxiety that is based upon underlying emotional conflict. A compulsion is an overpowering, repetitive, unwanted act which is a way of alleviating, controlling, or disguising the anxiety which comes from underlying emotional conflict. Obsessions stem from unacceptable desires, impulses, or feelings that the patient has tried unsuccessfully to repress. Often they involve feelings of an aggressive, hostile, murderous, or sexual nature. Compulsions are often exaggerations of socially acceptable rituals such as cleanliness, punctuality, politeness, orderliness. You may have heard the joking remark, "If a person is early for an appointment, he's anxious; if he's late, he's hostile; and if he's on time, he's compulsive."

In healthy behavior we see something similar to obsessions when the tune or the TV commercial or the jingle keeps running through our minds. Sometimes we have worries that are similar to obsessions. For example, we can't remember after we have left home if we turned off the stove, or the TV, or locked the door, and it may be necessary to return home to check on things. Sometimes the obsessions are similar to phobias, as when a person repeatedly thinks frightening thoughts of death, destruction, illness, assault, murder, obscene and lewd sexual acts. The overly-clean, punctual, or well-organized individual may be incorrectly labelled "compulsive," especially if we don't happen to agree with his way of doing things. When we don't want things to be so neat and clean, we say about someone else, "Oh, she's too compulsive." However, if we do want things to be neat and clean, we praise the other person for his orderliness. A certain amount of cleanliness and orderliness is necessary, even essential in life, but when it interferes with, rather than contributes to, one's comfort and safety, then we say it is sick behavior.

As in phobias, if the patient's obsessive-compulsive behavior is interrupted or prevented, he may become overwhelmed with anxiety. Also, he may realize that his behavior is inane or irrational or inappropriate, but still he is unable to control or stop it. Usually, he does not know why he behaves as he does, only that he must. If his obsessions or compulsions are not too bizarre, he may be able to live a fairly successful life, but the tendency is for the severity of the symptoms to increase. Since they do not resolve the underlying conflict, they often aggravate rather than relieve the person's anxiety.

Obsessive ideas result from the use of fantasy and displacement in response to anxiety. Those things which we are unable to accomplish in reality may come out in the form of fantasy. Unacceptable aggressive, hostile, sexual feelings may be unsuccessfully repressed and come out in the form of obsessions.

Compulsive acts result from the use of restitution or undoing in response to anxiety. We try to make up for the bad thought, or feeling, or deed by behaving in an exaggeratedly good way.

Handwashing is an example of symbolic behavior and a common symptom of obsessive-compulsive disorder. The person tries to rid himself of the dirt or guilt or responsibility for his thoughts, words, or deeds. In a symbolic act, Pontius Pilate washed his hands in public to absolve himself from responsibility in the crucifixion of Christ, saying, "I am innocent of the blood of this just person." In Shakespeare's play, *Macbeth,* Lady Macbeth repeatedly washes her hands in her sleep in an attempt to rid herself of the guilt she feels for participating in the death of the king, saying, "Out, damned spot!"

In illness, the idea and the act become exaggerated, inappropriate, and unhealthy, and they interfere with effective functioning. The obsessions make it impossible to think about or deal with the things at hand. The compulsions take precedence over other actions demanded by family, friends, society. For example, obsessive-compulsive patients become so controlled by their symptoms that they may spend most of the 24-hour day in the bathroom. They may repeatedly wash themselves until their skin is raw and bleeding. They may not be able to take time out from their activities to eat or sleep, let alone interact with other people (see Case Example No. 3).

Conversion Disorder. In conversion disorder, the neurotic patient uses the coping method of conversion to transform his underlying emotional conflict into specific kinds of motor and sensory dysfunction. The illness most commonly takes the form of paralysis of the arms and legs, blindness, or deafness. The symptoms both express and deny the unacceptable thought, desire, or impulse. For example, hysterical blindness, deafness, or muteness can be understood as a physical manifestation of the well-known admonition, "hear no evil, see no evil, speak no evil."

Often accompanying the illness is the patient's singular lack of concern about his physical condition, which is described as "la belle indifférence," literally translated as "the grand indifference." His physical condition then serves two purposes—the primary gain is the relief from the emotional tension, and the secondary gain is the advantage of the symptom. For example, hysterical paralysis or pain enables the individual to become a chronic invalid, which insures that he will be cared for, and at the same time it helps him avoid uncomfortable interpersonal or social situations.

Again, it is important to keep in mind that the individual does not consciously choose this neurotic illness. It is an unconscious, involuntary, faulty method of trying to effect some kind of adjustment in his life. He does not invent or imagine or fake his symptoms. He cannot see or hear or walk as the case may be, even though the structure of the involved sensory organs or muscles is intact. It is similar to the frightened speaker who has no saliva even though the salivary glands are intact, and no amount of logic will alter the condition. Physical pain, paralysis, or inability to function is just as real whether it is emotionally or organically caused.

In lay terms, the word "hysterical" is used to describe an exaggerated and senseless display of emotions. This kind of behavior is often associated with women rather than men. In fact, the prefix "hyster-" means uterus, and the older name of the illness, conversion hysteria, reflects the early belief that bodily functions or humor controlled emotions rather than the reverse. However, in psychiatric terms, this disorder may affect men, women, and children.

The deliberate feigning of illness or injury with the intent to deceive is called malingering, not a somatoform disorder (conversion disorder, psychogenic pain disorder, or hypochondriasis). It usually occurs in an attempt to avoid responsibility, work, or some kind of unpleasantness. For example, if a person calls in sick because he wants to go to the beach or attend to personal business instead of going to work, that is malingering. It is not to be confused with the unconscious, sick behavior of the neurotic patient. The malingerer knows that he is not sick, and usually so does everyone else.

Dissociative Disorders. In dissociative disorders, the neurotic patient uses the primary coping methods of conversion and dissociation. As a result, aspects of the individual's personality are split off from his awareness, and certain of his activities become unconscious and automatic. This type of illness includes psychogenic amnesia, psychogenic fugue, multiple personality, and depersonalization disorder. The symptoms represent an alteration in the individual's identity, awareness, and memory. Amnesia is the complete or partial loss of memory, temporary or permanent, which is due to emotional trauma. Fugue states are prolonged periods of amnesia, during which the individual behaves in an automatic fashion, and they are sometimes associated with petit mal seizures. Depersonalization refers to feelings of unreality and of estrangement from the self, body, or surroundings. Multiple personality refers to the existence within the same person of entirely different identities with different ways of functioning. Usually, there is one dominant personality and the other subpersonalities occur unconsciously and without reciprocal awareness. It is necessary to distinguish this neurotic illness from the psychotic illness of schizophrenia (see Chapter 11).

The intolerable state of anxiety causes the neurotic patient to split off those offending, unpleasant, or unacceptable parts of himself which result from internal conflict and which he cannot stand. He then proceeds to behave in ways outside of his conscious awareness and control which help to relieve as well as express the conflict. For example, the man who finds himself in an impossible life situation from which he cannot escape and which he cannot manage, develops amnesia, leaves behind him the responsibility of home and job, and takes up a new life somewhere else without ever knowing what has actually taken place.

Thigpen and Cleckley report the case of a young woman who, in reaction to the stress of her life, developed three distinct personalities, and with treatment, a composite fourth. (The student is referred to *The Three Faces of Eve* and its sequel *Strangers in My Body* listed in the chapter references.) Eve White represented her better self: retiring, calm, and self-controlled. Eve Black was her worst self: loud, boisterous, and provocative. Jane emerged as the more mature, capable, dominant personality. The final personality, Evelyn, was like Jane, yet more substantial and complete, and represented a resolution of the conflict and turmoil. The personalities emerged outside of the patient's conscious awareness and control.

Dysthymic Disorder. Dysthymic disorder or depressive neurosis usually occurs in relation to the loss of an important source of satisfaction—person, possession, or position. The patient represses the resulting feeling of hostility and turns it inward upon himself by the use of introjection. It is better to feel sad than to feel angry. The symptoms of the illness—despondency, guilt and despair—serve two purposes. They punish the individual for his "bad" feelings, and they punish others around him for disappointing him. No kind of behavior is more hostile or punishing than that of depression. Because of its threat to life, it exerts control and influence over other people in the environment.

This illness must be distinguished from psychotic depression (see Chapter 12). The distinction is usually made on the basis of the patient's pre-morbid personality, the nature of the precipitating life situation, and the extent, duration, and severity of disturbance in the patient's functioning. The development and dynamics of the illnesses are similar, and sometimes the distinction is a difficult and arbitrary one.

Hypochondriasis and neurasthenia are sometimes described as symptoms of all neurotic illness and sometimes as distinct types of neuroses (see Appendix B). Hypochondriasis is defined as morbid preoccupation with one's body functions, overconcern about one's health, and unreasonable fear of disease. Neurasthenia is characterized by complaints of chronic weakness, fatigue, and exhaustion resulting from continued frustration or ineffective adjustment.

CARE AND TREATMENT

Some of the most difficult and complex treatment problems are those related to the care of the neurotic patient. The patient may not be amenable to psychiatric treatment, in fact, may be insulted by the mention of it. As a result, the patient is usually treated in the office of the general practitioner. We need not be critical of the medical practitioners, nor underestimate the excellent care that some patients receive. However, it is a generally accepted fact that many neurotic patients are misdiagnosed and mistreated. They often go from one doctor to another, from one illness to another, from one operation to another. Only the most severely disturbed neurotic patient is admitted to the psychiatric hospital, and then usually in connection with some other aspect of mental illness. Unless the patient is fortunate enough to have sufficient insight of his own, friends or family to help him, or a private physician whom he respects, he seldom receives psychiatric care of any kind.

A second part of the problem is that the very nature of the illness may discourage a psychological approach to treatment. The neurotic patient often converts his emotional problems into physical complaints. He does this because he cannot stand to look at whatever it is that causes the emotional conflict in the first place. If he could, he would not need to go to all the trouble of developing a neurotic illness. In addition, although he often realizes that his solution (neurotic behavior) is not entirely satisfactory, he gets enough gratification that he is unwilling to trade the bird in the hand for the two in the bush. He doesn't know another way of resolving his problems, and he cannot give up the way he has found until he learns a better way.

A third facet of the problem is the reaction that neurotic behavior evokes in other people, including those who are in the helping professions. Because the illness or symptom is emotionally caused, rather than organic, we tend to discount its credibility. The patient's hypochondriacal symptoms are often ridiculed or rejected, and the patient himself punished or mistreated. For example, the private physician may try to pacify the patient by acceding to his demands, putting him in the hospital, or referring him to someone else. The office nurse may try to protect the busy physician by stalling the patient, trying to deal with the problem herself, or not giving the patient an appointment.

There are some facts which should be emphasized before talking more specifically about the care and treatment of neurotic patients. First, the illness, which includes the symptoms, is just as legitimate as any kind of illness. It is recognized and described as such. Second, one does not cure an illness by telling the patient that he is not sick. To do so denies the fact of the illness and the patient's right to have it. Third, acceptance of the illness and the patient who has it does not necessarily mean re-enforcement of the symptoms or that no attempt will be made to help the patient find better ways of solving his problems. Many people have tension headaches which result from the frustrations on the job, or at home, or with life in general, and they know the reality of the discomfort. To have someone tell them that the headache does not exist, or to imply there is something bad or peculiar about having such a headache is a humiliating and infuriating experience which usually makes the headache worse instead of better. Fourth, there are even more ineffective levels of adjustment than neurotic illness, including depression and suicide. It is essential that we have something better, not worse, to offer the patient before we ask him to give up what he has.

One of the first steps in the treatment process consists of relief of the patient's distress, which means, as well, relief of the symptoms of his illness since his symptoms are based upon his emotional distress rather than the other way around. Often this consists of the administration of one of the minor tranquilizers, or antianxiety drugs, such as Librium, Valium, Miltown, Equanil. Depending upon the nature of the distress, antidepressant drugs may also be given, such as Tofranil, Elavil, and Aventyl. The best physical approach to treatment is to relieve the anxiety and the symptoms at the same time, and if possible, with the same drug. For example, if the neurotic patient is complaining of nausea, the physical treatment of choice may be Compazine, which relieves both anxiety and nausea, the underlying cause as well as the symptom.

There is a great deal of controversy over the symptomatic treatment of the physical manifestations of neurotic illness. However, to deny a patient medication that he believes will help him and which is readily available to him does not seem particularly therapeutic. As we have suggested before, most of us have our own remedies for simple ills, and as long as they work in relieving our distress, we don't stop to worry about the physical or emotional origins of the distress or the chemical content of the drug. The same principles hold true for the general relief of human suffering, including neurotic illness. Medication or other physical treatment may relieve the neurotic symptoms although the relief may be temporary. However, physical treatment should not be carried to the extreme of over-medication or unnecessary surgery because these simply interfere further with the patient's adjustment rather than promoting his health or recovery. Obviously, to be successful, treatment of the neurotic patient must include some form of psychotherapy.

Many psychotherapists believe that the neurotic patient's physical symptoms and anxiety should not be relieved to the extent that he becomes so comfortable that the motivation for changing his ways is removed. In certain situations, it may be extremely important to the success of the psychotherapeutic effort that the neurotic patient not be given medication, but that he obtain his relief through his relationship with the therapist.

Sometimes placebos are used successfully in the treatment of neurotic patients. The success of the placebo depends primarily upon the success of the relationship between the therapist and patient. If the patient respects and trusts the judgment of the therapist, then placebos may work. However, often in such a relationship, suggestion alone is sufficient and a placebo is not needed. Furthermore, placebos often backfire. If a patient discovers he has been duped or tricked, especially by someone he has trusted, it often ends the effectiveness of the patient-therapist relationship and generally makes matters worse instead of better. I am not in favor of trying to fool the patient into thinking he is better when, in fact, he is not, as if the symptoms were something he made up in the first place. If, on the other hand, the patient believes that the therapist and the medication which he prescribes will help him, it is generally true that it will.

The psychological treatment of choice is psychotherapy. Psychotherapy must be aimed toward resolving the core problem—helping the patient increase his acceptance of himself, lessen his repression, increase his satisfaction, lessen his hostility, and in general, find better ways of satisfying his needs. The treatment begins with acceptance of the patient. Self-acceptance is something that one learns from his interactions with others. For the neurotic patient, self-acceptance comes about through his corrective emotional experiences with the therapist since he does not have it in his relationships with others. He must learn from his interactions with the therapist that he's not such a bad guy after all before he can make the necessary internal changes that result eventually in external changes in his behavior.

As he works with the therapist to revise his concept of himself, he needs to be surrounded with an environment which is accepting of him. If a girl wants to change the color of her eyes, she changes the things which surround and form the background for her eyes. She changes the color of her makeup, jewelry, and dress. Grey eyes can be made blue, and blue eyes green by such environmental changes. The patient needs the opportunity to try out some of his new ideas about himself and others. Since the neurotic patient is often an outpatient, it may be helpful to have significant members of the family in conjoint therapy—particularly, husband, wife, children, parents. The patient needs as many social outlets as possible to widen his perspective of himself and the world he lives in so that often social, recreational, vocational and educational activities are recommended. As many positive reenforcing experiences and new avenues of expression as he can tolerate are generally useful.

It is essential, too, that the neurotic patient have a thorough physical examination, including indicated laboratory and x-ray procedures, to rule out the possibility of some physical disease being present. Physical examination and psychotherapy may be combined by explaining the reasons for various procedures and going over the results with the patient. Often, this can be a kind of reality orientation for the patient whose primary problems include anxiety about himself and his physical health.

Now, let us look at three case histories of neurotic patients to see the clinical picture of what we have been discussing.

Case Example No. 1

The patient is a 46-year-old mother of two children who was admitted to the psychiatric hospital voluntarily on the recommendation of her private physician. For the past three to six months, she has had severe headaches with knifelike pains in her head. She has received Etrofon, Thorazine, and Dilantin for the headaches but they persist. She has had crying spells, has not slept well, and has had little appetite in recent weeks. A home visit from her mentally retarded son seems to have precipitated the present disturbance.

Patient's parents were 42 at the time of her birth. She is the youngest of four children. The family lived on a small ranch, and the father worked in nearby logging camps and later as a guard on an army transport. Her mother was a housewife. The patient recalls that the family was quite poor and money was in short supply. It was a rare treat to be given a nickel and to be told she could spend it all on candy. She refers to her father as "bull-headed," and says she felt much closer to her mother whom she describes as tender and understanding. Mother and father are both dead. Patient feels closest to her sister who is 14 years older than she.

School was difficult for the patient, but she recalls being good at typing. She had lots of friends, but had few outside activities and involvements with clubs and organizations. She was first married when she was 22. This marriage ended in divorce because of the husband's excessive sexual demands, excessive use of alcohol, and his failure to provide for her.

The patient married her present husband when she was 26. He is a factory worker whom she describes as a wonderful man, very understanding and a good supporter. She says that her frequent illnesses have caused financial problems. She enjoys sexual intercourse occasionally, but not as often as her husband desires it, and she says she is "kind of on the cold side." Two sons were born to this marriage. The oldest boy is seventeen and the patient feels she has somehow failed with him because he just gets by in school. He has lots of friends, enjoys shows, dances, sports. The youngest son is 13 and has been a patient in an institution for the mentally retarded for the past three years. They attempted to hospitalize him when he was six but had to wait until recently because there was no room. As a result of having him home, the family seemed to withdraw from neighbors and friends. The patient always seems to have a difficult time when this son visits at home, usually for a two-week period. The first week goes fine, but the patient insists upon keeping him home the second week, and things don't go so well.

The patient suffered a "nervous breakdown" when she was 14 years old which she remembers as extreme nervousness. She stayed out of school for a year. Her first hospitalization for mental illness was at a general hospital fifteen years ago when she received six ECTs. She sought help at this time because she was "feeling blue," and lost interest in things. Her husband found her with a butcher knife in her hand which he felt she intended to use upon herself. She has been admitted four times since to a psychiatric hospital: eight years ago she was hospitalized by court commitment, diagnosed as psychophysiological nervous system reaction, for a four-month period; four years later she was admitted voluntarily, diagnosed psychoneurotic depressive reaction, for about one month; one year later admitted again voluntarily, for about six weeks; and again two years later (one year ago) admitted voluntarily, diagnosed psychoneurotic reaction, anxiety type, for about one month.

Patient seeks admission at this time because of the severe headaches she has had for the past six months. These have necessitated hospitalization in the local general hospital every five or six weeks for a period of three to six days. Her physician states that she has had a number of complete physical examinations, including an eye, ear, nose and throat workup in which no significant physical disease was found. She has thought about suicide, but says she hasn't "the guts" to do anything about it.

On admission, the patient was described as clean and neatly dressed. She looked wan, pale, with red-rimmed eyes and an anxious facies. Her talk was coherent and relevant and she was cooperative throughout the interview. At the mention of her mentally retarded son, she began to cry, but rapidly controlled her tears. She smoked nervously and showed a fine tremor of hands and head.

She gave a history of a thyroidectomy in 1947, surgery for tubal pregnancy in 1959, and a hysterectomy in 1962. There is no history of neurological disorder, but she states she has had frequent headaches during most of her life. Her lab and x-ray work were normal. She related her nervousness and anxiety to her physical complaints. She had no insight into her problems on a psychological basis, but was motivated for relief from her physical symptoms including her sleeplessness. She was of average intelligence, showed no evidence of thought disorder; but she appeared depressed.

Patient was started on Sinequan 150 mg. h.s. She then became cheerful, alert, and eager to start planning her future.

After four days of hospitalization, she was put on self-medication of the above and was assigned to a nurse for counseling. She adjusted quickly, seemed relatively unbothered by headaches and complained of only minor physical symptoms, mainly stomach distress which was related to her home visits. She spent most of her mornings drinking coffee and smoking with a group of inactive patients.

Because her home was some distance from the hospital, it was four weeks before she could go home on a visit. The visit was not too successful. The patient could not eat, accused her husband of only wanting her home to cook and clean house. After another week back on the ward, she again asked for a home visit, and stated firmly that this time it would work because she would try harder.

The patient was seen in hour-long interviews twice weekly. She seemed to accept her counselor, and was generally friendly and open in her discussions, except that on one occasion, she accused the counselor of trying to keep her in the hospital for the rest of her life. Counseling was aimed at getting the patient to look beyond her physical complaints, and stop punishing herself with headaches, stomach aches, and admissions to the hospital. Specific activities that might be helpful to her were suggested. She was encouraged to learn to drive so that she would not be so confined to the house. She was urged to explore possible volunteer projects at the lodge where her husband was a member and at the institution for the mentally retarded where her son was a patient. Full-time employment was discussed so that she might help with the family financial burden. The problems with her mentally retarded son were discussed. She was encouraged to accept her mixed feelings as being those which most parents would experience in similar circumstances. It was suggested that she not keep him at home for longer than one week at a time, and that the family not take him along on their only vacation each year.

The patient's husband was seen on two occasions for hour-long sessions to discuss and make arrangements for the patient's return home. The patient was discharged on medications after seven weeks in the hospital and was referred to her family physician.

Diagnosis: Generalized anxiety disorder with somatoform and depressive features.

Case Example No. 2

Patient is a 45-year-old woman with one son by a previous marriage and one adopted daughter. Ten days prior to her admission to the psychiatric hospital, she drank an unknown amount of household cleaner while she was overmedicated from pills she had taken on her own, and was hospitalized in the general hospital. She denies that this was a suicidal attempt. She was transferred to the psychiatric hospital on the advice of her private physician. She has a long history of dependence on drugs of the analgesic, relaxant, and hypnotic type.

Patient was born in a logging camp, the youngest of three children. When the patient was three years of age, the family moved to a small town where she has lived ever since. She describes her father as a domineering, strict, volatile man, insistent upon being obeyed. She feels that he never showed her any affection and loved everyone else but her. Her mother she describes as a "doll." She felt close to her mother, and they spent considerable time doing things together and sharing problems. She did not get along well with her older brother and sister. She recalls that she was able to get what she wanted by playing one parent off against the other, generally undermining her father's strictness, and eliciting support and protection from her understanding mother.

She had considerable difficulty in her first year at school, characterized by difficulty concentrating and lack of interest. She failed the sixth grade because of "fooling around," daydreaming, not studying. She became more interested in high school, and began preparing for a career as a bookkeeper. She had many friends, participated in numerous social events, particularly dancing and skating. She began dating in high school and dated several different boys. During her junior year she met a young man two years older than she who was serving in the Navy. After a six-months' courtship in which the patient states she was "swept off her feet," they were married. The marriage was kept secret because she was still in school, and her parents did not know until six months later. A pregnancy occurred almost immediately but was interrupted by a miscarriage. The marriage lasted five years, although the patient began to have considerable trouble with her husband right after this miscarriage. The husband was away from home most of the time and refused to assume any responsibility. Upon graduation from high school, the patient worked to support herself as a clerk, waitress, and finally, as an accountant. Although separated from her husband, the patient tried to hold the marriage together; during one of their attempts at reconciliation, she became pregnant and a son was born nine months later. She finally filed for divorce when she discovered that her husband was unfaithful.

After her divorce, she renewed her acquaintance with the man who is her present husband. After three months of courtship, they were married. She was 25. She describes this marriage as "perfect" with no problems. She says her husband is a patient, loving, wonderful, hard-working, self-sacrificing man with a sense of humor. For the first year and a half of their marriage, she continued to work until the desire to remain home as wife and mother prompted her to quit. Over the next five years the patient and her husband shared an active and full life together. They were both eager to have a child of their own, although they shared the responsibility of raising her son, and they both saw several doctors when she did not get pregnant. Finally, when the patient was 34, they decided to adopt a little girl who is now ten years old. Although both parents were quite happy with this adoption, they still felt deeply the need to produce a child of their own.

Six years ago it was necessary for the patient to have a hysterectomy for reasons that are not quite clear. This was a great loss to the patient and her husband because it destroyed any hope of their having their own children. The patient's family life since then has centered around her illnesses. There was a marked, persistent change in her personality. She became irritable and apprehensive; her interests and activities declined; she developed several physical complaints requiring extensive medical evaluation and treatment. For two years there was prolonged physical discomfort and suffering. She complained of persistent, right-sided neck, shoulder, and arm pain, as well as trouble with her stomach, characterized by nausea, diarrhea, anorexia and weakness. At times her physical discomfort was so severe that she would cry from the pain, and at other times, she was unable to describe the nature of her complaints to her physician. She obtained no relief despite numerous medications. The patient's husband became increasingly concerned over her failure to respond to treatment, as well as his impression that she was taking increasingly larger amounts of medication.

Five years ago the patient ingested a large number of sleeping pills, became comatose and required treatment at a general hospital. Although the patient's physician and family speculated on the possibility of a suicidal attempt, this has been vigorously denied by her. Her explanation is that she took the medicine, became dopey and dazed, lost track of the amount, and accidentally took too much. While in the general hospital, she spent some time undergoing psychiatric evaluation and treatment. Diagnosis of depressive reaction was made and outpatient treatment was arranged. However, upon discharge, she did not seek psychiatric help. Instead, she returned home, again developed complaints of pain, sought out physicians for care and received medications in order to obtain relief from her discomfort. Three months later she underwent shoulder surgery for treatment of a possible scalenus anticus syndrome. As a result there was an increase in her pain, requiring more medication.

Over the next three years, the earlier cycle was again repeated. During this time the patient contacted at least seven private physicians in the community, and became increasingly dissatisfied with their attempts to alleviate her discomfort. Four months ago, as a part of an extensive medical workup to determine if neurosurgical intervention would help to alleviate her pain, a consultation with a private psychiatrist was obtained. He recommended that no further surgical procedures be performed, and that the patient be given psychiatric care on an outpatient basis. Again this recommendation was not followed by the patient.

By this time several physicians were independently involved in her medical treatment. She was taking increasing amounts of sleeping pills, tranquilizers, muscle relaxants, codeine and morphine. Then, ten days prior to admission, the patient swallowed the household cleaner. Again the possibility of a suicidal attempt was considered, and again the patient claimed this was strictly an accident. Nonetheless, she was referred for psychiatric treatment.

On admission, the patient was described as a well-oriented, appropriately-dressed, pleasant-looking, middle-aged woman, who looks older than her stated age. She spoke clearly and logically without pressure but in a whining tone. She has good recall, poor concentration, no evidence of a thought disorder. Her affect is a little shallow with a predominance of depression. She candidly reported the incidents which led up to her admission.

On physical examination, there was no evidence of physical illness. Neurological exam was essentially negative except for fine tremors of the hands. Lab exam negative. Chest x-ray revealed "blunting of the left costophrenic angle. The pulmonary parenchyma reveals no lesions." A barium swallow revealed a stricture of roughly 15 cm. in the distal end of the esophagus for which the patient received dilatation.

On admission the patient was put on Mellaril 25 mg. q.i.d. She adjusted well and had few complaints except for a sore throat.

The patient was assigned a counselor and an activity group. She immediately asked for an appointment with her counselor. When she was seen, she appeared tired, haggard, pale. She manifested a moderate amount of anxiety by a chewing motion of her mouth and wringing of her hands. She seemed to have some difficulty swallowing, and as she focused upon this somatic complaint in her discussion, it became more prominent. Her speech was normal in rate and content, but lacked enthusiasm or expression. Her facial expression, likewise, was limited to a fixed, drawn, somewhat tense appearance, broken only by an occasional smile as she attempted to deny the seriousness of events leading up to her hospitalization. She maintained that she had entered the hospital in order to deal with the problem concerning drugs, and that this problem no longer existed since withdrawal. She demonstrated a desire to leave the hospital as soon as possible. She stated that since she was no longer taking drugs and had come to realize the harmful effects that drugs have upon her, she would be able to return home and function satisfactorily on the basis of pure determination and will power. She repeatedly denied any emotional problems, personal problems, family problems, and claimed that she would be able to continue living despite her physical discomforts without the use of medicine and treatment if only allowed to leave the hospital.

Counseling consisted of increasing confrontation directed toward her marked denial of the obvious emotional problems involved in her illness. Time was spent in allowing the patient to work through her feelings in regard to the earlier hysterectomy. When this topic was discussed, she cried quite freely, related her disappointment and sense of failure, as if it were a current situation rather than something that happened six years ago. Joint sessions were held with the husband in which attempts were made to point out to the patient how her behavior was seen by others, and how she controlled and manipulated her husband and family with it. As a result, she successfully completed two weekend visits in which she and her husband went through the house and threw away all of the accumulated pills. The family, as a group, participated in social activities for the first time in years, and the patient experimented in relating to her husband in other areas than her physical symptoms.

After 23 days in the hospital, it was recommended that she be discharged and that she seek followup psychiatric care in the community on an outpatient basis.

Diagnosis: Generalized anxiety disorder with somatoform and depressive features.

Case Example No. 3

Patient is an 18-year-old single young lady living at home with her mother. For the past six months she has had the recurrent idea that she should kill her mother. This thought has upset her so that she has become increasingly anxious, tense, preoccupied. She would stand for long periods of time in the bathroom washing her hands.

The patient is the younger of two children with a brother two years older. Brother is apparently a happily married welder, and has been out of the home for several years. Patient and brother were never very close —he went with father and she with mother. Father died six years ago of a heart attack. He was a mild-mannered man who never disciplined the children and seemed to have little to do with the patient's upbringing. Mother is an aggressive, matronly woman who makes her living as a sales manager of a large women's wear store. She completely dominates the patient, making most of her decisions for her and even talking for her.

The patient is a small, doll-like girl with long red hair and large green eyes. She gives the impression of being fragile enough to break easily. She has always been fastidious in her dress and personal habits. Mother has encouraged this by being obviously pleased with her when she cleaned up a mess she had accidentally made or drew back from situations where she might get dirty. Mother has always chosen the patient's clothes, which add to her baby-doll appearance.

Patient completed high school with average grades. She never had many friends but always one or two close girl friends. When it came time for dating, she usually went with a group of youngsters rather than a particular boy. She states she has never really had a boyfriend. Mother has discouraged her in this regard and has become even more possessive (and restrictive) since father's death. The patient states she has never had any sexual relations or even any particular interest in sex. She feels it is all right for husband and wife, but there is something unpleasant about it, and she would rather not discuss it.

In the past few weeks, patient has gotten steadily worse until mother has had to stay home from work to care for her. She spends the greater part of her day in the bathroom washing and wiping herself. Her hands are rough, red, and in some places bleeding where she has rubbed away the outer layers of skin. She has difficulty thinking, eating, and sleeping. In fact, at the present time, she is unable to care for herself.

She was admitted to the psychiatric hospital and started on Serax 10 mg. t.i.d. and Navane 20 mg. h.s. A daily schedule was planned for her with strict time limits for her bathroom activities. After about a week, she became less tense, more able to concentrate and care for herself. She was continued on the above medications and assigned a counselor. She began to recognize and talk about some of her feelings toward her mother. It was thought she would benefit from discussing some of her problems with others her own age and she was assigned to therapy with a group of young patients. She became increasingly aware of the fact that she had other problems than her feelings about her mother, and she began to explore her inner conflicts regarding her identity. Her relationships with the other patients improved, and she spent considerable time with a young male patient who was shy and retiring.

Mother was also seen in counseling sessions and began to see her part in her daughter's illness. After three weeks in the hospital, the patient had a trial visit at home. Although there were some problems about her bathroom activities, she did not have a recurrence of her upsetting thoughts. She had increasingly long visits at home and things went fairly well. Medication was discontinued, and she was discharged six weeks after her admission with the recommendation that both she and her mother continue psychotherapy on an outpatient basis.

Diagnosis: Obsessive-compulsive disorder.

NURSING CARE AND TREATMENT

The nursing care and treatment of a patient with a neurosis fits within the general care and treatment plan. The physical nursing care should be appropriate to the particular illness and the individual patient.

Let us discuss here a few of the general points pertinent to nursing that should be emphasized.

Probably the most important single factor in effective nursing of the neurotic patient is the nurse's attitude of acceptance. Acceptance is based upon the fact that the patient has the right to be exactly what and who he is. Whether the nurse approves of the patient's behavior or likes him as a person is not the fundamental issue. The nurse must believe that the patient is sick, that if he could act differently he would, and that he desperately needs her help if he is to recover or change his way of doing things so that he is more successful. If she believes this, her attitude is apt to be more accepting, more positive, more therapeutic. If she believes the opposite, her attitude and, therefore, her approach to the patient is apt to be the opposite.

The nurse can best help relieve the patient's anxiety by her presence, her understanding, and her competence. Reassurance is like insight and motivation; one person does not give it to another. The nurse does not reassure the patient by telling him that he is not to worry, or that he is going to be all right, especially when his convictions tell him differently, but he is reassured when the nurse treats him with concern, respect, knowledge, and a sense of responsibility.

Often nurses have considerable difficulty handling the physical symptoms and complaints of the neurotic patient. The nurse's verbal and nonverbal interaction with the patient should neither confirm nor deny the patient's symptoms. The nurse who is overly concerned about or sympathetic toward the patient's symptoms will make him all the more anxious, and he will have all the more symptoms. The nurse who tells him there is nothing wrong with him or ignores his symptoms altogether will also make him more anxious and increase his complaints. Sometimes it helps to acknowledge how miserable the patient feels without talking about his symptoms at all, simply by saying something like, "You must feel miserable." Sometimes it helps to listen to what the patient has to say, and actually try to figure out what he is trying to tell you. Sometimes it helps to explain to the patient, instead of assuming that he already understands, such things as the workings of his body, various treatment procedures, or why things are done as they are in the hospital. Sometimes it helps to let the patient blow off steam about his doctor, the hospital, his next door neighbor, or his family. The important thing is to care for the patient, not the symptom.

It is important for the nurse to do for the patient what he cannot do for himself, either by giving him direct assistance or by manipulating his environment. If the neurotic patient cannot walk because of hysterical paralysis, it is up to the nurse to provide whatever is necessary in order for him to be ambulatory. It may be crutches, a wheelchair, or a walker. It may be necessary for her to teach him how to use these environmental aids. If a neurotic patient is having an anxiety attack, he often needs not only medication but someone to stay with him. There is nothing more frightening than to feel something terrible is about to happen to you, and leaving a patient alone in such a predicament can be cruel and inhuman.

It is important for the nurse to be as honest, realistic, and matter-of-fact with the neurotic patient as she can be. This takes great therapeutic skill as well as a basic desire to help the patient all she can. It often takes considerable self-control, strength of character, and emotional maturity on the part of the nurse. Otherwise, she is apt to expect more of the patient than he is able to achieve, and thus set up for him further failure, frustration, anxiety, and physical symptoms. She should care more for the patient than she does for his symptoms, and her relationship with him should take into primary consideration that he is a person who is ill. Sometimes this can be conveyed most clearly to the patient when the nurse does things for him before he asks for them, or spends time with him when he does not demand it, or agrees with him when he has a legitimate complaint about the world he lives in.

When we talked of normal anxiety, we said all of us experienced anxiety in reaction to the stress of any crisis situation we face in life. It is a natural component of growth and development, and moves a person in the direction of self-realization. However, in neuroses, the person is overwhelmed with feelings of helplessness stemming from his inadequate personality. Instead of accepting himself as he is, he establishes impossibly high goals for himself and thus sets up a repeated pattern of failure and frustration. His relationships with others are impaired because of his extreme dependency, diffuse hostility, and unrealistic demands. He represses rather than resolves his inner conflicts. When repression fails, he seeks other means of relief through the faulty use of auxiliary defenses—displacement, conversion, dissociation, restitution, and introjection.

Common to all neurotic illness, then, are the two basic conditions of overwhelming anxiety in response to threat and the development of neurotic symptoms aimed at protecting oneself.

Any illness has physical, emotional, and social aspects simply because the sick person is made up of these characteristics. Each aspect influences the other because they are interrelated, interwoven, interdependent to such a degree that they cannot be separated from one another in a person. Effective care and treatment of the neurotic patient is aimed toward the relief of anxiety and a change in the basic personality structure.

Effective nursing care and treatment is aimed toward the resolution of the core problem of the particular illness and the satisfaction of the needs of the individual patient. Whether or not it is achieved depends upon the technical and interpersonal competence of the nurse. It cannot be accomplished without the nurse's personal interest in and involvement with the patient.

REFERENCES

Barber, Theodore X., et al., eds.: *Biofeedback and Self Control: An Aldine Annual on the Regulation of Bodily Processes & Consciousness,* Aldine Publishing, Chicago, 1976.

Claggett, Marilyn Smith: "Anorexia nervosa: a behavioral approach," *American Journal of Nursing, 80* (August, 1980) pp. 1471–1472.

Ferland, Carol: *The Long Journey Home,* Knopf, New York, 1980.

Goldstein, Vide, et al.: "Caretakers and the whole problem of role fatigue," *Nursing Outlook, 81* (January, 1981) pp. 24–30.

Gordon, Barbara: *I'm Dancing As Fast As I Can,* Bantam Books, New York, 1980.

Jourard, Sidney: *The Transparent Self,* 2nd Edition, Van Nostrand Reinhold, New York, 1971.

Knowles, Ruth Daily: "Control your thoughts," *American Journal of Nursing, 81* (February, 1981) pp. 353–355.

Lancaster, Evelyn, and James Poling: *Strangers in My Body,* New American Library, New York, 1974.

Levin, Lowell Al: "Patient education and self-care: how do they differ?" *Nursing Outlook, 78* (March, 1978) pp. 170–175.
McNellis, Nancy Jean: "Are there true problem patients?" *American Journal of Nursing, 79*•(October, 1979) pp. 1742–1744.
Mullins, Anna C., and Ruth E. Barstow: "Care for the caretakers," *American Journal of Nursing, 79* (August, 1979) pp. 1425–1427.
Numerof, Rita E.: "Assertiveness Training," *American Journal of Nursing, 80* (October, 1980) pp. 1796–1799.
Stevenson, Robert Louis: *Dr. Jekyll and Mr. Hyde,* Penguin Books, New York, 1981.
Storlie, Frances J.: "Burnout: the elaboration of a concept," *American Journal of Nursing, 79* (December, 1979) pp. 2108–2111.
Thigpen, Corbett, and Hervey Cleckley: *Three Faces of Eve,* Popular Library, New York, 1974.

Chapter 16

Psychosomatic Reactions to Stress

As we have stated, emotions and the impact they have on a person are experienced in physical as well as psychological ways. Our emotions may affect the physical functioning of any organ or system of the body by increasing, decreasing, or distorting the way in which it is supposed to work.

Not only do emotions affect the physiology of the body in healthy reactions to stress, but they also affect the body in unhealthy patterns of adjustment. In neuroses, particularly in conversion disorder and hypochondriasis, emotional reactions are repressed and then converted or transformed into physical symptoms in an effort to resolve the crisis in a person's life. The result, however, is a further lack of balance, which adds to the stress rather than lessening it.

In life situations in which a person is faced with prolonged stress which he cannot master, he may develop physical illness. This kind of illness is generally referred to as psychosomatic, or psychophysiologic. All human illness might be defined as psychosomatic, since there are emotional (psychic) and physical (somatic), as well as social, aspects to anything which affects the person. This is one of the underlying views of holistic medicine, considering the person with the illness as a whole and treating him accordingly. Another underlying view is the concept of "wellness," focusing upon the degree of wellness rather than the degree of illness, and treating the patient accordingly. However, the term psychosomatic has come to mean a particular way of reacting to crisis situations which a person encounters in life. In psychosomatic disorders not only is the function of the organs and systems of the body disrupted, but there are actual changes in anatomical structure and demonstrable organic lesions.

The idea that factors other than physical ones influence man's functioning is not a new one. Folklore and literature are full of dramatic accounts of the impact of emotions on the physiology of the body. In pre-scientific times, malfunctions of the body were thought to be caused by evil spirits. The healing power of the medicine man, witch doctor, and priest are almost as well established as that of the physician. Their success may be attributed to the use of a combination of mental, spiritual, social, and physical approaches in the treatment of the ills of mankind. Cures of physical ailments on the basis of faith are a matter of record, such as those at the famous shrine of Lourdes.

In the nineteenth century the practice of medicine became increasingly scientific, as it was based upon the principles of physics and chemistry. As a result, the spiritual and mental aspects of disease were all but discarded. Emphasis was placed more upon the body parts and how they worked or didn't work than upon the whole man. Virchow's discovery of cellular pathology and tissue change in disease was one of the greatest achievements in medicine, while at the same time, it was one of the greatest deterrents to the recognition of the effects of stress and emotions upon physical functioning. It was left to psychiatry and, particularly, psychoanalysis to bring a new understanding to the treatment of the sick person. Some of Freud's major contributions to medical science come from his study and treatment of neurotic patients who had become the rejected and neglected people of the time.

Increasing clinical evidence of the physical effects of emotions upon body organs and systems was gathered in the fields of psychiatry, neurology, endocrinology, and biochemistry. Flanders Dunbar (see Chapter References) concluded from a series of studies of patients that people with certain personality traits developed characteristic organic diseases. Upon the basis of her discoveries, she described specific personality profiles in the development of psychosomatic disorders. W. B. Cannon established the view that specific emotions (specifically anxiety, rage, and fear) caused characteristic physiological responses in organs controlled by the autonomic and endocrine systems. Hans Selye expanded the knowledge about the physiology of stress and the body's adaptive reaction by introducing his General Adaptation Syndrome (GAS) (see page 60).

Some of these new ideas have stood the test of time and others have been discarded. Franz Alexander is credited with putting together the concepts which are generally accepted as the current basis of psychosomatic medicine. His investigations revealed that (1) emotional states are accompanied by internal physiological processes of an adaptive nature; (2) these physiological processes are generally under the control of the autonomic nervous system;

(3) prolonged emotional tensions cause chronic dysfunction in the body's responses; and (4) these pathological responses result in tissue damage which is accompanied by characteristic symptom formation.

Definition

The new diagnostic category for psychosomatic disorders is "Psychological Factors Affecting Physical Condition" (see Appendix B). We will follow Alexander's findings on psychosomatic disorders—that is, physical diseases can be caused by chronic emotional reactions to the stress of everyday living. The body systems and organs affected are usually innervated by the autonomic nervous system. The physical changes are similar to those we see in healthy reactions to stress, except that they are more intense and prolonged. These are sometimes called "diseases of adaptation," because they represent chronic or prolonged preparation of the body for emergency action. For some reason, action is not or cannot be taken, so that the emotional tension is not relieved. As a result, the body organ or system involved breaks down or wears out under the continued assault.

As we have seen in Chapter 5, if the individual is continually bombarded with the stimulus of stress, without relief or resolution, physiologically he reaches the stage of exhaustion; physical disease and sometimes death may result. These disorders represent, then, the individual's reaction to cumulative problems in his interpersonal relationships, situation difficulties and crises in his life, repression of his impulses, desires, and emotions, and chronic preparation for him to combat his anxiety without the relief of appropriate action.

Although these disorders are sometimes referred to as "organ neuroses" or "vegetative neuroses," they differ from the neurotic reaction of somatoform disorders in three fundamental ways. In conversion disorders, the physical symptoms are an attempt to relieve emotional tension and are a symbolic expression of the underlying conflict. The symptoms develop in the voluntary muscles and sensory organs as a substitute expression for repressed desires, impulses, emotions. On the other hand, in psychosomatic disorders, the physical symptoms are not substitute or symbolic expressions but are the physiological component of emotions. The symptoms develop in organs primarily under the control of the autonomic nervous system. The disease occurs when, under prolonged stress or unresolved conflict, the physical response becomes chronic and tissue damage occurs. Thus, in psychosomatic disorders, there is actual physical damage.

Types

Although anxiety or other reaction to stress can be an important part of any illness, it is a primary factor in the development of certain physical illnesses. The first group includes illnesses in which chronic stress or anxiety is thought to have a direct causative effect—essential hypertension, peptic ulcer, mucous and ulcerative colitis, bronchial asthma, rheumatoid arthritis, neurodermatitis, hyperthyroidism, dysmenorrhea, migraine headache. These are the diseases most commonly accepted as psychosomatic disorders and are described officially as Psychological Factors Affecting Physical Condition (see Appendix B). The second group includes illnesses or injuries in which one's way of life or way of handling anxiety are thought to have a contributing effect—obesity, diabetes, epilepsy, tuberculosis, accidents. In addition to these groups, certain physical illnesses which are life threatening, such as surgical operations, heart disease, cerebral vascular accidents (CVA), and cancer, may produce sufficient anxiety in the patient to cause further pathologic reactions.

PROCESS OF DEVELOPMENT

Psychosomatic disorders clearly demonstrate the close relationship between the individual's physical and emotional functioning. Furthermore, they call for the treatment of the whole person, rather than his parts or a particular disease. Unfortunately, such comprehensive treatment is seldom put into practice either in the medical or the nursing care of the patient with a psychosomatic disease. As a result, he often suffers recurrent bouts of the illness which necessitate his hospitalization.

Again, each patient and his particular illness is different from any other. However, there are some similarities in the development of psychosomatic disorders. Let us discuss these generalities, keeping in mind that all patients do not fit the characteristic development and symptomatology as we are discussing it.

The patient who develops a psychosomatic disorder is seen by some authorities as generally healthier in his personality and adjustment than the patient, for example, with a neurotic illness. For one thing, his way of reacting to stress is more acceptable to himself and others. If the patient has a demonstrable physical lesion, it is understood he should be cared for in whatever way is necessary in order for him to recover. This may include hospitalization, medication, rest or vacation, change of occupation, or even changes in the home situation. All of these involve a respite from the ordinary demands and responsibilities of the patient's life situation. The psychosomatic disorder, then, usually represents an interruption in the patient's way of satisfying his needs rather than a lack of satisfaction. For example, the successful businessman who comes to the hospital with a bleeding ulcer trades his independent way of getting satisfaction for a dependent way.

The psychosomatic patient may be a generally successful person at home, at work, at play. He is often described as responsible and giving while, at the same time, competitive and demanding. What sometimes happens in the process of growing up is that the individual never has been allowed, and thus does not allow himself, a sufficient amount of dependent gratification. He may have always been fiercely independent, too independent for completely successful living. This outer and conscious layer of independence serves to protect his inner, and mostly unacceptable, longings for dependence. Thus, his independence serves as a reaction formation to his dependent strivings. Often he takes on the problems and responsibilities of his family, friends, and business associates in addition to his own. This may be a contributing factor in the development of his illness. He may be the kind of person to whom many people turn for assistance and advice in their own lives and this adds to his already considerable load. When he is no longer able to tolerate the demands, many of which he takes upon himself, a physical illness develops which may require his removal (and thus relief) from the demanding circumstances.

The particular organ or system of the body that is affected may be of personal, psychological significance to the patient. He learns certain values from his interactions with significant others and these are expressed through certain body functions. For example, if he grows up in a family where love is expressed through the preparation, serving, and partaking of food, the gastrointestinal system takes on particular significance in his way of life. He may then react to strong emotions, of both love and hate, with symptoms of the GI tract. If he grows up in a family where respect and approval are given for intellectual achievement, he is apt to attach great significance to his cerebral functions, and react to strong emotions with brain dysfunction. He learns as well from those around him what kind of physical expression is most acceptable. So, he may grow up in a food-oriented family, but he learns that he gets the most desired response from significant others when he has respiratory distress. Then he may develop the symptoms of bronchial asthma in response to strong emotions. He also learns how to behave from the way he sees those around him behaving, so his physical symptoms may reflect the symptoms of his parents. Thus, he not only inherits his anatomy and physiology from his parents, but in addition, what he learns in interaction with them determines how he sees and expresses himself physically. In other words, he learns from his parents how to use his anatomy and physiology as well.

Frequently, in the history of patients with psychosomatic illness, there is some difficulty in handling hostility effectively. Often the individual has a great need to be liked by others, and he has learned that hostile feelings may cause him to lose the much needed parental love and approval. As a result, he may repress the hostility he feels in reaction to frustration, convert it into physical terms, and suffer from some physical disease. We can see a similarity between the development of psychosomatic disorders and depression. They are both a result of self-inflicted punishment meant to atone for hostile or other unacceptable feelings. In both, the significant people in the patient's life are also punished, as well as controlled, by the sick behavior. The essential difference is that in psychosomatic disorders, the patient relies upon conversion as a reaction to stress, whereas in depression the patient relies upon introjection. The results are different: in psychosomatic disorders the physical disease, and in depression the mood disorder. Often, however, there are alternating periods of psychosomatic illness and depression in the same patient. When he is depressed, he is not physically ill, and when he is physically ill, he is not depressed.

There are physical factors, too, that contribute to the development of psychosomatic disorders in people. Physical symptoms may develop in any body organ or system which is particularly vulnerable at the time. A person may have inherited some constitutional weakness in a particular organ or system. It may be that certain parts of his body are more susceptible to disease as a result of recurring bouts of illness affecting those parts. Because of his way of life, a person may have misused or even abused certain of his body organs or systems so that they are less capable of handling stress in healthy ways. Sometimes a person inherits or develops allergic reactions which make certain parts of his body more susceptible to breakdown under prolonged and intense emotional tension.

To review, the physiological reaction to stress is a result of the stimulation of the autonomic nervous system which prepares the person for defensive action (fight or flight). If the individual is unable to act in his defense, and if the stress does not cease or lessen, the body organs or systems affected become exhausted from overwork and break down. The result is some kind of physical dysfunction which we call a disease or a lesion or a syndrome. These physical diseases are often called diseases of adaptation or psychosomatic disorders.

SYMPTOMS OF PSYCHOSOMATIC DISORDERS

It is important for the student to remember that psychosomatic disorders have both physical and emotional causes and symptoms, and both must be treated to effect a cure. Although any body organ or system may be involved, we will discuss only the most commonly accepted psychosomatic illnesses.

Circulatory System. In reaction to prolonged stress and unresolved anxiety, a person may develop essential hypertension. This is a condition in which the patient's blood pressure is chronically elevated without any demonstrable organic lesion, and generally without other physical symptoms. It may be that his life situation presents a constant source of stress (such as extreme competitiveness in his job) which he cannot resolve, escape, or more adequately cope with. As a result inner tension builds up that may be attributed to mounting feelings of hostility and aggression which he dare not acknowledge, let alone express. It may be that he has learned to handle such feelings by repression and conversion rather than by more effective means. At any rate, the constant state of preparation for fight without the action to relieve it results in the chronically elevated blood pressure.

Another psychosomatic disorder is migraine headache, which must be distinguished from other tension headaches. The symptoms of severe headache, nausea, vomiting, and photophobia may be precipitated by emotional stress. The symptoms are caused by an initial constriction and subsequent dilation of the cerebral arteries, and involve the functions of the circulatory, endocrine, and nervous systems. The attack usually begins with feelings of malaise, irritability, and fatigue. Visual disturbances, such as photophobia and scotomata,* often accompany the attack. The headache is severe and usually starts on one side, although it may involve the whole head before it is over. The patient is often a perfectionistic, hard-working person who satisfies his needs for affection and approval by achievement. He may have difficulty expressing his hostility, so that his pent-up rage is turned upon himself in the form of the punishing headache.

Digestive System. These psychosomatic disorders include peptic ulcer and colitis. In peptic ulcer, the patient develops an ulcerated lesion in the mucosa of the stomach wall as a result of his chronic emotional state. The stimulation of the autonomic nervous system in reaction to stress is to prepare the GI tract for action—hyperemia, hypermotility, hypersecretion. When there is no intake of food, the engorged mucosa, increased peristalsis, and hyperacidity serve as a source of irritation to the lining of the gut. If this is a frequent or constant reaction to the stresses of life, the lining wears out (or is digested) and a lesion in the form of an ulcer may result. Often the patient's exterior is that of the go-getter—aggressive, ambitious, independent—to counteract the interior (and unacceptable) desire to be taken care of (see Case Example No. 1, page 332).

*Island-like gaps in the visual field.

In ulcerative and mucous colitis, the lesions form in the lower part of the digestive tract rather than in the beginning. The development of the symptoms is much like that of peptic ulcer except for the location of the lesion. As the ulcerated lesions become inflamed and infected and scarring takes place, there may be serious complications such as perforation, hemorrhage, nutritional and fluid imbalance, and even secondary carcinoma. Mucous colitis is probably a more common reaction to chronic anxiety and often includes alternating symptoms of diarrhea and constipation, accompanied by abdominal discomfort and anorexia. The emotional component of the illness is often related to the individual's attempt to handle such unacceptable feelings as chronic rage and dependent longing. He rids himself of these feelings, frees himself from the discomfort of anxiety, and is taken care of, all at the expense of his visceral functioning.

Respiratory System. Bronchial asthma is a psychosomatic illness in which the attack is precipitated by sudden, intense emotional crises. The existence of allergic tendencies and chronic emotional stress and tension combine to produce spasms of the bronchioles. Often the patient has an excessive, unresolved, resented dependence upon his mother. His unmet needs for love and approval may be expressed by the asthmatic attack as a "cry for help" or as a substitute for tears.

Musculoskeletal System. Rheumatoid arthritis is a psychosomatic disorder in which chronic fatigue, aches and pains of the muscles and joints result from the patient's chronic preparation for defensive action. Often the patient has difficulty expressing his feelings, and he tends to relate to others through action of either a physical or intellectual nature. He may meet his needs for love and affection by performing services which make others dependent upon him, rather than he upon them.

Skin. In psychosomatic disorders of the skin, we may see the syndromes of neurodermatitis, urticaria, eczema, psoriasis, herpes, and pruritus. Skin changes commonly demonstrate reactions to strong emotions. We may see changes in color, temperature, and texture in response to stress and anxiety. The symptoms may include rash, sensitivity, itching, and lesions. Often the patient reacts to the skin condition by scratching or rubbing which serves to irritate it further, and sometimes results in infection. Common factors in the development of skin disorders are the presence of allergic as well as interpersonal problems. Often the patient is an insecure, passive person with strong dependent needs, who is afraid of experiencing rejection or hostility at the hands of significant people in his life.

Endocrine System. In hyperthyroidism, the symptoms of increased metabolism are due to excessive secretion of the thyroid hormone as a result of pituitary dysfunction. The condition is often precipitated by some disturbing emotional experience in which the patient is faced with the actual or threatened loss of an important source of satisfaction in his life. The patient is often an insecure, anxious individual with strong, unmet, dependent needs. He may be eager to please others, but at the same time, deeply and unconsciously resentful of having to do so. Generally, he is extremely sensitive, especially to the possibility of rejection, and tends to overreact to situations with characteristic restlessness, excitability, and agitation.

Reproductive System. The symptoms of dysmenorrhea, or painful menstruation, may result from chronic emotional turmoil or distress. Premenstrual tension, accompanied by edema, is common in many women, and the discomfort may be severe enough to cause incapacitation. Often the patient experiences repeated frustration in her relationships with people and in the fulfillment of her sexual role in life. The result may be increased tension, irritability, fatigue, and pain during her menstrual period.

EMOTIONAL FACTORS IN PHYSICAL CONDITIONS

Obesity. Overeating may become a way for the patient to relieve his feelings of anxiety or insecurity. He may substitute eating for other sources of satisfaction and comfort. Thus, he establishes a pattern that becomes a faulty method of adjustment. There are many factors that contribute to the accumulation of excess weight, but in general the person takes in more calories than the number he utilizes in his daily activities. Love and food are closely interwoven in most people's lives, as is demonstrated in their relationships with others—parents, family, friends, society, church. However, the obese patient goes to an extreme by his excessive and inappropriate intake of food, and not much can be said in favor of the resulting obesity. Like other kinds of faulty behavior, instead of making things better for the patient, it often makes things worse; it may also lead to cardiovascular disease, social rejection, or an early death.

Diabetes. Although diabetes is not considered a true psychosomatic condition, that is, emotionally caused, the diabetic patient's emotional state directly influences the disease process. Emotional stress causes an increase in blood sugar to equip the individual to handle the emergency situation. In the diabetic patient, this may produce an oversupply or hyperglycemia, and result in diabetic coma. If the stress is prolonged, it may result in a lowering of blood sugar or hypoglycemia and result in insulin shock. If he becomes discouraged or depressed because of his lack of success in life, the diabetic patient may not eat or take medication properly, and this can cause him serious problems. If he reacts to the frustrations of life by open rebellion or by manipulative behavior, he can be seriously ill in a matter of hours. Thus, emotions directly affect the onset, course, and response in the diabetic patient's illness and must be considered in any comprehensive treatment program.

Epilepsy. Epileptic seizures are generally caused by disturbances in the electrical discharges of the brain, or brain waves, as demonstrated in the EEG. They may be a result of injury, infection, malformation, or malfunction. Although it may not be a direct cause of the condition, emotional stress may precipitate a seizure in an epileptic patient. Interpersonal situations which produce strong feelings of anger, fear, disappointment, or grief may trigger a discharge of nervous impulses in the brain stem which aggravate the disturbance in the higher brain centers, and set off a seizure—grand mal, petit mal, or furor.

Tuberculosis. Although tuberculosis is caused by a microorganism, the tubercle bacillus, the onset, course, and response in the illness are closely correlated with the emotional state of the patient. The presence of organisms in the environment is a fact of life to which we make certain adaptations. Anything that lowers the individual's resistance to the ever-present germs makes him more susceptible to disease. Therefore, anxiety, tension, and unhappiness all contribute to an individual's lack of well-being and make him more susceptible to disease. Specifically, strong emotions of any kind may interfere with proper nutrition, rest, hygiene, and general physical well-being. Often the patient contracts tuberculosis as a result of emotional excesses or a particular period of emotional strain. Sometimes accompanying tuberculosis is the excessive use of alcohol or drugs.

For some people, tuberculosis may represent an unconscious desire to be dependent and cared for; for others, an opportunity to act out their hostilities toward life; for still others an escape from an intolerable life situation. Because of the serious nature of the illness and its necessary restrictions and confinement in the carrying out of effective treatment, many people react with increased anxiety. For most patients, the illness and its treatment regime represent a serious disruption in every aspect of personal, family, and social life. It may be extremely difficult for the patient to accept the curtailment of physical activities, or the isolation from his family, or the lack of many social activities, any or all of which may be major sources of satisfaction for him. He may react to the frustration of the illness with open hostility, rebellion, withdrawal, or depression, and his reactions may interfere with the treatment process and his rate of recovery.

Accidents. Accidents often are the direct result of emotional turmoil. The housewife gets angry at her husband while she is preparing supper, but instead of shouting at him, she cuts her finger. The irate father stomps out of the house after an argument with his son and slips on the walk and falls. The young man preoccupied with thoughts of his recent date gets too close to the car in front of him and bangs into the rear end. These are common occurrences which happen to most of us. For some people, however, accidents become a way of life. We call these people "accident-prone" because they are so frequently involved in some kind of accident. They are much more apt to hurt themselves than be hurt by some outside force. These people are not awkward or clumsy, nor do they deliberately inflict injury upon themselves. Often they are independent, self-reliant, impulsive people. They usually have some difficulty expressing their negative feelings, particularly hostility, and they tend to turn it inward upon themselves. Instead of punishing themselves with their feelings by depression, they punish themselves with physical wounds.

Insurance companies estimate that 80 per cent of all major accidents are due to personality factors, and further, that only about 10 per cent of the people are responsible for over 75 per cent of all accidents. Accidents are not ordinarily considered a disease yet they represent a major threat not only to health but to life. In the United States, accidents are listed as one of the top three causes of death, and the major cause of death in young people. In addition, many more people are temporarily incapacitated or permanently disabled from accidents.

Not only do emotions play a part in the cause, but accidents provoke emotional reactions which must be taken into consideration when caring for a patient. Any threat to the person's body image or personal competence invokes anxiety so that accidents which cause disfigurement, dismemberment, or dependency are particular sources of stress. The patient may react to the accident with any of the kinds of behavior we have discussed so far; most frequently, however, we see open hostility, depression, or withdrawal.

Surgery. An individual may use surgical procedures as a means of adapting to his life situation, so that, like accident-proneness, this becomes a pattern of behavior. That is to say, he may have multiple operations for a variety of physical complaints until this becomes a way of life. Women, more frequently than men, resort to this method of adjustment in an attempt to satisfy their needs, escape from an intolerable life situation, or punish themselves and others for unacceptable feelings, wishes, impulses, behavior.

Surgical procedures may also provoke anxiety to which patients respond with depression, open hostility, or withdrawal. Any surgical procedure which requires general anesthesia fills the patient with apprehension becauses he loses control over his behavior, does not know what is going to happen to him, and believes he may die without regaining consciousness. In addition, surgery which represents a threat to the person's body image or personal competence may provoke additional anxiety. Surgery involving the reproductive organs or sexual functions, such as a prostatectomy, hysterectomy, or mastectomy, is often accompanied by depression or other severe emotional reaction in the patient. Surgery which necessitates major changes in the patient's way of life, such as an amputation, lobectomy, or colostomy, is commonly accompanied by severe and prolonged emotional reactions.

REACTIONS TO LIFE-THREATENING ILLNESS

Coronary Heart Disease. The patient's emotions play an important role in the precipitation, course, and response in this illness. People generally worry about having a heart attack, and worry more after they have had one, with good reason. Heart disease is the number one cause of death among adults in this country and accounts for more chronic invalids than any other illness.

Cardiac patients are all separate and distinct individuals, but there are some things that they seem to have in common. They are usually hard-working, conscientious people who drive themselves, and they seem to particularly enjoy doing something useful. Often they have difficulty expressing their hostile feelings, and tend to keep them bottled up inside themselves. Frequently, they are careless about their physical health. They may eat irregularly, smoke too much, drink too much coffee, get insufficient rest and relaxation. They may not be particularly capable people, but their ambition and apparent enjoyment of hard work often carry them a long way down the road to success.

A patient's overwhelming fear of heart disease may cause him to become a chronic, helpless invalid, unless he can understand and accept the limitations of his organic illness. There is so much that is unknown about the heart and its illnesses, and so many beliefs that are contrary to fact, that a cardiac patient may literally be scared to death unless things are explained thoroughly to him.

Cerebral Vascular Accidents. A particular kind of cardiovascular disease that has become increasingly prevalent in the United States among elderly adults is the CVA or "stroke." As in heart disease, emotions play an important role in the patient's illness and treatment. A stroke is anxiety-producing not only because of its threat to life, but also because it so often seriously interferes with the patient's ability to interact effectively with his world and the people in it. Often a stroke renders the patient helpless, hopeless, and extremely frightened. His inability to speak or move or even swallow may overwhelm him and commonly does. Even as he begins to recover, his fear and frustration may prevent him from doing what he is physically capable of.

One of the most important aspects of the treatment process is that of rehabilitation. Rehabilitation cannot take place unless the patient is able to deal realistically with his feelings—fear, anger, despair, loneliness. It takes great emotional as well as physical strength to recover from a stroke.

Cancer. Another major disease which threatens the life, body image, and personal competence of the patient is cancer. No diagnosis strikes more fear in the hearts of patients or their families. People worry so much about getting cancer or having cancer that they are often afraid to go to the doctor for a regular checkup or for a particular symptom for fear the doctor will confirm their fear of the illness.

One of the best known ways to combat the illness is early diagnosis and prompt treatment. Yet many a woman has delayed consulting her physician for months when she is confronted with one of the well-known warning signs—vaginal bleeding. Likewise, many a man has put off seeing his physician for another well-known warning sign—pain on urination. Patients often say they had hoped the symptom would go away and instead it got worse. They have actually contributed to the seriousness of the illness by their emotional reactions.

Any of the body systems or organs may be involved—reproductive, urinary, circulatory, respiratory, digestive, nervous. Frequently, the disease involves those parts of the body that have particular significance for the patient such as the sexual organs, brain, stomach, and intestines. Also, the malfunction which results from the effects of the illness and its treatment may require that the patient change his whole way of life. For example, cancer of the lung which results in a lobectomy, or cancer of the breast which results in a radical mastectomy, may make it necessary for the patient to find a new kind of employment.

The patient's emotions are involved as well in the constant fear of recurrence even though he may recover from a particular episode. We do not know how cancer is caused, or exactly how it progresses, or what its eventual outcome will be, so it is accompanied by dread of the disease, fear of the unknown, and all of the common misconceptions. There is, in addition, the fear of pain and death, and the possibility that one may not be able to handle the stress in an adequate, reasonable, or courageous way.

CARE AND TREATMENT

In psychosomatic disorders, as with other kinds of illness, the best treatment is a combination of physical, emotional, and social approaches. The first order of the day is the treatment of the physical disease. Often the psychosomatic patient comes under our care with an emergency condition such as a bleeding ulcer. Following emergency care, there is often a need for long-range medical treatment such as diet, medication, establishing hygienic personal habits. In addition, the patient needs relief from anxiety which may be accomplished physically with the antianxiety tranquilizers. Often the medication which is given for the physical disease may also relieve the anxiety. For example, Compazine relieves both the physical symptoms of nausea and vomiting in peptic ulcer and the psychological symptom of anxiety. In the use of Donnatal for colitis, the hyoscine relaxes the smooth muscle of the gut, and the phenobarbital acts as a sedative to decrease the stimulation of the nervous system. Corticosteroids reduce pain in rheumatoid arthritis and enhance the patient's sense of well-being as well. Reserpine reduces blood pressure in essential hypertension and is a tranquilizer as well. Antidepressants may be used in cases where there are elements of depression, or where the physical disease is associated with underlying depression. (As the physical illness subsides, sometimes the depression is laid bare.)

In neurosis, the psychological approach may take precedence over the exclusion of physical treatment, whereas in the psychosomatic disorders, the physical approach may take precedence. Sometimes the patient is treated for the emergency condition and released without long-term medical or psychological treatment. Again, the most effective treatment combines the physical, psychological, and social approaches that are appropriate to the individual patient and his particular illness.

Whatever kind of psychotherapy is employed, it should be aimed at resolving the core problem by helping the patient to allow himself greater dependence upon others, while still maintaining a degree of independence. The goal is to help the patient move in the direction of a state of interdependence rather than either extreme of dependence or independence. This is accomplished by the attitude, words, and actions of the therapist in corrective interaction with the patient. Sometimes the patient's dependence upon the therapist is encouraged so that he may gain the satisfaction of his dependent needs as well as experience a change in attitude toward them. In other words, he learns through his relationship with the therapist that dependence is not so bad after all, and independence is not so great as he had thought.

The social approach to therapy is directed toward relieving the load of responsibility that the patient shoulders for his family, friends, business, and associates. Often, family therapy helps other members assume more of the shared and individual responsibility for the family's welfare. Sometimes a change of jobs is indicated, particularly when the work situation contributes significantly to the patient's stress and seems unlikely to change. Sometimes it is necessary for the patient to cut down on his activities, delegate some of his responsibility to others. The patient should be encouraged to discover new social outlets in order to increase his sources of satisfaction and relaxation.

In the other physical diseases in which anxiety may play a significant part, it is just as essential to treat the whole person as it is in the specific categories of emotional illness or mental disorder. Treatment should consider all the aspects of comprehensive care—prevention, treatment, and rehabilitation. Although the physical approach takes precedence, the emotional and social approaches should not be neglected. Their use may make it possible for the patient to recover optimum functioning sooner, they may lessen the severity of the illness and promote healing, and they may prevent the illness and its incapacitating effects from recurring.

It might be possible to decrease significantly the incidence of diabetes, epilepsy, tuberculosis, and accidents if people were helped to find more constructive ways of relieving their anxiety or solving their problems in living. If more counseling were available to youngsters in school, there would probably be a considerable decrease in the accident rate, which accounts for the majority of deaths in youngsters from age 1 to 24.

Counseling or psychotherapy would probably not eliminate physical illness, but it certainly would cut down on the severity of the illness and the individual's reaction to it. A patient's emotional reaction to surgery, heart disease, CVA, or cancer—worry, despair, depression—can and seriously does interfere with his recovery. The old saying, "the operation was successful but the patient died," has a basis in fact. Sometimes there seems to be no medical or physical reason why the patient should not improve and eventually recover, but he may be so fearful, so certain, or desirous of death, or so resigned to it, that he does indeed die. A person has to have something or someone to live for, and if that is missing, he may not have sufficient strength, desire, or will to survive (see Kubler-Ross, 1974).

Certainly, counseling or psychotherapy may be essential in helping a patient adjust to major changes in his way of living which come as a result of any of the physical illnesses discussed. It is a crucial part of the treatment in patients with heart disease, CVA, and cancer. Without it, the patient may not survive the shock of disability, the threat to his life, the necessity for changing his whole way of living. With it, the patient may enjoy a life of even greater security, peace and harmony despite, or perhaps because of, his illness.

Now let us look at some clinical examples.

Case Example No. 1 (Peptic Ulcer)

The patient is a 52-year-old widow who has been taking care of her invalid parents and a mentally ill sister for the past several years. Over the past two years, she has had many problems at home which kept her in a state of constant anxiety and worry. An ulcer developed in the lower part of her stomach, breaking down the lining of the stomach, and creating a lesion.

The patient was hospitalized for three weeks and treated medically with a bland diet and medications. Her medications consisted of Tagamet 300 mg. q.i.d., Combid Spansule 1 q. 12 h., and Riopan 400 mg. q.i.d. and p.r.n. Although the ulcer had not healed completely, she was much better and was discharged on the above medications.

A month later her father died of a CVA. Shortly after this, the sister had an acute psychotic episode, was hospitalized in a mental hospital, and discharged again to her sister's care. The patient began to suffer again from the symptoms of peptic ulcer—pain, nausea, vomiting. Just prior to admission, she was vomiting violently and frequently. She was dehydrated and malnourished, weighing only 87 pounds, and suffering from almost constant pain.

She was admitted to the hospital for possible surgery. Gastric analysis revealed excess free hydrochloric acid in the stomach. Pre-operatively she was treated with bland diet, antacids, multivitamins, and the medications mentioned above. Gastric resection was done and about 50 per cent of her stomach was removed. A nasal-gastric tube was inserted to remove excess acid and other fluids and she was given I.V. fluids for about four days.

The patient has assumed the responsibility for the other family members all of her life. Her mentally ill sister has lived with her for years. After her husband died, she brought her elderly parents to live with her, too, and recently she has been taking care of her father who was partially paralyzed from a prior stroke. She is described as a dutiful daughter, conscientious and hard-working. She does not complain about her lot in life, even though the demands made upon her by her family leave her little time for herself.

During her hospitalization, she expressed great concern about her sister's illness, as well as her own fear of becoming mentally ill. Because of this, it was suggested she might like to talk with someone about her problems. She agreed and a psychiatric consultation was arranged.

She met a total of six times with the psychiatrist and in her counseling sessions resolved some of her problems. She talked freely about the tremendous burden of responsibility she carried for her family and her own needs to be cared for. After counseling, she decided to sell most of her property, build a small home where she and her sister could live, and which she could manage comfortably. She also made plans to place her invalid mother in a nearby nursing home where she would be adequately cared for and where the patient and her sister could visit frequently.

Case Example No. 2 (Coronary Heart Attack)

The patient was a 49-year-old married man, father of six children. He was employed as chief of police in a small town. He worked hard at his job, was coach of a little league baseball team, and found time to work in his garden. He was well-liked by the townspeople and his neighbors, and many people came to him for advice.

At the end of a particularly busy summer, he suffered a heart attack which was diagnosed as a mild coronary. He spent five days in the hospital and was advised by his physician to take things easier and get more rest. However, he returned to work the next day and resumed his community and family activities as well.

The patient had always been an extremely independent person. He had not taken any sick time from the job except the five days he spent in the hospital. He had been a very active person and resented restrictions upon his freedom of movement. He was the oldest boy in a family of seven and spent much of the time while growing up caring for his younger brothers and sisters. When he was twelve he got a job after school to help out with the family finances and most of what he earned went for food and clothing for the family. He was described as a friendly, good-natured, warm-hearted man who loved activities. He was ambitious, hard-working, and generous. His favorite recreation was competitive sports.

Two months after he resumed his normal activities, a particularly bad fire occurred in the community when he was on duty. He answered the call with the volunteer fire department and spent several hours fighting the blaze. He drove back to the police station by himself and on the way, he experienced severe chest pain and difficulty breathing. However, he continued on to the station, climbed a flight of stairs to his office, and telephoned his wife. She, in turn, called their doctor and the ambulance and drove to the station. By the time the ambulance arrived, the patient was in extreme difficulty, although still conscious. He did not respond to emergency care and died on the way to the hospital.

Case Example No. 3 (Accident)

The patient is a 21-year-old single man who was admitted to the hospital as a result of an automobile accident. He suffered severe compression fractures of the lumbar vertebra and his legs were partially paralyzed at the time of admission.

Patient lives with his father and mother, and he is the center of attention, being the only child. He has finished high school and is employed as an unskilled laborer. His father is employed as a logger and works only in the summertime. The mother and father seem to get along well and provide a secure home environment, although their standard of living is in the low-income bracket. They seem to be able to cope with everyday problems and stress quite easily.

Patient has been given everything his parents could afford. He has his own room, his own car, and mother tries to cook everything he likes. The night of the accident he had an argument with his father about the crowd he was running around with. Father didn't approve of some of their actions, and when he questioned their morals, the patient "blew up" and told his father to mind his own business, that he was twenty-one, and was old enough to pick his own friends. He slammed out of the house and then crashed into a car, four blocks from home.

Patient has had no previous hospitalization or significant past medical history. His present illness consists of fractures of the 1st and 4th lumbar vertebrae. Although his legs are partially paralyzed, he will be able to get around with a leg brace, but he will not be able to work for six months.

He had some difficulty urinating so a 3-way Foley catheter was inserted. He was nauseated, unable to keep food down until about the third day; then he asked for food and was given a general diet as tolerated. He was very anxious and had difficulty following directions. He was given Urecholine Chloride for urinary retention, Valium to calm his anxiety, and Dalmane for sleep.

He had considerable difficulty doing things for himself and was often irritable and demanding. It was hard for the nurses to be patient with him and not get angry when he asked them to do things for him that they were sure he could do for himself. However, the nurses became aware of the fact that he was afraid he would never walk again, so they decided to drop in to his room whenever they could just to say hello, and this seemed to help a great deal.

He was given a chance to talk with a psychiatrist and worked out some of his dependency problems as well as his resentment towards his parents for treating him like a little boy. The psychiatrist saw the whole family together in several sessions, in order to help them relate to one another in a more adult and realistic fashion.

His parents visited the patient daily and frequently took him for a ride in his wheelchair, or supported him while he took short walks around his room. He was referred to physical therapy and responded well, began to do things for himself, and became increasingly cheerful as he was able to get around better. He was discharged after four weeks with one leg in a brace.

Case Example No. 4 (Cancer, Surgery, Depression)

Patient is a 64-year-old married man who came to the doctor's office complaining of prostate trouble and difficulty urinating. His urine was checked and it was clear, yellow, with a trace of sugar. Upon physical examination, the prostate gland was enlarged and there was considerable tenderness surrounding it.

Ten days later he was admitted to the hospital and a cystoscopic examination and biopsy were done. The cystoscopy showed a heavily fibrous bladder tissue but not a visible tumor. Microscopic examination of the biopsy revealed malignant cells. Two days later a transurethral resection of the prostate gland was performed.

He tolerated the surgery well and was returned to his room with a 3-way retention catheter in place. He was given a diabetic diet and put on insulin. His postoperative course is described as uneventful and he was discharged one week after surgery.

Two weeks following his discharge, he made a serious suicidal attempt and was admitted to the psychiatric hospital. He felt that life was over for him, and there was no use going on. He was put on regular insulin, diabetic diet, Tofranil 50 mg. t.i.d., chloral hydrate 0.5 gm. h.s.

The patient is described as a very independent person, but a worrier. He worried about finances, getting old, not being able to earn a living, and so on. Most of his worries are not realistic, since he and his wife are well-covered by a retirement plan. In fact, his wife has always been well taken care of. Most of his life has been spent working, either at his job or in his workshop. He is very proud of his carpentry ability and likes to make things for other people.

He was assigned a counselor in the hospital and began to talk about his feelings of loneliness and despair. He felt he was going to die anyway and should be "put out of his misery." Gradually, he began to accept the fact that his death was not imminent and he might have many years left to enjoy life. His wife was seen in conjoint therapy and they began to make plans for his return home. These included plans to continue working, at least for another year. He was discharged from the hospital after three weeks on Elavil 10 mg. t.i.d. and returned for weekly outpatient counseling.

NURSING CARE AND TREATMENT

Psychosomatic Disorders. First of all, effective treatment of the psychosomatic patient should consist of the nursing action appropriate to the particular physical disease and the needs of the individual patient involved. The nurse relieves the patient's suffering by diminishing his fear, tension, and anxiety. She accomplishes this by applying her technical and interpersonal competence to the problem at hand.

Second, she meets the patient's dependent needs by caring for him, and allowing him to be dependent upon her when the circumstances call for it. For example, she may provide the ulcer patient with between-meal snacks—milk, ice cream, eggnog. With the asthmatic patient, she may spend more time in conversation or services. She may assist the arthritic patient in walking or exercising his affected joints. An important part of meeting the patient's dependent needs is the nurse's attitude. If she is accepting of the patient's disability, she will encourage his acceptance of his illness, and thus reduce his anxiety. If she is critical of his lack of ability to help himself, she may further add to his independent-dependent conflict and increase his anxiety. For example, I have heard nurses say to an ulcer patient, "Here's your baby food." How do you suppose he feels about that? Certainly, it doesn't make him feel better. In fact, it makes me uncomfortable just telling about it.

Third, the nurse must allow the patient as much independence as he can tolerate. This can be done by allowing the patient to make as many decisions about himself and his care as he is capable of. Also, he should be encouraged to do for himself those things which he can successfully manage. Sometimes simple respect and recognition of the person that he is, the position that he holds, or the success that he has achieved in life may be all that is possible or required in order to satisfy his independent needs. It is important that the nurse not encourage or allow him to be more independent than his illness allows. For example, the physician with a bleeding ulcer should not be expected to tell the nurse when he needs assistance, or what kind of assistance he needs. Nor should he be given whatever assistance is required with the attitude that he is imposing upon the nurse, or that he is being childish or incompetent. Nor should he be expected to give consultation or medical advice to the nurses or other patients. He is the patient and he is the one to be cared for.

Fourth, it is often necessary for the nurse to prevent the patient from assuming more social responsibility than he is capable of while he is sick. He should be relieved of as many decisions about business, family, associates, and friends as possible. Sometimes this can be done by the nurse or social worker making the necessary calls or contacts for him. Sometimes the nurse can encourage members of the family to assume more responsibility for decisions, particularly while the patient is sick. Sometimes the nurse can report the problem to the physician and he can help the patient and his family handle the difficulty. Sometimes it is necessary for the nurse to limit or restrict the patient's phone calls, visitors, or activities while he is sick. For example, the nurse may help reduce the demands upon the patient, by saying, "Here, let me make that phone call for you."

Physical Illness. Probably the single dimension that makes the difference between effective and mediocre nursing care is that in effective care, primary consideration is given to the person who is sick rather than to the illness he has. It is not infrequent to hear nurses referring to "the gall bladder in Room 200" or "the appendectomy down the hall" or "the hip fracture in intensive care." Many nurses, and therefore their nursing care, lack the necessary personal interest and involvement to be really helpful or therapeutic. Very often, nurses are completely unaware that their patients are frightened, angry, depressed, or lonely. Their observations, communication, and care are so focused upon the patient's physical condition that they often do not even see him as a person. Such an impersonal attitude on the part of the nurse often adds to the patient's feeling of discomfort, reduces his sense of well-being, and even interferes with his recovery.

In addition, nurses often have a tendency to interpret and judge behavior in superficial terms. For example, if a patient laughs a lot, the nurse may judge him to be happy, whereas he may be trying desperately to cover up a fear that he is going to die. Or if a patient complains, he may be judged cantankerous, rather than angry at the blow life has dealt him. If he is quiet, he may be judged to be cooperative rather than sad.

Patients who are physically ill need the interpersonal competence of the nurse as well as her technical competence. They need understanding, compassion, acceptance, personal interest and concern. They need to have people around them who listen to them, figure out what they are asking for, and satisfy as many of their requests as possible. It is often true that a person who is well can get far better personal service at a hotel than a sick person can get at a hospital. Certainly the sick person needs it more than the well person, and just as certainly, he pays as much for it. Yet, for many treatment personnel, it has become customary to withhold as much personal involvement as possible. It does not seem likely that a nurse can be of much help to a dying patient, for example, if she is not personally involved, if she is not compassionate, if she does not feel the impending loss.

In an illness the patient reacts in physical, emotional and social ways which are both characteristic of the illness in general and of him as a person. Thus, any illness might be seen as psychosomatic, a combination of psychological and somatic symptoms. However, the term psychosomatic has come to mean something more specific in medical diagnosis and treatment. It generally refers to those organic disorders in which chronic stress and anxiety are thought to have a direct causative effect. The patient encounters prolonged crisis situations in his life which he is unable to master. The body organ or system which is stimulated by the accompanying anxiety simply wears out or breaks down from repeated or continual action, or preparation for action which, for some reason, is not taken. Sometimes these disorders are called "diseases of adaptation" because they are an attempt to adjust to life even though unsuccessful.

The most effective way to treat patients with psychosomatic disorders is, of course, to treat the whole person—physically, emotionally, socially. One of the most important aspects of the treatment is the relationship between patient and therapist (physician, nurse, social worker, psychologist). In the long run, the patient with a psychosomatic disorder can be treated successfully only if he is helped to make some changes in the way in which he reacts to the crisis situations in his life which produce the stress, anxiety, and physical illness.

REFERENCES

Adams, Margaret, et al.: "Psychological response in critical care units," *American Journal of Nursing, 78* (September, 1978) pp. 1504–1512.

Ames, Beatrice: "Art and a dying patient," *American Journal of Nursing, 80* (June, 1980) pp. 1094–1096.

Bayles, Michael D.: "The value of life—by what standard?" *American Journal of Nursing, 80* (December, 1980) pp. 2226–2230.

Cousins, Norman: *Anatomy of an Illness,* W. W. Norton, New York, 1979.

Drapo, Peggy J.: "A hostel for the handicapped," *American Journal of Nursing, 78* (September, 1978) pp. 1530–1531.

Dunbar, Flanders: *Mind and Body: Psychosomatic Medicine,* Rev. Ed., Random House, New York, 1955.

Eland, Joann M.: "Living with pain," *Nursing Outlook, 78* (July, 1978) pp. 430–431.

Fuller, Sarah S.: "Holistic man and the science and practice of nursing," *Nursing Outlook, 78* (November, 1978) pp. 700–704.
Hagerty, Genevieve: "Growing more balmy each day—love, Mom," *American Journal of Nursing, 80* (December, 1980) pp. 2173–2175.
Hodgins, Eric: *Episode,* Simon & Schuster, New York, 1971.
Kübler-Ross, Elisabeth: *Questions and Answers on Death and Dying.* Macmillan, New York, 1974.
Otto, Herbert, and James Knight: *Dimensions in Wholistic Healing: New Frontiers in the Treatment of the Whole Person.* Nelson-Hall, Chicago, 1979.
Smith, Dorothy W.: "Survivors of serious illness," *American Journal of Nursing, 79* (March, 1979) pp. 440–443.
Trockman, Gordon: "Caring for the confused or delirious patient," *American Journal of Nursing, 78* (September, 1978) pp. 1495–1499.
Wieczorek, Rita Reis, and Bernice Horner-Rosner: "The asthmatic child: preventing and controlling attacks," *American Journal of Nursing, 79* (February, 1979) pp. 258–262.
Wilkinson, Olive: "Out of touch with reality," *American Journal of Nursing, 78* (September, 1978) pp. 1492–1494.

Chapter 17

Community Mental Health and Psychiatric Nursing

We talked in Chapter 7 about the importance of treating the whole person—physically, emotionally, and socially. Community mental health is an attempt to put that concept into real practice, to deal with problems as they exist in a person's life, without removing him from the resources that surround him. It is an alternative to the kind of isolation and alienation that often occurs with hospitalization in a state mental hospital. In addition, it mobilizes the forces in the community to resolve their own health problems at the first level of occurrence, as they do in China and other countries. Community mental health also emphasizes the preventive and rehabilitative aspects of psychiatric services, as well as the phase of acute treatment.

THE COMMUNITY MENTAL HEALTH MOVEMENT

The community mental health movement has evolved over a number of years and is a result of changing times and changing ideas about human services. Two sets of circumstances occurred during and after World War II that gave great impetus to the development of these services. First, it became evident from the numbers of young men of draft age who were rejected and discharged from the service because of psychiatric disabilities that mental illness was a significant health problem in this country. Second, servicemen who became psychiatrically ill were treated with brief psychotherapy and sent back to the front lines as soon as possible—a departure from the traditional long-term psychotherapy.

Following the war two other developments made significant contributions to the changes in psychiatric treatment. General hospitals began to accept psychiatric patients for treatment, which made it possible for people to receive treatment closer to home and for psychiatrists to put short-term therapy into wider practice. In addition, the advent of psychoactive drugs decreased the length and violence of mental illness and made the patients more accessible for other kinds of treatment. This promoted the ease of treating psychiatric patients and the general public's acceptance of the mentally ill as treatable people.

Despite these advances, by 1955 the nation's mental hospitals housed over half a million patients. Deplorable conditions in many of the hospitals became a public issue through the efforts of authors, journalists, legislators, and the general public. As a result, Congress passed the Mental Health Study Act of 1955, which created the Joint Commission on Mental Illness and Mental Health. The report of this commission, *Action for Mental Health*, appeared in 1961. Among the things emphasized by the commission's report was the provision of mental health services on a local basis in such places as general hospitals and psychiatric clinics. It also recommended that large state hospitals be reduced in size and that no new ones be built.

This was followed by President Kennedy's message to Congress in 1963 concerning the treatment of the mentally ill and mentally retarded. In it he called for "a bold new approach" to the care of the mentally ill, that of community-based services. He also introduced the idea of federal assistance in the care of the mentally ill, which had previously been primarily each state's responsibility, and proposed joint support from federal, state, and local government and private funds.

Then came the Community Mental Health Centers Act of 1963 for the construction of mental health centers. Each state was allocated a certain amount of money based on a formula established by the Hill-Burton program of matching funds. However, requests for federal assistance had to come from local sponsors and had to fit within an approved state-wide plan for mental health services. Since then, amendments in 1965, 1967, and 1970 have broadened federal support both for construction and staffing.

The community mental health center program is based upon the underlying concept of providing all citizens with accessible and comprehensive mental health services close to home. It requires each center to provide five essential services: (1) inpatient care; (2) outpatient care; (3) emergency services around the clock;

(4) partial hospitalization (day and night care); and (5) community consultation and education. Five additional services are recommended for a comprehensive care program: (1) precare and aftercare for patients hospitalized in long-term care facilities; (2) diagnostic services; (3) rehabilitation services; (4) research and evaluation programs; and (5) training and education programs.

The original intent was to establish 2000 such centers to serve the nation's entire population. As of 1971, approximately 400 had been funded and approximately half of these were in operation. We obviously have a long way to go before we can guarantee every citizen of the United States adequate community mental health services. The community mental health movement has not been without problems. Not all patients released from state hospitals have found adequate support in community centers. In the larger cities a class of street people or "bag ladies" (who sleep in parks or doorways and carry all their possessions with them in shopping bags) has developed, many of whom are believed to be former state hospital residents who are unable to establish other living arrangements.

In the meantime, many improvements have been made in the services offered by state mental hospitals. In fact, many of the 10 essential services just listed for community centers are now provided by state hospitals, including emergency services, partial hospitalization, community consultation and education, diagnostic and rehabilitation services, and aftercare. In addition, there has been a drastic reduction in the patient population of many state hospitals. For example, in one state hospital the patient population was reduced from 2000 to 500 in less than 10 years, while at the same time nearly four times as many patients were treated on a short-term basis. There has been a general upgrading of staff, both in numbers and in training, in many state hospitals. Also, there has been an effort to develop diversified treatment programs to meet the needs of the communities served by the hospitals. The state mental hospitals will continue to provide vital services as part of the total comprehensive mental health care program for some time to come.

CRISIS INTERVENTION

Probably the main method of treatment in community mental health services today is that of crisis intervention. As we have seen in Chapter 7, crisis as we define it refers not to a catastrophe but to a turning point in a person's life. It is like the Chinese word for danger, which is the same as the Chinese word for opportunity.

How the person reacts to the crisis determines whether it is dangerous to the individual or an opportunity for personal growth.

There are generally two types of crises—developmental and situational. Erikson, as we have seen in Chapter 4, describes the life cycle in terms of eight ages or stages of psychosocial development, from infancy to old age. In each of these stages a person faces certain crises or problems that he must master. Developmental crises, such as the identity crisis of adolescence, are universal; they affect all people. On the other hand, situational crises are life experiences peculiar to an individual that represent, as Caplan puts it, obstacles to important life goals that are for a time insurmountable. Situational crises include life-threatening experiences, such as serious illness or injury; personal loss, such as divorce or death of a loved one; and threats to personal security, such as loss of status or life savings.

What is a situational or life crisis for one person may not be for another. Furthermore, a similar experience may not be a crisis for the same person if it occurs at a different time in his life or under different circumstances. What then determines an individual's crisis? Aguilera and Messick in *Crisis Intervention* say that three factors affect the equilibrium or adjustment of the individual: his perception of the experience, the support systems available to him, and the methods he has learned to use to cope with stress.

At this point, let us review some of the things we have already discussed in Chapters 4, 5, and 6. As each person progresses through the various stages of life, he changes physically, emotionally, and socially. He is expected to master certain tasks and meet certain expectations. In order to survive and feel secure, he must adapt and adjust to the changes, tasks, and expectations of each stage of his life. We call this healthy growth and development. He must learn as well ways of handling stress and anxiety that not only protect and defend him, but at the same time promote the satisfaction of his basic needs. The more versatile or flexible a person he is, the more adaptable, better adjusted, and more appropriate or realistic in his behavior, the better prepared he is to meet and master the stress of different life experiences. Also, such a person is more likely to be able to learn new methods, new competencies, and new ways of behaving that help him accommodate himself to changes in expectations that accompany the various stages in the life cycle. He reacts to life experiences, in other words, from a position of strength rather than of frailty. However, if the stress is too great, if his defenses are not strong enough, if he cannot find new ways to master the stress and does not have sufficient support from significant people around him, the stress becomes a crisis situation, and he is apt to react with maladaptive or disturbed or unhealthy behavior, unless he is helped.

Caplan in *Preventive Psychiatry* describes four phases in the development of a crisis. He says that in the first phase the person responds to the stress situation by an increase in tension and an attempt to use his usual methods of solving problems. If these methods fail, then what we see in phase two is a greater increase in tension and anxiety, and a feeling of ineffectiveness. In phase three, the person calls forth all the resources he has within himself and approaches others around him and even tries new ways of handling the problem. As a result, one of these three possibilities is likely to happen: (1) the problem is solved to the satisfaction of the individual; (2) the problem is redefined or the person's goals are altered; or (3) the problem is avoided by giving up one's goals altogether. If there is no resolution, then phase four takes place, in which the person reacts with maladaptive or disturbed behavior.

Crisis intervention therapy may be instituted at any number of intervals. The therapist may act as an important source of support for the individual, so that the stress is handled and a crisis situation never develops. Or the therapist may become an important part of the resources to be utilized in phase three of the crisis and the problem may be solved satisfactorily. It is also possible that the therapist may not appear on the scene until after the disturbed reaction has occurred. Obviously, the earlier the intervention can take place, the less threatening or damaging the crisis is to the person.

Crisis intervention operates on the principles of problem-solving (see Chapter 8, The Nurse-Patient Relationship): (1) identification of the problem; (2) decision about a course of action; (3) implementation of the selected plan; and (4) evaluation of the effectiveness of the selected plan and modification of that plan. In comparison, Aguilera and Messick identify the following steps: (1) *assessment* of the events leading up to the crisis, the factors contributing to the crisis, the individual's strengths and weaknesses in meeting the crisis, and the support systems available to him; (2) *planning* for what is needed to restore equilibrium, what the possible alternatives are, and how the support systems can best be utilized; (3) *intervention,* the form of which depends upon the needs of the client, the circumstances, and the nature of the crisis; and (4) *resolution and anticipatory planning,* including reinforcement of the client's adaptive methods, introduction to new methods, and helping him see his progress, make realistic plans for the future, and see how this present experience may help him in future crises.

PSYCHIATRIC NURSING

Changes in psychiatric nursing occurred simultaneously with the changes in psychiatric treatment. The role of the psychiatric nurse prior to 1955 was that of assistant to the psychiatrist and administrator of a ward or unit. Her functions were those of observing and recording patients' behavior, assisting the physician with medical care or physical treatment of the patients, management of ward functions, and supervision of nursing staff. She generally worked in a state mental hospital because that is where most mentally ill patients were treated.

In the 1960s, with the development of university programs for advanced training in psychiatric nursing, we saw the development of the psychiatric nursing clinical specialist. The primary function of the psychiatric nurse expanded from the one-to-one relationship with the mentally ill patient to include group therapy, family therapy, and milieu therapy. The setting for treatment then became the general hospital and other community facilities, as well as the psychiatric hospital.

The community mental health movement had a great impact upon psychiatric nursing. It changed the direction of psychiatric nursing and expanded the practice of the psychiatric nurse. Patients became clients, asking the nurse for mental health care services. She became a primary therapist, directing the treatment of a client, as well as participating in it. As a nurse, she is uniquely qualified to provide home and family care as well as individual care. Clients generally find the nurse less threatening and are therefore apt to be more open in the discussion of their problems. Caplan in *An Approach to Community Mental Health* describes this specialized function of the nurse in terms of closeness—physical, emotional, and social. The nurse has traditionally been at the patient's side at home or in the hospital, and for longer periods of time than any of the other therapists. She is generally less formal and distant in her interactions with clients and expresses her feelings more freely. She is perceived by the client as being on the same status level, rather than as an authority figure. She is concerned with physical health as well as mental health, and she generally has a sense of reality that makes it possible for her to help people in a practical, down-to-earth fashion. All this makes her more accessible to people in trouble, and they can utilize her as a special source of support. For example, in my experience as a community mental health nurse, families and individuals would often accept my help, although they freely expressed the feelings that they wanted nothing to do with psychiatry or the mental health clinic.

In defining psychiatric nursing in Chapter 8, we said it was that kind of nursing practice that provides the therapeutic relationship and environment necessary in order to help patients meet their needs and when necessary to correct the unhealthy aspects of their behavior. In community mental health nursing, the primary method of treatment is crisis intervention. The community mental health nurse makes an assessment of the client's needs, his ability to meet them, and the circumstances surrounding him. With the patient, she decides what is required in order for his needs to be met, and what resources can best be utilized. The nurse helps the client utilize these support systems himself and does for him what he cannot do for himself. She helps him see what has been accomplished, what works for him and what does not, what alternative methods might be more effective, and what kind of realistic plan he can make for the future. To accomplish all this, she employs individual, group, and family therapy and learning techniques, as they are appropriate to the individual client and the circumstances he finds himself in at the time.

Not only is she engaged in direct therapy, but an extremely important aspect of the work of the community mental health nurse is that of consultation and education. She is a mental health consultant, advocate, and teacher to her individual client, his family, community service agencies and organizations, and other health care facilities and professionals; in fact, she is a teacher and consultant for the total community that she serves. The psychiatric nurse works very closely with other service agencies in providing for the health, education and welfare of members of the community. She must be in a position to consult with them about her clients and with her clients about what services these agencies provide. Working with the nursing staff in general hospitals and nursing homes, she gives them expert advice and assistance in meeting the emotional needs of all patients, as well as working with special psychiatric problems. She collaborates with public health nurses and other clinical specialists to provide the nursing care necessary for the clients she serves and participates with other professionals in planning for and providing the most comprehensive health care services possible for the community.

REAL LIFE SITUATIONS IN COMMUNITY MENTAL HEALTH NURSING

Let us look now at some real situations in which a community mental health nurse provided the kind of services we have discussed. The first situation describes her work with an individual client who is mentally ill, but living in the community. It also points out the necessity of working with the family—the husband in this case.

Situation 1

Mary Lou, a 37-year-old housewife, lived in a remote section of the county. She spent most of the time alone, except for her faithful collie. Her husband left for work early in the morning and did not return until late at night. Her oldest son was out of the home on his own. Her youngest son was away at school during the day and had a job in the evening, so he was seldom home. There was one fairly close neighbor, but Mary had alienated her by accusing her of trying to seduce her husband. She had no telephone, and no one visited her, so that she spent hour after hour without human contact.

Mary had been hospitalized several times at the state mental hospital with episodes of manic and depressed behavior. Over the years she had become increasingly suspicious, experiencing delusions and hallucinations of a persecutory nature. She was on heavy doses of medication: Thorazine 50 mg. q.i.d. and p.r.n., Stelazine 5 mg. b.i.d., Cogentin 1 mg. b.i.d., and Prolixin 75 mg. I.M. q. 2 wks. Her husband put her medications out for her every morning before he went to work, with each dose in a separate container.

The community mental health nurse visited her regularly once a week to check on her medications, give her intramuscular medication, and establish a therapeutic relationship with her that would enable her to talk about her feelings and concerns. At first she cried frequently and displayed a great deal of anxiety, especially on the days she was to receive her intramuscular medication. She expressed the fear that the shot would put her to sleep, and she would be taken back to the state mental hospital. It took several weeks before Mary could trust the nurse enough to be somewhat relaxed when she visited. She began to straighten up the house a bit before the nurse arrived, and sometimes she served instant coffee during the visit.

One day during the cold weather Mary did not greet the nurse at the door as usual. After the nurse had called and banged around on both doors, Mary finally came to the door in her night clothes. The house was a mess and extremely cold. Mary told a mixed-up story about having no fuel, going to bed and turning on the electric blanket to keep warm. The nurse found an old axe, chopped some wood, and lit a fire to warm up the house. Mary was encouraged to get dressed and make some hot coffee to warm them both up.

The nurse went back that night to talk with both Mary and her husband. The husband was frustrated and angry because Mary was not getting better and blamed the doctor and the mental health clinic for this. After letting him express his feelings, the nurse told him his feelings were certainly understandable, but it didn't help the situation to leave Mary abandoned without sufficient wood for the fire. He admitted this, and said he just felt fed up and didn't care any more, but that he would chop some wood that very evening, which he did. The nurse suggested that he and Mary come to the clinic one evening a month to see the psychiatrist and talk about their problems, and an appointment was made for them to do this.

Situation 2 describes the collaborative work of the nurse and other therapists and agencies in meeting the needs of clients. It identifies the practical kind of help that people in crisis often need. It also brings out the combination of physical, emotional, and social needs that people experience in crisis.

Situation 2

The Taylors were an elderly couple who lived in an old trailer house in the country. Marie was confined to a wheelchair with both legs amputated just above the knee. John had had a stroke and was paralyzed on the right side, could not see, and could help himself very little. Marie and John had promised each other they would not let the other be put in a nursing home as long as they could possibly avoid it.

Marie took very good care of John and the house, but required assistance in getting John up in the morning and back to bed at night. She depended upon a young man who lived in the vicinity to help her. However, the young man got a full-time job in town, so he was no longer available, resulting in a crisis situation for the Taylors.

The community mental health nurse had been visiting regularly because Marie had occasional episodes of depression and needed continued supportive therapy. A physical therapist from the Public Health Department had also been visiting regularly, teaching Marie to walk with prostheses. The nurse and physical therapist collaborated in giving assistance to both Marie and John.

It was extremely difficult to find a replacement for the young man because of the peculiar hours during which assistance was needed—a couple of hours in the morning and a couple of hours at night. In addition, it was some distance from town, so it would hardly pay someone for the travel time. The son and daughter-in-law lived close by and they helped for a time, but they felt it was too much of a burden for them. Therefore, the community agencies were alerted and everyone began looking for someone to help the Taylors.

Finally a response came from a young girl who had been working at a local nursing home. She was interested in doing some creative work on her own, which meant leaving the full-time job at the nursing home, but she needed a part-time job. She lived in the neighborhood, understood quite a bit about people in stress, and seemed ideal for the job, so she was hired. One of the most helpful things she did during the time she worked there was plant a garden. Marie wanted a garden very much, but was unable to do the necessary work herself. Since the hired girl had never planted a garden before, Marie had to instruct and supervise her in the project. This gave Marie a tremendous source of satisfaction, and although she complained about the girl's ignorance, she thoroughly enjoyed the role of supervisor.

Situation 3 describes the use of the nurse-patient relationship and behavior modification in treating a mentally ill patient in a nursing home. It demonstrates the community mental health nurse's role in consultation and education, as she works with the nursing home staff. It also brings out the interrelationship between physical and psychiatric treatment.

Situation 3

Kathryn was a 28-year-old single woman who was a patient in a nursing home. She was a regressed and dependent person, who had never been able to function on her own. She had periods during which she could do very little for herself and was difficult for the nursing staff to handle because of her negativistic and hostile behavior.

The community mental health nurse made weekly visits to the nursing home to consult with the staff about special problems they had in coping with certain kinds of behavior. It was suggested that the mental health nurse spend some individual time with Kathryn to see if she could help her become more self-sufficient. The nurse saw her weekly and spent about an hour with her each time. Most of the visits consisted of trips to town for shopping and dining out. Kathryn became increasingly responsive to these visits and would get herself all fixed up and be waiting when the nurse arrived. There was no question about her general improvement during this time.

It became necessary for the nurse who had been working with Kathryn to leave, and she was replaced by another nurse. Despite the second nurse's efforts to be supportive and caring, Kathryn became increasingly distrustful and felt the nurse was going to harm her. She became disruptive in the nursing home, particularly at night, growing delusional and having hallucinations. The staff were asked to be accepting and supportive of her during this time because of her reaction to the loss of her friend, the first nurse.

Then she began spending considerable time in the bathroom, complaining of having to void frequently and of a burning sensation when she did void. The next three days she was a constant care to the nursing home staff, spending hours in the bathroom or, when confined to bed, on the bedpan. It was impossible to distract her. It was difficult to tell whether she was suffering from an acute physical illness, such as a urinary infection, or severe anxiety and accompanying agitation, or a combination of the two. At any rate, the psychiatrist and the physician were both consulted, and it was decided to transfer her to the local general hospital for treatment. She was put to bed and cared for both physically and psychiatrically. The mental health nurse made daily visits to the hospital. At the end of five days, she was much better and returned to the nursing home.

At that point, the supervising nurse in the nursing home and the mental health nurse met with the patient and staff and set up with her a simple daily schedule. She was to take care of her own personal needs—eating, grooming, making her bed, and so on. If she did these tasks successfully, she would be rewarded by a ride or a trip to town when the mental health nurse visited. Kathryn responded slowly at first, but when she was denied a trip out of the nursing home a time or two because she had not fulfilled her part of the bargain, she began to do the tasks expected of her. She gradually established a trust relationship with the mental health nurse and her behavior began to improve slowly.

Situation 4 describes the nurse's use of individual and family therapy in the treatment of a mentally ill client at the Mental Health Center. It demonstrates how easily the whole family can become embroiled in a crisis situation regarding the behavior of one member. It also brings out how some crises can be resolved by finding a simple, practical solution, like a job outside of the home.

Situation 4

Leon was a 21-year-old man who lived at home with his parents and two younger brothers. Leon had always been "different" according to mother, and she had felt she had to defend him from the criticism of others most of his life. He had little ambition, and although he was physically fit, he did very little work around the farm. By contrast, his younger brothers not only did their regular chores around the farm, but earned considerable money doing extra work for the neighbors.

Over the years considerable resentment had built up in the brothers and father toward Leon because of mother's protective attitude toward him. The crisis situation developed when father contracted to do some extra planting and needed Leon's help. Because Leon either did not help him or "goofed up" when he did, father became increasingly angry and short-tempered with him. The oldest brother, now about Leon's size, began to threaten to beat up Leon if he didn't help more around the farm. Mother was afraid there would be a brawl in which someone (probably Leon) would get hurt, so she appealed for help.

Leon and his mother had been visiting the Mental Health Center every two weeks. The community mental health nurse gave Leon an intramuscular injection of Prolixin at that time and talked with both of them to foster a healthier relationship between mother and son. After a discussion with mother, it was decided to meet with father and then with the whole family to help them resolve the problems. Father and the rest of the family voiced a lot of hostility toward Leon, and he reacted to this by saying he would move out. Since he had no job and no place to go, this was not a realistic decision, and he was helped to see this. It was possible, however, to help him move in the direction of becoming more independent by helping him find a job through one of the community agencies. Once he had gotten the job outside of the home, the tension in the family eased considerably.

The mental health nurse continued to meet with father and mother to help them understand some of Leon's limitation, to help them handle their own feelings of frustration and guilt more constructively, and to help them interact in a more positive way with Leon.

Situation 5 describes the nurse's role in direct care of an extremely dependent client. It demonstrates the educational function of the nurse in teaching daily living skills to the client. It also brings out the use of other community resources, such as the day care center.

Situation 5

Alice was a 30-year-old mother of six children. She was married to a serviceman for 10 years and apparently got along fairly well in a very protected environment. However, the husband found somebody more to his liking and divorced her. He was awarded the children by the court, and he moved to another state, taking the children with him. Alice spent some time after this visiting an aunt, but soon returned to her hometown without money or any means of support.

She was referred to the mental health clinic by the authorities because of her inability to care for herself. Furthermore, she seemed unconcerned about her state of affairs. She was emotionally flat in her responses, extremely dependent, and ignorant of even the simplest ways of going about caring for herself.

It was necessary for the mental health nurse to meet with Alice daily and literally take her by the hand and teach her how to do the necessary tasks of independent living. First thing was to help her find a place to live. The nurse took her around to various places that were advertised until they found a place that was livable and that she could afford. The nurse helped her apply for public assistance and food stamps. Next, it was necessary for the nurse to help her sell the furniture that she did not need and that she had to pay storage on. The nurse took her grocery shopping and to the laundromat, helped her open a checking account, and showed her how to balance her checkbook.

Gradually, as she became more capable of daily living activities, she was referred to a day care center where she could be with other people and learn something about how to interact successfully with others. She showed gradual but continued improvement until it was possible for her to do many things by herself, although she still relied heavily on others for help.

Situation 6 describes the nurse's application of individual psychotherapeutic principles in the treatment of a client with somatic reactions to stress. It demonstrates the collaboration between family physician and psychiatric nurse. It also brings out the uniqueness of the nurse as a nonthreatening treatment agent, as perceived by the client.

Situation 6

Evelyn was a 58-year-old housewife whose husband was a retired machinist. She was a meek, mild-mannered person who had always been dominated by her husband. As he began to show some signs of cerebral arteriosclerosis, she became increasingly anxious and finally wound up in the hospital with a peptic ulcer.

The community mental health nurse was asked by her physician to see Evelyn and try to alleviate some of the anxiety. On her first visit to the Mental Health Center, Evelyn wanted to make it clear that she didn't want "anyone fooling around with [her] mind!" She was willing, however, to see the nurse at regular weekly intervals to "talk about her concerns and problems."

Her major source of difficulty seemed to be her husband and the fact that she got so angry with him for treating her in an authoritarian fashion. At the same time she had difficulty taking over from him some of the responsibility (such as the finances) that he obviously could no longer handle. Her anxiety was expressed physically by her inability to sleep and her difficulty with the digestive process. The sleep problem was treated with medication, and the peptic ulcer with medication and diet, prescribed by her physician.

Evelyn was encouraged by the nurse to assert herself more in the management of the household. She was also encouraged to express her feelings to her husband before they got to a destructive stage, and at the same time to try to understand how he must be feeling with the periods of confusion and loss of memory that assailed him.

As she became less like a child and more like a partner to her husband, two things happened. Evelyn's anxiety, tension, and physical problems began to subside, and her husband seemed to appreciate her taking over more responsibility, so his anxiety, tension, and irritability began to lessen. As they both improved, the nurse's help was needed less and less, and the visits became bimonthly and then monthly.

As the practice of psychiatric nursing broadens, many areas of specialization for the nurse develop. She may become a clinical specialist in psychiatric nursing, focusing upon a certain age group, such as autistic children, or disturbed adolescents, or disabled elderly people. She may specialize in a certain clinical area, such as medicine and surgery, pediatrics, geriatrics, orthopedics, or obstetrics. Her work may be confined to one aspect of the health services spectrum by specializing in prevention, acute care, chronic illness, or rehabilitation. She may specialize in a certain kind of treatment, such as individual, group, family, or milieu therapy. The psychiatric nurse may function as a mental health consultant to general hospitals, nursing homes, public health departments, or other community agencies, such as police departments. She may be an independent practitioner set up in private or group practice, or an educator or administrator in psychiatric nursing.

Whatever kind of job she holds, she performs at least one of two broad functions. She is either a primary therapist giving direct care to a variety of patients, or she is a consultant, educator, or administrator helping others give direct care to patients. In many kinds of practice, such as community mental health nursing, the psychiatric nurse does both.

REFERENCES

Aguilera, Donna, and Janice Messick: *Crisis Intervention: Theory and Methodology,* 3rd Edition, C. V. Mosby, St. Louis, 1978.

Barton, Gail M., and Carolyn H. Krone: "Creation of an aftercare program," *American Journal of Nursing, 78* (May, 1978) pp. 864–867.

Bernal, Henrietta: "Levels of practice in a community health agency," *Nursing Outlook, 78* (June, 1978) pp. 364–369.

Brofman, J. Lynn: "An evening home visiting program," *Nursing Outlook, 79* (October, 1979) pp. 657–661.

Caplan, Gerald: *Support Systems and Community Mental Health,* Human Sciences Press, New York, 1974.

Caplan, Gerald: *Principles of Preventive Psychiatry,* Basic Books, New York, 1964.

Caplan, Gerald: *An Approach to Community Mental Health,* Grune & Stratton, New York, 1961.

Chaisson, G. Maureen: "Correctional health care—beyond the barriers," *American Journal of Nursing, 81* (April, 1981) pp. 737–738.

Clark, Carolyn Chambers: "Inner dialogue: a self-healing approach for nurses and clients," *American Journal of Nursing, 81* (June, 1981) pp. 1191–1193.

Lentz, Judith, and Elsa Meyer: "The dirty house," *Nursing Outlook, 79* (September, 1979) pp. 590–593.

Lyon, Glee Gamble, and Emily A. Hitchens: "Ways of intervening with the psychotic individual in the community," *American Journal of Nursing, 79* (March, 1979) pp. 490–493.

Morgan, Arthur, and Judith Morena: *The Practice of Mental Health Nursing,* J. B. Lippincott, Philadelphia, 1973.

Norris, Catherine M.: "Self-care," *American Journal of Nursing, 79* (March, 1979) pp. 486–489.

Putt, Arlene M.: "A biofeedback service by nurses," *American Journal of Nursing, 79* (January, 1979) pp. 88–89.

Ray, Dixie W., and Beverly C. Flynn: "Competition vs. cooperation in community health nursing," *Nursing Outlook, 80* (October, 1980) pp. 626–630.

Reinhardt, Adina, and Mildred Quinn: *Family Centered Community Nursing,* C. V. Mosby, St. Louis, 1973.

Ward, Barbara J.: "Hospice home care program," *Nursing Outlook, 78* (October, 1978) pp. 646–649.

Appendices

Appendix A

GLOSSARY OF PSYCHIATRIC TERMS

Addiction—Physiological and emotional dependence upon the effects of drugs, such as narcotics, LSD, alcohol, barbiturates, resulting in typical symptoms when the drug is withdrawn.

Adjustment—The relationship between an individual and his environment as measured by the degree of satisfaction of his basic needs and the acceptability of his behavior.

Adolescence—The transitional stage of development during which the youth is moving away from childhood through puberty toward adulthood.

Affect—Sustained feeling, emotion, mood, or emotional response.

Alcoholism—Physiological and emotional dependence upon the effects of alcohol; intake of alcohol in sufficient amounts to damage the individual's health or functioning.

Ambivalence—The existence within the individual of opposing emotions, impulses, or desires.

Amnesia—Complete or partial lack of memory, either temporary or permanent, due to physical or emotional trauma.

Antidepressant—A psychoactive drug used to elevate the mood, level of activity, and thought process, and increase the individual's sense of well-being.

Anxiety—An unpleasant subjective experience composed of fear and tension in response to a perceived physical or psychological threat.

Apathy—Lack of interest or feeling response in situations that usually provoke such reactions.

Attitude—An enduring, learned predisposition to behave in a consistent way toward a certain class of objects, situations, or people.

Autism—Thinking unduly directed toward one's self, to the exclusion of reality.

Behavior—The sum total of an individual's reaction to stimuli, consisting of internal and external responses. External behavior is observed objectively as what a person does; internal behavior such as thinking and feeling can only be observed by introspection or inferred from external behavior.

Biofeedback–The use of instruments to provide information about physiologic responses to stress. Used to help patient learn to control these responses.

Bipolar disorder–Major affective disorder in which there are episodes of manic and depressed behavior; formerly called manic-depressive psychosis. It is subdivided into three types—manic, depressed, and mixed.

Blocking—Sudden interruption of thought, action, or speech as a result of emotional conflict.

Body language—A method of nonverbal communication in which a person's thoughts, feelings, and attitudes are expressed through physical means such as tone of voice, facial expression, gestures, posture, movement, and touch.

Catatonia—A type of schizophrenia characterized by periods of excitement or stupor or both.

Comatose–A state of abnormal deep stupor, associated with organic brain damage, from which an individual cannot be readily aroused by external stimuli.

Compensation—A coping method whereby an individual makes up for his real or imagined deficits or inadequacies in one area by excelling in another.

Compulsion—An overpowering, repetitive, unwanted act which is meant to relieve anxiety based upon underlying emotional conflict.

Confabulation—Symptom of mental confusion consisting of replacing memory loss by fantasy.

Conflict–A psychological struggle in which the individual is faced with simultaneous opposing or mutually exclusive impulses, drives, desires, or needs, as a result of internal or external forces.

Confusion—A state characterized by bewilderment, lack of clear thinking, or clouding of conscious awareness, making it difficult for an individual to distinguish, recognize, or restore order to his surroundings.

Conscience–That part of the personality, made up of incorporated parental attitudes, prohibitions, and commands related to standards, values, and mores, which guides the social behavior of an individual.

Conversion—A coping method whereby an individual denies, disguises, or relieves emotions by converting them into physical symptoms.

Coping method—A mental process which operates automatically and unconsciously to determine behavior; a method of protecting one's self from anxiety and helping to meet one's needs; sometimes called defense or mental mechanisms.

Counseling—A form of psychotherapy generally directed toward a specific problem area of an individual's life—vocation, marriage, education, religion, interpersonal relations—using guidance, advisory, and sometimes healing techniques.

Crisis intervention–A form of psychiatric treatment that utilizes problem-solving techniques to resolve the existing threat to the individual.

Delirium tremens (D.T.'s)—An acute brain syndrome precipitated by excessive use of alcohol, characterized by overwhelming anxiety, coarse tremors, and frightening visual hallucinations.

Delusion—An idea contrary to reality that an individual has not previously held, that is not commonly held, that is not changed by logic, and that is based upon his underlying emotions.

Dementia—Progressive decline in intellectual ability and appropriateness of emotional response.

Depersonalization–Feelings of unreality or strangeness related to identity, self, or situation.

Depression—Pathological condition characterized by despondency, despair, and often suicidal ideas. It may be a factor in many illnesses or a more specific syndrome in neuroses and psychoses.

Deprivation—Severe frustration from prolonged, intense, widespread interference in the satisfaction of an individual's basic needs.

Deterioration—Qualitative impairment of a physiological or mental function, or the personality as a whole.

Disorientation—Lack of normal ability to identify person, place, or time.

Displacement—A coping method whereby a person transfers emotions associated with one idea, object, or person to another.

Dissociation—A coping method whereby a person detaches himself, his emotional investment, or certain aspects of his personality from interactions with his environment.

Dissociative disorder–A neurotic condition in which there is a sudden, temporary alteration in consciousness, identity, or behavior. It includes psychogenic amnesia, psychogenic fugue, multiple personality, and depersonalization disorder.

Drive—Tendency initiated by shifts in the inner balance of the individual which propels him toward attainment of a certain goal.

Dysthymic disorder–A neurotic condition in which there is a depressed mood or lack of interest or pleasure in usual activities. It is less severe and shorter in duration than a major depressive episode.

ECT–Electroconvulsive therapy; a method of treatment used in certain kinds of mental illness, such as depression, in which a controlled amount of electric current is passed through the temporal region of the brain; sometimes called Electroshock therapy (EST).

Elation—Transcending or exultant joy or happiness.

Emotion—A strong feeling with both psychological and physiological components.

Empathy—Ability to comprehend how another person feels in his situation and to communicate that acceptance and understanding to him.

Euphoria—An exaggerated, unrealistic sense of well-being.

Exhibitionism—Deriving sexual satisfaction from exposing one's body, usually the genitals, to others, particularly in public places.

Extrovert—A person who directs his interest and emotions outward toward the environment, and finds pleasure in external things.

Fantasy—A coping method whereby a person substitutes a more pleasant, satisfying or rewarding situation of his own for the real one.

Fear—An emotion of violent agitation in the face of danger.

Fixation—A coping method whereby an individual stops at a particular stage of development or way of behaving because of too much or too little satisfaction.

Flight of ideas—Rapid succession of verbal expressions that jump rapidly from one topic to another, that are only superficially related, and that may fail to reach a goal.

Frustration—Interference with the satisfaction of an individual's basic needs.

Fugue—A prolonged period of amnesia, during which the individual behaves in an automatic fashion; sometimes associated with petit mal seizures.

Functional disorder—Malfunction of an organ, body, or person, based upon underlying emotional, rather than organic, causes.

Gender identity–The inner sense of maleness or femaleness that identifies the person as being male, female, or ambivalent.

Geriatrics—The science of diseases of the aged.

Grandiose—Characterized by unrealistic, imposing plans, or unrealistic notions of one's own ability or importance.

Habit—An acquired act that has become, through repetition, relatively fixed.

Hallucination—A sensory perception without external stimulus, based upon underlying emotions, which is not commonly experienced by a group of people, not previously experienced by the individual, and not changed by logic.

Hallucinogenic—Originating or producing hallucinations; usually refers to drugs or toxic conditions capable of producing hallucinations.

Hallucinosis, acute—A psychotic disorder associated with excessive use of alcohol, characterized by auditory hallucinations of an accusatory or threatening nature in a state of relatively clear consciousness.

Heredity—The genetic process of passing on certain endowments or traits from parent to child.

Heterosexuality—Interest in and deriving sexual satisfaction from persons of the opposite sex.

Homosexuality—Interest in and deriving sexual satisfaction from persons of the same sex.

Hostility—Tendency to feel angry and act antagonistically toward people or situations.

Hypochondriasis—Morbid preoccupation with one's own body functions, over-concern about one's health, and an unreasonable fear of disease.

Hypomanic—Exhibiting increased activity, above the general or individual's usual level, but below that characteristic of manic behavior.

Identification—A coping method whereby an individual thinks, feels, or acts like another person or group of people who are important or significant to him.

Illusion–A misperception of external stimulus based on emotional needs or conflict.

Impulse—The force associated with instinctual behavior which prompts a response performed without delay, reflection, voluntary direction, or control.

Inhibition—Unconscious check or restraint upon the expression of basic impulses, desires, or emotions.

Insight—Ability on the part of the individual to correctly evaluate himself and his behavior in relationship to reality.

Instinct—A tendency to act in an organized and biologically adaptive way that is characteristic of a given species.

Intoxication—Depression of the CNS function, characterized by blurred speech, ataxia, impairment of mental function, loss of emotional control, vomiting, and stupor, in reaction to some toxic substance taken into the body.

Introjection—A coping method whereby a person incorporates the ideas, objects, persons of his environment; feeling response directed inward toward one's self.

Introvert—A person who directs his interest and emotions inward toward himself, and derives pleasure from internal sources.

I.T.—Intensive treatment.

Korsakoff's syndrome—Chronic brain syndrome due to vitamin deficiency, often associated with long-standing excessive use of alcohol, characterized by memory impairment, confabulation, disorientation, and peripheral neuropathy.

Major affective disorders–Psychotic conditions in which there are marked disturbances in mood, resulting in inappropriate emotional responses of elation or despair, over- or underactivity, and severe disruption in relationships with others. Includes major depression and bipolar disorders.

Malingering—Deliberately feigning illness or injury with the intent to deceive others.

Manic behavior—Pathological increase in an individual's functioning—thinking, feeling, and doing.

Masochism—Deriving sexual satisfaction from suffering pain, ill-treatment, or humiliation, inflicted by one's self or others.

Maturity—The state of fulfillment or realization of an individual's potential in which he is able to accomplish what is expected of him, hold positive attitudes toward himself and others, and master the stress of his life situation.

Milieu—The physical, emotional, and social aspects of an individual's immediate environment which may be utilized in the psychiatric treatment of patients.

Mood-Sustained and persuasive emotion that colors one's perception of oneself and the world.

Motivation—The process within the individual which prompts him to behave as he does in order to achieve certain goals.

Multiple personality-A dissociative reaction in which the person adopts two or more personalities.

Narcissism-Self-love, representative of the early stage in human development.

Negativism—A generalized resistance to suggestion from outside one's self, and a tendency to behave in the opposite way from what is requested or expected.

Neologism—A newly coined word, a symptom of some types of psychosis.

Neurasthenia—A symptom of neurosis characterized by feelings of generalized weakness and fatigue.

Neurosis (psychoneurosis)—A functional mental disorder, characterized by anxiety which may be felt and expressed directly, or unconsciously controlled and expressed in the form of symptoms.

Obsession—An overpowering, repetitive, unwanted idea, which is meant to relieve the anxiety based upon underlying emotional conflict.

Organic disorder—Impairment of function attributed to pathological lack or defect of organic structure.

Organic mental disorder-Those psychotic conditions in which there is evidence of brain or CNS dysfunction. Causes are associated with aging, toxic substances, or a variety of physical disorders.

O.T.—Occupational therapy; a method of treatment for the sick or injured using planned occupational activities, directed toward the individual patient's needs and abilities.

Panic—An attack of overwhelming anxiety, associated with unreasonable terror which impels a person to blind, frantic action.

Paranoid—A type of schizophrenia, characterized by delusions of persecution and grandeur, and marked suspiciousness.

Paraphilia—Sexually deviant behaviors involving sexual stimulation or gratification in ways considered unusual or unacceptable by society.

Pedophilia—Deriving sexual satisfaction from visual or physical contact with children.

Perception—Part of the thinking process in which the individual receives and recognizes internal or external sensations which guide his behavior.

Personality—The organization of the sum total of the behavior patterns of the individual; the whole person.

Personality disorders—Inflexible, maladaptive ways of thinking, feeling, and doing that interfere with successful interaction with others and the environment.

Phobia—An abnormal, unreasonable, overwhelming fear of an object or situation, caused by underlying emotional conflict.

Projection—A coping method whereby a person attributes his own thoughts, feelings, and actions to the external environment; feeling response directed outward toward the environment.

Psychoactive drugs—Drugs used to relieve anxiety and counteract its manifestations, specifically tranquilizers and anti-depressants.

Psychoanalysis—A body of psychiatric principles and methods of treatment set forth by Freud, based upon the concepts of unconscious motivation, conflict, and symbolism.

Psychogenic—Originating in the mind or emotions.

Psychology—The science of the mind; the scientific study and explanation of human behavior.

Psychoneurosis—See **Neurosis.**

Psychosexual development—The concept of growth and development in which the individual progresses through stages from infancy to maturity.

Psychosis—Severe mental disorder in which there is a marked interference with the individual's functioning, affecting his thinking, feeling, and doing; serious disturbance in his ability to distinguish reality from his own subjective experience; and severe disruption in his relationships with others and his environment.

Psychosomatic disorder—A physical disease with changes in structure and function caused by chronic emotional reactions to everyday life.

Psychotherapy—A planned psychological procedure undertaken by a professionally trained person to restore an individual to mental health.

Puberty—The period during adolescence in which the reproductive organs become capable of functioning and the individual develops secondary sex characteristics.

Rapport—The harmonious feeling experienced by two people who hold one another in mutual respect.

Rationalization—A coping method whereby a person finds a more acceptable or plausible reason for his behavior than the real one.

Reaction formation—A coping method whereby a person denies certain unacceptable aspects of his behavior by developing the extreme opposite kind of behavior.

Regression—A coping method whereby a person returns to earlier, more comforting, but less mature ways of behaving.

Rehabilitation—Use of physical, emotional, social treatment approaches to restore maximum or optimum functioning in an individual so that he may achieve the fullest life possible.

Repression—A coping method whereby an individual excludes from his awareness unpleasant or unwanted experiences, emotions, or ideas.

Retardation—Pathological decrease in an individual's functioning, particularly in thinking; slowing down of function.

Retrospective falsification—Distortions in remembering or reporting past experiences, based upon the emotional needs of the individual.

Restitution—A coping method whereby an individual atones for his unacceptable ideas, feelings, or actions.

R.T.—Recreational therapy; a method of treatment for the sick or injured using planned leisure activities directed toward the individual's needs and abilities.

Rumination—Repetitive process in which an individual goes over and over the same thoughts, such as in depression.

Sadism-Deriving sexual satisfaction from torturing others by inflicting pain, ill-treatment, or humiliation upon them.

Schizophrenia—A functional psychosis characterized by marked distortions in thinking, interference in the ability to distinguish between reality and fantasy, and emotional withdrawal which usually results in inappropriate and sometimes bizarre behavior.

Self—That part of an individual's personality which constitutes his perception of himself and the world around him, and which controls and directs his methods of adjustment and ways of interacting with others.

Senile, Senility—Having the characteristics of old age; state resulting from the aging process.

Senile dementia-A mental disorder of the elderly, characterized by serious disturbances in the functioning of the individual, and pathological physical conditions which add to his general lack of well-being.

Sensorium—The individual's state of mental clarity or conscious awareness of his surroundings.

Siblings—Children born of the same two parents, usually excluding twins, half-brothers and sisters, and step-brothers and sisters.

Sociopathic disorder—Mental illness which is characterized by life-long maladjustment resulting from the individual's inability to control and direct his behavior in socially acceptable ways; also called personality or character disorder.

Somatic—Pertaining to the body rather than emotions, intellect or environment.

Somatoform disorders—Neurotic disorders with physical symptoms for which there are no demonstrable organic findings or known organic causes. Presumably based on emotional or psychological factors.

Stress—Physical or psychological force sufficient to cause strain or distortion in a system or when very great, to alter the system.

Sublimation—A coping method whereby a person directs his unacceptable impulses into constructive channels.

Substitution—A coping method whereby a person replaces unacceptable ideas, objects, or persons with more acceptable ones.

Tension—Physical preparation of the body for action, particularly affecting the muscles, which is the physical reaction to anxiety and stress.

Therapeutic—Pertaining to or consisting of treatment; healing, curative.

Tranquilizer—A psychoactive drug which is used to reduce anxiety, distortions in thinking, level of activity, and increase the individual's sense of well-being.

Trauma—Any experience that inflicts serious damage upon the individual, either physical or psychological.

Unconscious—That part of an individual's mind which is not open to his direct scrutiny, control, or awareness, but which nevertheless affects his behavior.

Appendix B

CLASSIFICATION OF MENTAL DISORDERS*

ORGANIC MENTAL DISORDERS

Dementias arising in the senium and presenium
  Primary degenerative dementia, senile onset
    with delirium
    with delusions
    with depression
    uncomplicated
  Primary degenerative dementia, presenile onset
  Multi-infarct dementia
Substance-induced
  Alcohol
    Intoxication
    Idiosyncratic intoxication
    Withdrawal
    Withdrawal delirium
    Hallucinosis
    Amnesic disorder
  Barbiturate or similarly acting sedative or hypnotic
  Opioid
  Cocaine
  Amphetamine or similarly acting sympathomimetic
  Phencyclidine (PCP) or similarly acting arylcyclohexylamine
  Hallucinogen
  Cannabis

SCHIZOPHRENIC DISORDERS

Disorganized
Catatonic
Paranoid

*Taken from Appendix C, "DSM III Classification: Axes I and II Categories and Codes," *Quick Reference to the Diagnostic Criteria, DSM-III,* American Psychiatric Association, 1700 18th St., N.W., Washington, D.C., 20009, 1980.

SCHIZOPHRENIC DISORDERS *(Continued)*

Undifferentiated
Residual

AFFECTIVE DISORDERS

Bipolar disorder
  Mixed
  Manic
  Depressed
Major depression
  Single episode
  Recurrent
Dysthymic disorder (neurotic depression)

ANXIETY DISORDERS

Phobic disorders
Anxiety states
Obsessive compulsive disorder
Post-traumatic stress disorder

SOMATOFORM DISORDERS

Somatization disorder
Conversion disorder
Psychogenic pain disorder
Hypochondriasis
Atypical somatoform disorder

DISSOCIATIVE DISORDERS

Psychogenic amnesia
Psychogenic fugue
Multiple personality
Depersonalization disorder
Atypical dissociative disorder

PSYCHOSEXUAL DISORDERS

Gender identity disorders
Paraphilias
Psychosexual dysfunctions

PSYCHOLOGICAL FACTORS AFFECTING PHYSICAL CONDITION

Specify physical condition

PERSONALITY DISORDERS

Paranoid
Schizoid
Schizotypal
Histrionic
Narcissistic
Antisocial
Borderline
Avoidant
Dependent
Compulsive
Passive-aggressive
Atypical, mixed, or other personality disorder

Appendix C

COMMON PSYCHOACTIVE DRUGS

Group 1. The Antipsychotic Drugs

Trade or Brand Name[1]	*Generic or Non-proprietary Name*	*Usual Adult Dosage*[2] *and Administration*	*Therapeutic Action and Uses*	*Adverse Reactions*	*Nursing Actions and Responsibilities*
Butyrophenone: Haldol	Haloperidol	*Range 1–100 mg. daily* 0.5–2 mg. b.i.d. or t.i.d.—usual dosage. *I.M.* – 2–5 mg. q. 1–4 h. for severely disturbed.	*Actions:* Antipsychotic Tranquilizer Sedate without impairing cortical function Depress subcortical area of brain Inhibit function of hypothalamus, limbic and reticular activating systems	*Cardiovascular:* Hypotension *Allergic:* Skin–photosensitivity, pigmentation, dermatitis Liver–jaundice, hepatitis, damage Blood–agranulocytosis, leukocytosis, leukopenia, anemia	1. Observe any physical, emotional, behavioral reactions of the patient and report to physician, charge nurse and other staff 2. Observe patient for skin changes–jaundice, dermatitis, flushing, perspiration, sunburn 3. Watch for symptoms of motor restlessness, muscular twitching, rigidity, tongue rolling, lipsmacking, chewing movements, grimacing, drooling, weakness, fatigue, drowsiness
Phenothiazines: Compazine	Prochlorperazine	*Range 15–150 mg. daily* 5–10 mg. t.i.d. or q.i.d.–usual dosage *I.M.* – 10–20 mg. q. 1–6 h. for severely disturbed			
Mellaril	Thioridazine	*Range 20–800 mg. daily* 20–60 mg. daily–usual dosage			

[1]Trade names listed are for identification purposes only and do not constitute either an endorsement or criticism of any drug.

[2]Dosage is adjusted upward or downward according to each patient's individual response and clinical condition. The lowest effective dosage for each individual patient should always be used.

Table continued on following pages

Group 1. The Antipsychotic Drugs *(Continued)*

Trade or Brand Name	*Generic or Nonproprietary Name*	*Usual Adult Dosage and Administration*	*Therapeutic Action and Uses*	*Adverse Reactions*	*Nursing Actions and Responsibilities*
Prolixin	Fluphenazine	*Range 1–20 mg. daily* 1–10 mg. daily–usual dosage *I.M.* – Decanoate 12.5–100 mg. q. 2 wks.	*Uses:* **1. To reduce agitation, tension, apprehension, anxiety in:** a. Mental illness, particularly hospitalized psychotic patients b. Somatic conditions with emotional stress c. Alcoholism with agitation or withdrawal symptoms d. Illness with severe pain such as cancer	*Neuromuscular:* (Extrapyramidal) Dyskinesia–involuntary muscular movement, twitch Akinesia–muscular fatigue, weakness Akathisia–motor or muscular restlessness Parkinsonism–marked drowsiness, muscular rigidity, fixed stare, masked facies, drooling, ataxic gait	4. Observe patient's behavior for signs of: a. Desired effects–calmer, more in control of behavior, more easily directed b. Undesirable effects–increased anxiety, agitation, depression 5. Watch for signs of URI, pneumonia
Stelazine	Trifluoperazine	*Range 2–30 mg. daily* 1–2 mg. b.i.d. or t.i.d.–usual dosage *I.M.* – 1–2 mg. q 4–6 h. 10 mg. daily maximum			
Thorazine	Chlorpromazine	*Range 30–1200 mg. daily* 10–25 mg. b.i.d. or t.i.d.–usual dosage *I.M.* – 25–50 mg. q. 1–4 h.			

Trilafon	Perphenazine	*Range 6–64 mg. daily* **2–4 mg. t.i.d. or q.i.d.–usual dosage**		*Autonomic* Dry mouth Nasal congestion Constipation Urinary retention Dehydration Dizziness	
		I.M. – 5–10 mg. q. 6 h.	2. To reduce nausea and vomiting in somatic conditions such as pregnancy		6. Protect patient from exposure to direct sun
Quide	**Piperacetazine**	**10 mg. 2–4 times a day** **Up to 160 mg. daily**	3. To reduce narcotic, sedative and anesthetic requirements in surgery		7. Have patient lie down during and following administration of high dosage or I.M. injection
Tindal	**Acetophenazine**	**20 mg. t.i.d. – usual dosage** **80–120 mg. daily–hospitalized** **400–600 mg. daily–severe**	4. To reduce blood pressure such as in essential hypertension	*Behavioral* Apathy Inertia Depression	8. Check patient's B/P for hypotension; TPR for fever; I&O for dehydration, constipation, urinary retention
Vesprin	**Triflupromazine**	**100–150 mg. daily–usual dosage** ***I.M.* – 60–150 mg. daily**		*Potentiates* other CNS depressants such as alcohol, barbiturates, narcotics	
Serentil	**Mesoridazine**	**100–400 mg. daily** **50 mg. t.i.d.–usual dosage** ***I.M.* – 25–200 mg. daily**			

Table continued on the following pages

Group 1. Antipsychotic Drugs *(Continued)*

Trade or Brand Name	*Generic or Nonproprietary Name*	*Usual Adult Dosage and Administration*	*Therapeutic Action and Uses*	*Adverse Reactions*	*Nursing Actions and Responsibilities*
Phenothiazine-like:					
Navane	Thiothixene	*Range 6–60 mg. daily* 2 mg. t.i.d. or q.i.d.–usual dosage		May be *complicated* by upper respiratory infection or pneumonia	
Taractan	Chlorprothixene	*Range 30–600 mg. daily* 25–50 mg. t.i.d. or q.i.d. –usual dosage *I.M.* – 25–50 mg. t.i.d. or q.i.d.			9. Withhold medication, have patient lie down, notify physician or charge nurse if B/P unusually low such as: 90 systolic 60 diastolic
Dibenzoxazepine:					
Loxitane	Loxapine	20–60 mg. daily–usual dosage Up to 60–100 mg. daily Over 250 mg. daily not recommended		May be *contraindicated* in: Arteriosclerosis Cardiovascular disease Liver disorders Coma Shock	10. Protect patient from injury such as falling, hazardous activities, suicide
Dihydroindolone:					
Moban	Molindone	50–75 mg. daily–usual dosage Up to 225 mg. daily			

Lithium: Eskalith Lithane Lithonate	Lithium carbonate	*Range 900–1800 mg. daily* *Acute:* 1800 mg daily in 3 doses to maintain serum level of 1.0 to 1.5 mEq/liter. *Maintenance:* 900 mg daily in 3 doses to maintain serum level of 0.5 to 1.0 mEq/liter.	*Uses:* 1. To control manic and hypomanic states in manic-depressive psychosis. 2. Some prophylactic value in chronic illness.	*Mild:* Anorexia, nausea, malaise, thirst, fatigue, fine hand tremor *Cardiovascular:* Arrhythmias, hypotension *Neuromuscular:* tremor, ataxia, twitching, muscle weakness, lack of coordination *CNS:* dizziness, incontinence, drowsiness, restlessness, confusion, retardation *ANS:* blurred vision, dry mouth *GI:* nausea and vomiting, diarrhea, weight loss *GU:* albuminuria, oliguria, polyuria, glycosuria	11. In addition to the Nursing Actions and Responsibilities listed previously, the patient receiving lithium should be observed for the following: a. Symptoms of depression or toxicity, nausea and vomiting, diarrhea, thirst, malaise, fatigue. Withold medication with toxic effects—hypotension, ataxia, nausea and vomiting, somnolence, polydipsia, polyuria. b. Adequate fluid intake, 2500–3000 c.c. per day. c. Check serum lithium levels twice a week to conform with acute and maintenance levels under dosage.

Group 2. The Antianxiety Drugs

Trade or Brand Name	*Generic or Non-proprietary Name*	*Usual Adult Dosage and Administration*	*Therapeutic Action and Uses*	*Adverse Reactions*	*Nursing Actions and Responsibilities*
Atarax Vistaril	Hydroxyzine	*Range 75–400 mg. daily* 25–100 mg. t.i.d. or q.i.d. –usual dosage *I.M.* – 50–100 mg. q. 4–6 h.	*Action:* *Antianxiety Tranquilizer* *Uses:* 1. To relieve relatively mild anxiety and tension in: a. Mental illness, particularly neuroses and alcoholism b. Stressful life situations, such as menopause c. Psychosomatic conditions, such as peptic ulcer	*Different From Phenothiazines:* 1. Less potent, less toxic. 2. Less autonomic imbalance or extrapyramidal symptoms. 3. Seldom cause postural hypotension or Parkinsonism. 4. Lower incidence of sensitivity.	1. Observe any physical, emotional, behavioral reactions of the patient and report to the physician, charge nurse, other staff. 2. Observe patient's behavior for signs of: a. Desired effects – calmer, more in control, more easily directed b. Undesirable effects – increased anxiety, agitation, depression. 3. Watch for symptoms of drowsiness, incoordination, dizziness, weakness. 4. Protect patient from injury – falling, hazardous activities, suicide.
Equanil Miltown	Meprobamate	*Range 200–2400 mg. daily* 400 mg. t.i.d. or q.i.d. –usual dosage			
Librium	Chlordiazepoxide	*Range 15–300 mg. daily* 5–10 mg. t.i.d. or q.i.d. –usual dosage *I.M.* – 50–100 mg. q. 2–6 h. up to 300 mg. daily			
Valium	Diazepam	*Range 4–40 mg. daily* 2–10 mg. b.i.d. or q.i.d. –usual dosage *I.M.* – 2–10 mg. q. 2–6 h. up to 30 mg. q. 8 h.			

Tranxene	Clorazepate	*Range 15–60 mg. daily* 30 mg.—usual daily dose Up to 90 mg. daily		*Similar to Phenothiazines:* Drowsiness, lethargy Incoordination, ataxia	5. Check patient's B/P for hypotension, TPR for fever; I&O for vomiting, dehydration, constipation, urinary retention.
Ativan	Lorazepam	*Range 1–10 mg. daily* 2–6 mg. daily–usual dosage	2. Combined with other drugs to relieve physical and emotional symptoms, such as in cancer or or psychosis	Dizziness, headache Weakness, fatigue Epigastric discomfort, nausea, and vomiting.	
Serax	Oxazepam	10–15 mg. 3–4 times daily–usual dosage Up to 120 mg. daily		Hypotension Paradoxical excitement Tachycardia, dry mouth, hypersensitivity	6. Withhold medication, put patient to bed, notify physician or charge nurse if B/P is unusually low.
Verstran	Prazepam	*Range 20–60 mg. daily* 30 mg. daily–usual dosage			

Group 3. The Antidepressant Drugs

Trade or Brand Name	*Generic or Non-proprietary Name*	*Usual Adult Dosage and Administration*	*Therapeutic Action and Uses*	*Adverse Reactions*	*Nursing Actions and Responsibilities*
Aventyl **Pamelor**	Nortriptyline	*Range 20–100 mg. daily* 10–25 mg. t.i.d. or q.i.d. – usual dosage			
Elavil	Amtriptyline	*Range 75–300 mg. daily* 25 mg. t.i.d. or q.i.d. – usual dosage *I.M.* – 20–30 mg. q.i.d.	*Action:* *Antidepressant* *Nonenzyme* *Inhibitor* Mood elevator Psychostimulant Psychic energizer	Dry mouth Blurred vision Perspiration Restlessness Generalized tremor Tachycardia	1. Observe any physical, emotional, behavioral reactions of patient and report to physician, charge nurse, other staff.
Norpramin Pertofrane	Desipramine	*Range 75–200 mg. daily* 25 mg. t.i.d. or q.i.d. – usual dosage	Atropine-like Adrenergic blocking Gastric antisecretory	Insomnia Weakness, fatigue Headache Mental confusion Dizziness, vertigo Epigastric discomfort	2. Observe patient closely for suicidal clues. 3. Watch for symptoms of overactivity, restlessness, tremor; or drowsiness, confusion, fatigue.
Tofranil **Imavate**	Imipramine	*Range 75–300 mg. daily* 25 mg. t.i.d. or q.i.d. – usual dosage *I.M.* – 100–150 mg. daily in divided doses up to 300 mg.	*Uses:* 1. Treatment of depression—moderate-severe	Drowsiness Constipation Urinary retention Urethral or ureteral spasm Skin rash	4. Protect patient from injury—falling, hazardous activities, suicide.

Vivactil	Protriptyline	*Range 10–60 mg. daily* 5–10 mg. t.i.d. or q.i.d. –usual dosage			
Adapin Sinequan	Doxepin	*Range 75–150 mg. daily* 25 mg. tid–usual dosage Up to 300 mg. daily			
Deprol	Meprobamate 400 mg. plus benactyzine 1 mg.	1 tab 3–4 times daily–usual dosage Up to 6 tabs. daily	2. Treatment of anxiety-tension states 3. Treatment of psychosomatic disorders such as gastro-intestinal	*May be contraindicated* for patients with: Glaucoma Epilepsy Cardiovascular disease Urinary retention	5. Check patient's B/P for hypertension, TPR for fever, I&O for perspiration, dehydration, constipation, urinary retention.
Asendin	Amoxapine	200–300 mg. daily–usual dosage Up to 600 mg. daily		Or patients receiving other drugs such as: Anticholinergic, MAOI, Sympathomimetic, Thyroid	6. Watch for signs of increased anxiety, agitation, depression.
Ludiomil	Maprotiline	75–150 mg. daily–usual dosage Up to 300 mg. daily	4. Combined with tranquilizer for agitated depression		
Surmontil	Trimipramine	75–150 mg. daily–usual dosage Up to 300 mg. daily			

Group 4. The Antiparkinsonism Drugs

Trade or Brand Name	*Generic or Non-proprietary Name*	*Usual Adult Dosage and Administration*	*Therapeutic Action and Uses*	***Adverse Reactions***	*Nursing Actions and Responsibilities*
Akineton	Biperiden	*Range 2–8 mg. daily* 2 mg. t.i.d. or q.i.d. – usual dosage *I.M.* – 2–5 mg. q. 6–12 h.	*Action:* *Antiparkinsonism* Antispasmodic Antihistamine *Autonomic Blocking Agent*	Dry Mouth Blurred vision Skin dryness, rash Fever Palpitations, tachycardia Constipation	1. Observe any physical, emotional, behavioral reactions of patient and report to physician, charge nurse, other staff
Artane	Trihexyphenidyl	*Range 1–15 mg. daily* 2 mg. t.i.d. or q.i.d. – usual dosage	Parasympatholytic Anticholinergic Antimuscarinic	Nausea, vomiting Urinary retention Drowsiness Mental confusion	2. Watch for symptoms of excitement, nervousness, dry skin; or headache, dizziness, confusion
Cogentin	**Benztropine mesylate**	*Range 0.5–8 mg. daily* 1–2 mg. daily or b.i.d. – usual dosage *I.M.* – 1–2 mg. q. 6–12 h.	Reduce number of nerve impulses passing to peripheral effector cells by way of post-ganglionic nerve fibers Keep acetylcholine	Headache Dizziness Excitement Weakness Incoordination	3. Protect patient from injury – falling, hazardous activities, suicide. 4. Check patient's B/P, TPR, I&O as indicated.
Kemadrin	Procyclidine	*Range 5–60 mg. daily* 2.5 mg. b.i.d. or t.i.d. – usual dosage	molecules from fulfilling their impulse-transmitting functions at tissues and organs innervated by post-ganglionic cholinergic nerve fibers		5. Watch for signs of increased anxiety, agitation, depression, distorted thinking.

Trade or Brand Name	*Generic or Non-proprietary Name*	*Usual Adult Dosage and Administration*	*Therapeutic Action and Uses*	*Adverse Reactions*	*Nursing Actions and Responsibilities*
			Uses: To relieve the extra-pyramidal symptoms caused by pheno-thiazines—drug-induced pseudo-parkinsonism		

1. AMA *Drug Evaluations*, 4th Ed. American Medical Assoc. Chicago, Ill., 1980.
2. *Physicians Desk Reference*, 36th Ed., Medical Economics, Oradell, N. J., 1982.

Appendix D

PATIENT RIGHTS*

Facilities shall support and protect the fundamental human, civil, constitutional, and statutory rights of each patient.

The facility shall have a written plan or policies and procedures that describe the rights of patients and the means by which these rights are protected and exercised. These rights shall include the following:

Each patient shall have impartial access to treatment, regardless of race, religion, sex, ethnicity, age, or handicap.

Each patient's personal dignity shall be recognized and respected in the provision of all care and treatment.

Each patient shall receive individualized treatment, which shall include at least the following:

a. the provision of adequate and humane services, regardless of sources of financial support;
b. the provision of services within the least restrictive environment possible;
c. the provision of an individual treatment plan;
d. the periodic review of the patient's treatment plan;
e. the active participation of patients over 12 years of age and their responsible parent, relative, or guardian in planning for treatment;
f. the provision of an adequate number of competent, qualified, and experienced professional clinical staff to supervise and implement the treatment plan.

Each patient's personal privacy shall be assured and protected within the constraints of the individual treatment plan.

The patient's family and significant others, regardless of their age, shall be allowed to visit the patient, unless such visits are clinically contraindicated.

Suitable areas shall be provided for patients to visit in private, unless such privacy is contraindicated by the patient's treatment plan.

Patients shall be allowed to send and receive mail without hindrance.

Patients shall be allowed to conduct private telephone conversations with family and friends, unless clinically contraindicated.

If therapeutic indications necessitate restrictions on visitors, telephone calls, or other communications, those restrictions shall be

*From "Consolidated Standards Manual For Child, Adolescent, and Adult Psychiatric, Alcoholism, and Drug Abuse Facilities," 1981, Joint Commission on Accreditation of Hospitals.

evaluated for therapeutic effectiveness by the clinically responsible staff at least every seven days.

If limitations on visitors, telephone calls, or other communications are indicated for practical reasons (for example, expense of travel or phone calls) such limitations shall be determined with the participation of the patient and the patient's family. All such restrictions shall be fully explained to the patient and the patient's family.

Each patient has the right to request the opinion of a consultant at his or her expense or to request an inhouse review of the individual treatment plan, as provided in specific procedures of the facility.

Each patient shall be informed of his or her rights in a language the patient understands.

Each patient shall receive a written statement of patients rights, and a copy of this statement shall be posted in various areas of the facility.

As appropriate, the patient, the patient's family, or the patient's legal guardian shall be fully informed about the following items:

a. the rights of patients;
b. the professional staff members responsible for his or her care, their professional status, and their staff relationship;
c. the nature of the care, procedures, and treatment that he or she will receive;
d. the current and future use and disposition of products of special observation and audiovisual techniques, such as one-way vision mirrors, tape recorders, television, movies, or photographs;
e. the risks, side effects, and benefits of all medications and treatment procedures used, especially those that are unusual or experimental;
f. the alternate treatment procedures that are available;
g. the right to refuse to participate in any research project without compromising his or her access to facility services;
h. the right, to the extent permitted by law, to refuse specific medications or treatment procedures;
i. the responsibility of the facility, when the patient refuses treatment, to seek appropriate legal alternatives or orders of involuntary treatment, or, in accordance with professional standards, to terminate the relationship with the patient upon reasonable notice.
j. as appropriate, the cost, itemized when possible, of services rendered;
k. the source of the facility's reimbursement, and any limitations placed on duration of services;
l. the reasons for any proposed change in the professional staff responsible for the patient, or for any transfer of the patient either within or outside of the facility;
m. the rules and regulations of the facility applicable to his or her conduct;
n. the right to initiate a complaint or grievance procedure and the appropriate means of requesting a hearing or review of the complaint;
o. the discharge plans;
p. the plans for meeting continuing mental and physical health requirements following discharge.

In accordance with the requirements of any applicable law or any other standard in this Manual, a written, dated, and signed informed consent form shall be obtained from the patient, the patient's family, or the patient's legal guardian, as appropriate, for the participation in any research project and for use or performance of the following:

a. surgical procedures;
b. electroconvulsive therapy;
c. unusual medications;
d. hazardous assessment procedures;
e. audiovisual equipment;
f. other procedures where consent is required by law.

The maintenance of confidentiality of communications between patients and staff and of all information recorded in patients' records shall be the responsibility of all staff.

The facility shall provide continuing training for all staff and specific orientation for all new personnel in the principles of confidentiality and privacy.

The patient shall be allowed to work for the service provider only under the following conditions:

a. the work is part of the individual treatment plan;
b. the work is performed voluntarily;
c. the patient receives wages commensurate with the economic value of the work;
d. the work project complies with local, state, and federal laws and regulations.

A patient may be required to perform personal housekeeping tasks without compensation.

Appendix E

ANA STANDARDS OF PSYCHIATRIC AND MENTAL HEALTH NURSING PRACTICE*

PROFESSIONAL PRACTICE STANDARDS

STANDARD I. Theory

The nurse applies appropriate theory that is scientifically sound as a basis for decisions regarding nursing practice.

STANDARD II. Data Collection

The nurse continuously collects data that is comprehensive, accurate, and systematic.

STANDARD III. Diagnosis

The nurse utilizes nursing diagnoses and standard classification of mental disorders to express conclusions supported by recorded assessment data and current scientific premises.

STANDARD IV. Planning

The nurse develops a nursing care plan with specific goals and interventions delineating nursing actions unique to each client's needs.

STANDARD V. Intervention

The nurse intervenes as guided by the nursing care plan to implement nursing actions that promote, maintain, or restore physical and mental health, prevent illness, and effect rehabilitation.

STANDARD V–A. Psychotherapeutic Interventions

The nurse uses *psychotherapeutic interventions* to assist clients to regain or improve their previous coping abilities and to prevent further disability.

STANDARD V–B. Health Teaching

The nurse assists clients, families, and groups to achieve satisfying and productive patterns of living through health teaching.

STANDARD V–C. Self-Care Activities

The nurse uses the activities of daily living in a goal-directed way to foster adequate self-care and physical and mental well-being of clients.

STANDARD V–D. Somatic Therapies

The nurse uses knowledge of somatic therapies and applies related clinical skills in working with clients.

STANDARD V–E. Therapeutic Environment

The nurse provides, structures, and maintains a therapeutic environment in collaboration with the client and other health care providers.

STANDARD V–F. Psychotherapy

The nurse utilizes advanced clinical expertise in individual, group, and family psychotherapy, child psychotherapy, and other treatment mo-

---

*From American Nurses' Association, "Standards of Psychiatric-Mental Health Nursing Practice," ANA, 2420 Pershing Rd., Kansas City, Mo., 64108, 1982.

dalities to function as a psychotherapist, and recognizes professional accountability for nursing practice.

STANDARD VI. Evaluation

The nurse evaluates client responses to nursing actions in order to revise the data base, nursing diagnoses, and nursing care plan.

PROFESSIONAL PERFORMANCE STANDARDS

STANDARD VII. Peer Review

The nurse participates in peer review and other means of evaluation to assure quality of nursing care provided for clients.

STANDARD VIII. Continuing Education

The nurse assumes responsibility for continuing education and professional development and contributes to the professional growth of others.

STANDARD IX. Interdisciplinary Collaboration

The nurse collaborates with interdisciplinary teams in assessing, planning, implementing, and evaluating programs and other mental health activities.

STANDARD X. Utilization of Community Health Systems

The nurse participates with other members of the community in assessing, planning, implementing, and evaluating mental health services and community systems that include the promotion of the broad continuum of primary, secondary, and tertiary prevention of mental illness.

STANDARD XI. Research

The nurse contributes to nursing and the mental health field through innovations in theory and practice and participation in research.

Index

(Page numbers in *italics* indicate illustrations; (t) refers to tables.)